Essential
Pediatric Oncology

Editor

Rakesh Mondal
MD(PGI) DNB PDSR (SGPGI) MNAMS MRCPCHI
Pediatric Immuno-Oncologist
Professor, Pediatric Medicine
Medical College and Hospital
Kolkata, West Bengal, India

Editorial Assistance

Sumantra Sarkar MD
Associate Professor
Pediatric Medicine
IPGMER and SSKM Hospital
Kolkata, West Bengal, India

Madhumita Nandi MD
Associate Professor
Pediatric Medicine
NRS Medical College
Kolkata, West Bengal, India

Forewords
Tapas Sabui
Utpal Chowdhury

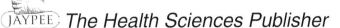

JAYPEE *The Health Sciences Publisher*

New Delhi | London | Philadelphia | Panama

Jaypee Brothers Medical Publishers (P) Ltd

Headquarters

Jaypee Brothers Medical Publishers (P) Ltd
4838/24, Ansari Road, Daryaganj
New Delhi 110 002, India
Phone: +91-11-43574357
Fax: +91-11-43574314
Email: jaypee@jaypeebrothers.com

Overseas Offices

J.P. Medical Ltd
83, Victoria Street, London
SW1H 0HW (UK)
Phone: +44-2031708910
Fax: +44(0)20 3008 6180
Email: info@jpmedpub.com

Jaypee-Highlights Medical Publishers Inc
City of Knowledge, Bld. 237, Clayton
Panama City, Panama
Phone: +1 507-301-0496
Fax: +1 507-301-0499
Email: cservice@jphmedical.com

Jaypee Medical Inc
The Bourse
111 South Independence Mall East
Suite 835, Philadelphia, PA 19106, USA
Phone: +1 267-519-9789
Email: jpmed.us@gmail.com

Jaypee Brothers Medical Publishers (P) Ltd
17/1-B Babar Road, Block-B, Shaymali
Mohammadpur, Dhaka-1207
Bangladesh
Mobile: +08801912003485
Email: jaypeedhaka@gmail.com

Jaypee Brothers Medical Publishers (P) Ltd
Bhotahity, Kathmandu
Nepal
Phone: +977-9741283608
Email: kathmandu@jaypeebrothers.com

Website: www.jaypeebrothers.com
Website: www.jaypeedigital.com

Essential Pediatric Oncology

First Edition: **2016**

ISBN 978-93-5152-978-1

Printed at Sanat Printers

Dedicated to

Those who are involved in fighting battles against
Pediatric Cancer and the Supreme Surety

Contributors

Abhisekh Roy
Assistant Professor
Department of Pediatrics
North Bengal Medical College
Darjeeling, India

Agni Sekhar Saha
Senior Resident, Pediatric ICU
Medical College Kolkata
Kolkata, India

Ajay Ghosh
Professor, Department of
Applied Optics and Photonics
University of Calcutta
Kolkata, India

Alok Shobhan Datta
Associate Professor, Orthopediatrics
IPGMER and SSKM Hospital
Kolkata, India

Amitava Chandra
Neurosurgeon
Rabindra Nath Tagore Institute of
Cardiac Sciences
Kolkata, India

Anirban Chatterjee
Assistant Professor
Department of Pediatrics
IPGMER and SSKM Hospital, Kolkata
NBMC Hospital, Darjeeling, India

Anjan Das
Assistant Professor, Pediatric Medicine
NRSMCH, Kolkata, India

Anup Kumar Roy
Professor (Principal), Pathology
North Bengal Medical College
Darjeeling, India

Anup Majumdar
Professor
Department of Radiotherapy
IPGMER and SSKM Hospital
Kolkata, India

Arnab Chattopadhyay
Assistant Professor
Department of Hematology
Institute of Hematology and Transfusion
Medicine, MCH, Kolkata, India

Arpita Bhattacharya
Pediatric Hematologist and Oncologist
Apollo Gleneagles Hospital
Kolkata, India

Ashish Mukherjee
Director, NSCBI
Kolkata, India

Astha Tiwari
Senior Resident
Department of Pediatric Medicine
IPGMER and SSKM Hospital
Kolkata, India

Avijit Hazra
Professor
Department of Pharmacology
IPGMER and SSKM Hospital
Kolkata, India

Biman Roy
Assistant Professor, Physiology
IPGMER and SSKM Hospital
Kolkata, India

Bishwanath Mukhopadhyay
Professor and Head
Department of Pediatric Surgery
NRS Medical College and Hospital
Kolkata, India

Dipankar Gupta
Associate Professor
Department of Pediatrics
IPGMER and SSKM Hospital
Kolkata, India

Diptendra Sarkar
Professor, General Surgery
IPGMER and SSKM Hospital
Kolkata, India

Dipti Bhattacharya
Professor, Nursing Education
College of Nursing
Kolkata, India

Goutam Mukherjee
Associate Professor
Department of Obstetrics and
Gynecology
North Bengal Medical College
Darjeeling, India

Indira Banerjee
Fellow, Pediatric Cardiology
Rabindranath Tagore Institute of
Cardiac Sciences
Kolkata, India

Jayanta Dasgupta
Professor
Department of Gastroenterology
IPGMER and SSKM Hospital
Kolkata, India

Jayanta Ghosh
Associate Professor
Department of Pediatric Medicine
North Bengal Medical College
Darjeeling, India

Jaydeep Chowdhury
Associate Professor
Institute of Child Health
Kolkata, India

Kakoli Chowdhury
Senior Resident
Department of Radiotherapy
IPGMER and SSKM Hospital
Kolkata, India

Kalpana Datta
Professor
Department of Pediatrics
CSS Hospital
Kolkata, India

Krishnendu Mukherjee
Professor, Pathology
IPGMER and SSKM Hospital
Kolkata, India

Madhumita Nandi
Associate Professor
Department of Pediatrics
IPGMER and SSKM Hospital
Kolkata, India

Madhusmita Sengupta
Professor
Department of Pediatrics
CNMCH Hospital
Kolkata, India

Mousumi Nandi
Professor
Department of Pediatrics
NRSMCH Hospital
Kolkata, India

Nibedita Chatterjee
Associate Professor
Department of Obstetrics and
Gynecology
IPGMER and SSKM Hospital
Kolkata, India

Pradip Kumar Mitra
Professor, Pathology
Director, IPGMER and SSKM
Hospital, Kolkata
India

Pragya Pant
Assistant Professor
Department of Pediatric Medicine
North Bengal Medical College
Darjeeling, India

Pranab Sahana
Assistant Professor
Department of Endocrinology
Medical College Hospital
Kolkata, India

Prantar Chakrabarti
Professor
Department of Hematology
Institute of Hematology and
Transfusion Medicine, MCH
Kolkata, India

Rajib De
Post-Doctoral Resident
Department of Hematology
Institute of Hematology and
Transfusion Medicine, MCH
Kolkata, India

Rakesh Mondal
Pediatric Immuno-Oncologist
Professor
Pediatric Medicine
Medical College and Hospital
Kolkata, India

Sanat Ghosh
Professor
Department of Pediatrics
BC Roy Memorial Hospital for Children
Kolkata, India

Sandip Samanta
Assistant Professor
Dr BC Roy Memorial Hospital for
Children
Kolkata, India

Subhayan Mandal
Assistant Professor
Department of Surgery
North Bengal Medical College
Darjeeling, India

Suhas Ganguly
Resident Pediatrician
Flushing Hospital Medical Center
New York, USA

Sumantra Sarkar
Associate Professor
Department of Pediatric Medicine
IPGMER and SSKM Hospital
Kolkata, India

Sunil Natha Mhaske
Professor and Head
Department of Pediatrics
Vithalrao Vikhe Patil Foundation's
Medical College and Hospital
Ahmednagar, Maharashtra, India

Supratim Datta
Professor
Department of Pediatrics
IPGMER and SSKM Hospital
Kolkata, India

Tapan Dhibar
Professor
Department of Neuro-Radiology
BINP Hospital
Kolkata, India

Toshibananda Bag
Assistant Professor
Department of Pediatrics
North Bengal Medical College
Darjeeling, India

Foreword

I am very glad to write the Foreword for the book *Essential Pediatric Oncology*. Today all the pediatricians should know about detailed clinical approaches in different pediatric oncology issues, regarding patient management for better child care service. This knowledge will help us to render better care to our children suffering from childhood malignancies.

It is very difficult to cover all guidelines, but it is a sincere effort of great compilation on highly relevant topics. I hope that the relevant topics would be of great help to the undergraduates, postgraduates, practicing pediatricians and pediatric oncologists to improve the health of our society and the country at large.

Lastly, I must appreciate the great effort of Dr Rakesh Mondal to make this initiative a great success.

I am hopeful that we would be witnessing more such editions in the future.

Tapas Sabui MD
Professor and Head
Department of Pediatric Medicine
Medical College, Kolkata
President Rheumatology Chapter
Indian Academy of Pediatrics (2013–2014)
Kolkata, West Bengal, India

Foreword

It gives me great pleasure to write the Foreword for the book *Essential Pediatric Oncology.*

In this millennium of globalization, it is very important for the pediatricians to be abreast with the clinical approaches in different issues of pediatric oncology for proper management. They also require to know using medication very clearly and also should be aware of recent evidence regarding management of different childhood malignant cases. Though this has not covered all the issues, but it is a great compilation on highly relevant topics. I hope that these rational topics would be of great help to the undergraduates, postgraduates, oncology consultants, pediatric oncologists and practicing pediatricians to deliver optimal health care to their patients suffering from different types of childhood cancer.

I am hopeful that we would be able to manage our cases better and update our knowledge in a day-to-day practice.

Utpal Chowdhury MD
Director
Institute of Hematology and
Transfusion Medicine
Kolkata, West Bengal, India

Preface

The specialty of pediatric oncology continues to grow over the decades for better understanding of the diseases and advanced management of the ailments. Even though a significant number of children from the developing countries are suffering from malignancies, the concise and updated compilation was lacking. We have tried to give a precise description of those problems related to childhood cancer. We are fortunate enough to have learned contributors from different parts of India and the world. Wherever appropriate, we have included different angles of approach in relevant issues. In this book, all the chapters are meticulously written, however, there are areas of controversy existing which require debate as applicable for any other scientific write-up. It is best to follow institutional guidelines, if necessary. Several chapters encompassing different aspects have been added to make it more comprehensive. Certain special issues like parents' perspective, technology related to cancer, biomedical statistics, management in the resource constraint settings and resident-friendly protocols are highlighted. Change is only constant in science so any suggestion, comments and constructive criticism for this compilation are most welcome for future progress in the interest of child health improvement.

Rakesh Mondal

Acknowledgments

We sincerely thank the learned contributors for sharing their valuable information exchange for this endeavor. We specially mention the help from Almighty for his spiritual guidance. We sincerely thank Prof P Mitra (Director, IPGMER), Prof Ashok Ghosh (MSVP-IPGMER), Prof JB Ghosh, Prof U Chowdhury, Prof Anup Mazumdar, Prof Bishwanath Mukherjee, Prof Amitava Sen, Prof Shyamal Das, Prof Krishendu Mukherjee, Prof Alakendu Ghosh, Prof Swati Chakravorti, Prof PK Chandra, Prof AK Roy, Prof P Tripathy, Prof Surjit Singh (PGI, Chandigarh), Prof SK Kabra (AIIMS), Prof Amita Aggarwal (SGPGI, Lucknow), Prof RK Marwaha (PGI, Chandigarh), Dr Ashish Mukherjee (Director, NSCBI), Dr Supratim Datta, Dr Mrinal Kranti Das, Dr Dipankar Gupta, Dr Mousumi Nandi, Dr Priyankar Pal, Dr Amitava Chandra, Dr Jaydeep Chowdhury, Dr Prantar Chakrabarti, Dr Arnab Chatterjee, Dr Arpita Bhattacharya, Dr Tapan Dhibar, Dr Kalyan Mondal, Dr Tapas Sabui, Dr Tapan Ghosh, Dr Madhumita Nandi, Dr Anirban Chatterjee, Dr Niloy Das, Dr Sekhar Roy, and Dr Pravanjan Chatterjee for their pertinent advice, valuable opinion and help. Dr Biman Roy, Dr Anjan Das, Dr Suhas Ganguly, Dr Manasi Purkait, and our junior colleagues, also helped us in all possible ways whenever required. At last, we thank our parents, our all-junior and senior colleagues, the children and their parents; and our friends, Mr Pannalal Ghosal and Mr Jaydev Sardar for their support. We are grateful to Master Ivan Mondal for kind help for sparing so much time in this dedicated job. We also acknowledge the sincere cooperation of Tania Ghosh Sarkar and Rita Mondal during our laborious hours.

We also express our gratitude to Mr (Adv) S Chakravorty, Mr (Adv) Dipak Mukherjee, and Hon'ble Retd Judge SP Sengupta, in this opportunity who have helped in difficult times. We hope that the collection would be of great help to undergraduates, postgraduates, pediatric practitioners, oncologists, pediatric oncologists and pediatric consultants alike and we should be waiting for their comments and suggestions for improvement in future. We are also fortunate to have collaborated with a number of colleagues from our own and other institutions that remained named or unnamed to bring out this book.

We highly appreciate the all-round cooperation and genuine support of Ms Jaypee Brothers Medical Publishers (P) Ltd., New Delhi, India, to finish the assignment in time and for the excellent outcome of this book.

Introduction

Pediatric Oncology is a newly specialized entity in clinical horizon for the last few decades. Pediatricians of today are expected to know more than the clinical skills with accurate clinical approach in managing pediatric oncology cases. These issues are truly inter-sectoral. This should help to deliver efficient patient care in childhood cancer patients. This book is aimed at increasing the awareness regarding basics of clinical approach in pediatric oncology practice and related issues. It does not give all possible issues regarding that in this small collection, however, we have attempted to cover only some of the important topics required in a day-to-day pediatric oncology practice.

"Nothing in life is to be feared; it is only to be understood".....Marie Curie.

Contents

Plate 1

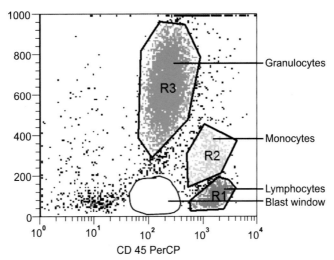

Fig. 5.1: CD 45 vs Side scatter histogram from a normal peripheral blood

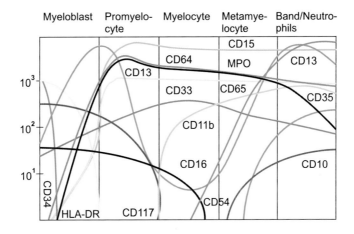

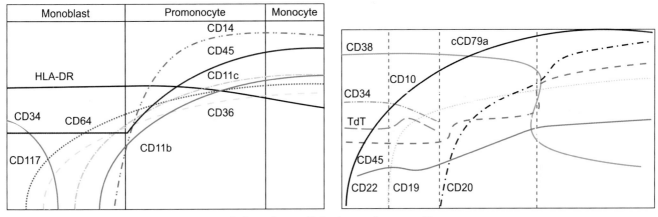

Refer to Appendix in chapter 5 on page 33

Plate 2

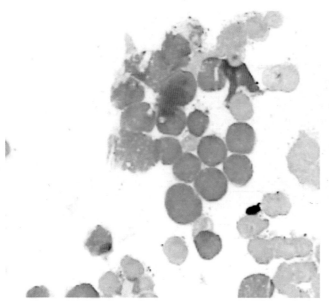

Fig. 7.2: Bone marrow slide of acute lymphoblastic leukemia

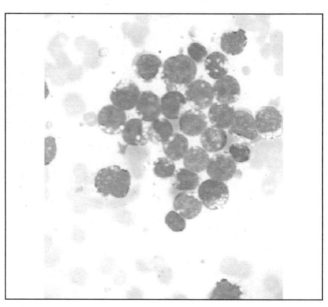

Fig. 9.1: Microphotograph showing lymphoblast proliferation suggestive of Burkitt's lymphoma

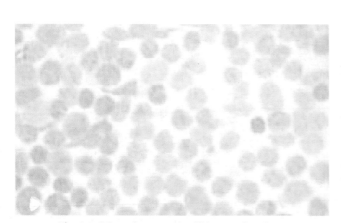

Fig. 9.7: Microphotograph of biopsy taken from enlarged lymph node of NHL

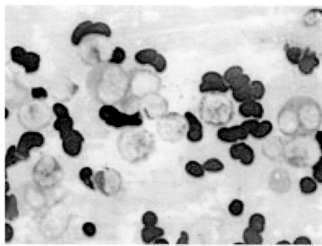

Fig. 10.4: Bone marrow picture of MPO positive myeloblast with Auer rod

Plate 3

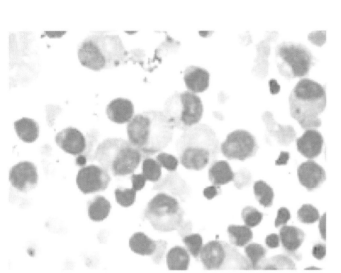

Fig. 10.5: Bone marrow photograph of AML M4

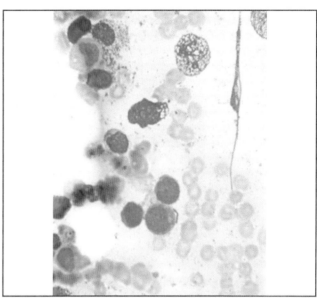

Fig. 11.1: Bone marrow microphotograph of a child with myelodysplastic syndrome

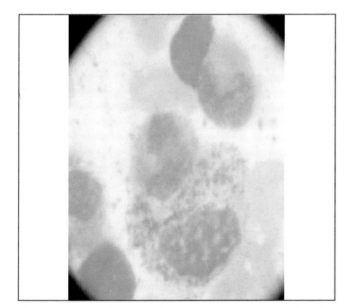

Fig. 12.3: Microphotograph of bone marrow slide showing phagocytosis of neutrophils in hemophagocytic lymphohistiocytosis (HLH)

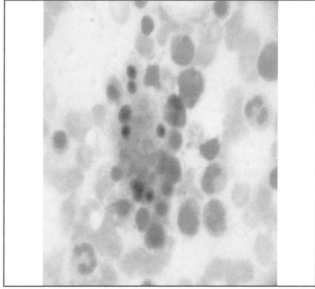

Fig. 12.4: Microphotograph of bone marrow slide showing phagocytosis of erythrocytes in hemophagocytic lymphohistiocytosis (HLH)

Plate 4

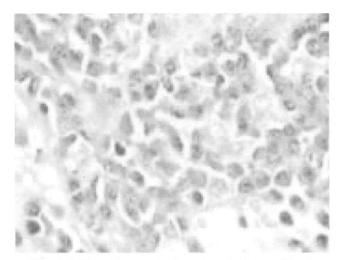

Fig. 12.7: Microphotograph of lymph node biopsy of Rosai-Dorfman's disease

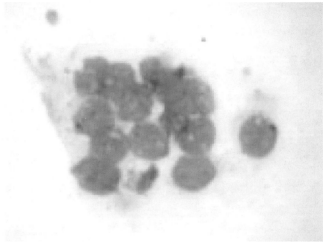

Fig. 13.6A: Neuroblastoma metastatic cell cluster in bone marrow

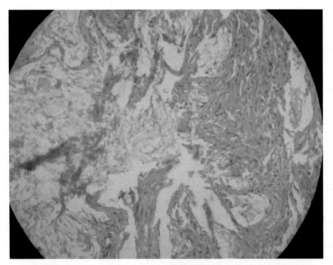

Fig. 24.4: Microphotograph of adenocarcioma of intestine

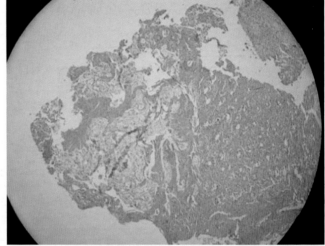

Fig. 24.5: Microphotograph of adenocarcioma of intestine

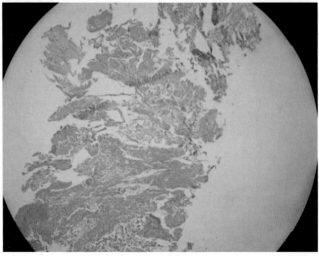

Fig. 24.6: Microphotograph of adenocarcioma of intestine

1 History of Pediatric Oncology

Sunil Natha Mhaske

The history of medicine is a continuous evolution of progress from basic inventions to today's ongoing researches in its various branches. Likewise the history of oncology especially related to child has very important responsibility over the medical fraternity. Progress in Pediatric Oncology is one of the biggest success stories in oncology in the last millennium. Now we will see the pioneer work done by various great persons in this success path in year-wise manner.

2650 to 1950 BC: The first reference of cancer goes back to this time, when in three Egyptian papyri detected the breast tumor together with a uterine carcinoma. (Opera omnia. Vol. XI, II, 12. Kuhn CG, editor. Leipzig, Germany; 1826. p. 139-41).

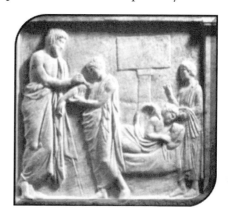

25 BC to 50 AD: Aurelius Cornelius Celsus translated carcinos into the Latin cancer, meaning crab. Also he described the phenomenon of metastatic process in malignancies.

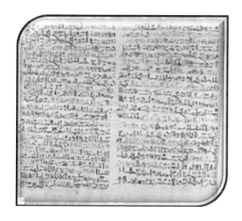

1900 to 1600 BC: The earliest evidence of tumor was found in the skull of a female from Bronze Age period.

460 to 370 BC: Hippocrates was first to describe various kinds of cancer. As per Greek words 'carcinos' means- crab or crayfish. He described the appearance of cut malignant tumor as the veins stretched on all sides like the crab has its feet, so the name was kept. Also in Greek words swelling is known as oma, so he later added suffix and named as carcinoma.

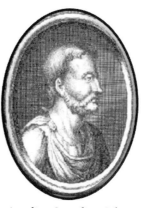

Aurelius Cornelius Celsus

129 to 199 AD: Claudius Galenus (Galen): He was Greek, who described benign tumors as "oncos" meaning as swelling. Also he was pioneer to introduce the term 'sarcoma' from the Greek word 'sarca' (flesh).

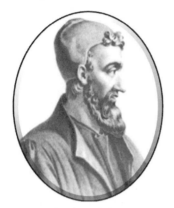

Claudius Galenus

Jun 25, 1560 to Feb. 1634: Wilhelm Fabry: He was a German professor, who believed that breast cancer was caused by a milk clot in a mammary duct.

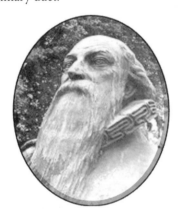

Wilhelm Fabry

Oct 09, 1593 to Sept, 1674: Nicolaes Tulp—believed that cancer was a poison that slowly spreads and it was contagious (Marilyn Yalom "A history of the breast" 1997. New York: Alfred A Knopf. ISBN 0-679-43459-3).

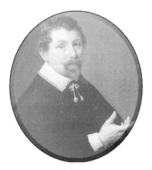

Nicolaes Tulp

May 11, 1614 to Nov 10, 1672: Francois de la Boe Sylvius: He was a Dutch professor, who believed that all diseases were the outcome of chemical processes and acidic lymph fluid causes the cancer.

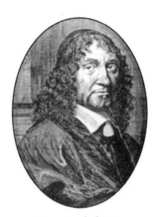

Francois de la Boe

1661 to 1749: Jean Godinot: He was a pioneer in starting the first cancer hospital in the world in Rheims (1740), which was dedicated to the cancer patients.

January 6, 1714 to December 22, 1788: Sir Percivall Pott: He was an English surgeon, first to demonstrate that a cancer may be caused by an environmental carcinogens (Dobson J Percivall Pott in Annals of the Royal College of Surgeons of England, vol. 50, 1972, pp. 54–65).

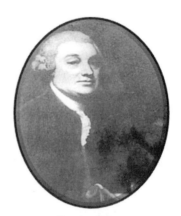

Percivall Pott

*1787: John Hunter: He was reported to be the first to operate on metastatic melanoma in 1787.

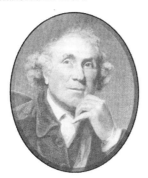

John Hunter

*1804: René Laennec: He was the French physician, who was first to describe melanoma as a disease entity. His report was initially presented during a lecture for the Faculte de Medecine de Paris and then published as a bulletin in 1806.

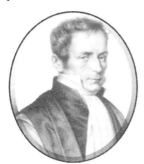

René Laennec

*November 22, 1811 to April 12, 1876: Campbell Greig De Morgan: He was a British surgeon who first mentioned that cancer arose locally and then spreads first to the lymph nodes and then more widely in the body (Campbell De Morgan's 'Observations on cancer'—John M Grange, John L Stanford, Cynthia A Stanford SRN, Journal of the Royal Society of Medicine, 2002;95:296–9).

1832: Thomas Hodgkin: He was a pathologist, first to described a form of lymphoma, which was named as of Hodgkin's disease (Amalie M Kass, Edward H Kass. Perfecting the World: The life and times of Dr Thomas Hodgkin, 1798–1866, Harcourt Brace Jovanovich 1988).

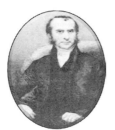

Thomas Hodgkin

*1857 to 1940: John Templeton Bowen: He was an American dermatologist, who named Bowen's disease and Bowenoid papulosis.

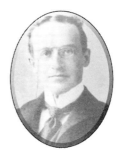

John Templeton Bowen

*January 12, 1862 to April 16, 1936: William Coley: He was an American bone surgeon and cancer researcher, pioneer of cancer immunotherapy. In 1968, a protein related to his work was identified as alpha tumor necrosis factor (Terlikowski SJ. Tumour necrosis factor and cancer treatment: a historical review and perspectives.)

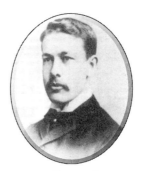

William Coley

*1864: Rudolf Virchow: A German physician who was first to describe an abdominal tumor in a child as a "glioma" The characteristics of tumors from the sympathetic nervous system and the adrenal medulla were then noted in 1891 by German pathologist Felix Marchand (Rutherford, Dr Adam, August 2009—"The Cell: Episode 1 the Hidden Kingdom". BBC4.)

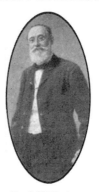

Rudolf Virchow

December 25, 1866 to May 16, 1943: James Stephen Ewing: He was an American pathologist, who discovered a form of malignant tumor which is known as Ewing Sarcoma.

1868 to 1944: Ludwig Pick: He coined the term Pheochromocytoma in 1912 and described the chromaffin color change in tumor cells associated with adrenal medullary tumors.

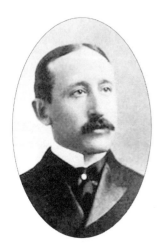 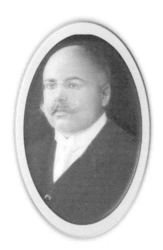

James Stephen Ewing   Ludwig Pick

April 8, 1869 to January 3, 1928: James Homer Wright: He was an American pathologist, who was chief of pathology at Massachusetts General Hospital. He is the same "Wright" for which Wright's stain, and the "Homer Wright rosettes" associated with neuroblastoma [Lee RE, Young RH, Castleman B. James Homer Wright: a biography. Am J Surg Pathol. 2002;26(1):88–96].

January 01, 1875 to March 26, 1960: Emil Herman Grubbe: He was the first American to use X-rays for the treatment of cancer (Pioneer in X-Ray Therapy. Science, New Series, 125, 3236—18–19. 4 January 1957. JSTOR 1752791).

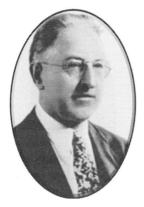

Emil Herman Grubbe

*1886: Frankel made the first description of a patient with pheochromocytoma.

19th century: Marie Curie and Pierre Curie discovered radiation, the first effective non-surgical treatment of cancer patients ("charitynavigator.org").

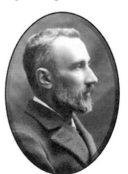

Pierre Curie

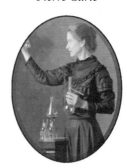

Marie Curie

1902: Theodor Boveri: He was a German professor of zoology at Munich, who identified the genetic basis of cancer. He studied that mutations of the chromosomes can generate a cell with unlimited growth potential, which passes onto its descendants. He proposed the existence of tumor suppressor genes and oncogenes, also mentioned that cancers might be caused or promoted by radiation, physical or chemical insults or by pathogenic microorganisms (*Journal of Cell Science 121-Supplement 1: 1–84*).

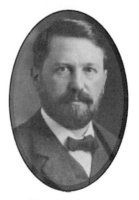

Theodor Boveri

1903: JJ Thomson: He discovered the presence of radioactivity in well water. That's why preparations of radium salt in bath water was suggested as a way for patients to be treated at home, as the radioactivity in the bathwater was permanent. Radium baths became used experimentally to treat arthritis, gout, and neuralgias.

1903 to 1973: Dr Sidney Farber: He was a pediatric pathologist, who is regarded as the **Father of Modern Chemotherapy.** He evaluated the role of aminopterin as a folate antagonist in childhood acute lymphoblastic leukemia. He showed for the first time that induction of clinical and hematological remission in this disease was achievable (Miller, Denis R. A tribute to Sidney Farber—the Father of Modern Chemotherapy, British Journal of Hematology. July 2006;134).

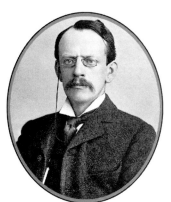 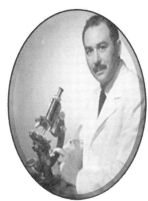

JJ Thomson   *Sidney Farber*

1905: Niels Finsen: He discovered that lupus was amenable to treatment by ultraviolet rays when separated out by a system of quartz crystals, and thereafter created a lamp to sift out the rays. The Finsen lamp became widely used in for phototherapy. Finsen was soon awarded a Nobel Prize for his research.

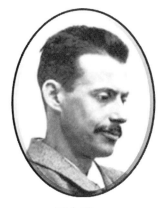

Niels Finsen

1910: Max Wilms: He was pioneer in the study of tumor cells originating during the development of the embryo, known as "nephroblastoma" or Wilms' tumor. This is a malignant tumor of the kidney. He did extensive work in the field of radiology, using radiation therapy for treatment of tumors and tuberculosis.

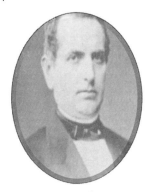

Max Wilms

1926: Roux (in Switzerland) and Mayo (in USA) were the first surgeons to remove pheochromocytomas.

1926: Janet Lane-Claypon: She observed that the bone marrow of victims of the atomic bombs of Hiroshima and Nagasaki was completely destroyed. From these observations, she concluded that diseased bone marrow could also be destroyed with radiation and this led to the development of bone marrow transplants for leukemia.

1950: Charles Heidelberger: He synthesized the fluoro-pyrimidine 5-fluorouracil, which had a broad-spectrum activity against various types of solid tumors (Skipper HE, Schabel FR, Jr, Wilcox WS. Experimental evaluation of potential anticancer agents. XII. Cancer Chemother Rep, 1964;35:1–111.)

October 21, 1956: Patrick S Moore: He was an American virologist who co-discovered together with his wife, Yuan Chang, two different human viruses causing the AIDS-related cancer Kaposi's sarcoma and the skin cancer Merkel cell carcinoma (Schmidt C Yuan Chang and Patrick Moore: teaming up to hunt down cancer-causing viruses. Journal of the National Cancer Institute, 2008;100–8:524–5, 529).

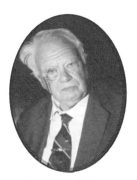

Charles Heidelberger

November 17, 1959: Yuan Chang: She was an American virologist and pathologist who co-discovered the two human cancer viruses—Kaposi's sarcoma associated herpes virus and Merkel cell polyomavirus (Antman K, Chang Y. Kaposi's sarcoma. New Engl J Med, 2000;342–14:1027–38).

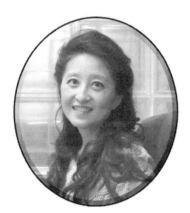

Yuan Chang

1962: Copp and Cheney: They purified calcitonin and was considered as a secretion of the parathyroid glands, later identified as the secretion of the C-cells of the thyroid gland (Copp DH, Cheney B -January 1962-Nature 193, 4813: 381–2).
1965: DeVita VT, Moxley JH, Brace K, Frei E III: They developed for the first time the MOMP program for intensive combination chemotherapy and X-irradiation in the treatment of Hodgkin's disease (Proc Am Assoc Cancer Res, 1965;6:15)
*1968: Anthony Epstein, Bert Achong and Yvonne Barr identified the first human cancer virus, called the Epstein—Barr virus (Epstein MA, Achong BG, Barr YM. Virus particles in cultured lymphoblast from Burkett's lymphoma. Lancet, 1964;1:7335: 702–3).
1973: HeLa Gold, Michael: He discovered oncoviruses (A Conspiracy of Cells: One Woman's Immortal Legacy and the Medical Scandal it Caused. ISBN 978-0-88706-099-1.)
1984: Harald Zur Hausen: He discovered first human papillomaviruses—HPV16 and HPV18, which were responsible for cervical cancers. For this discovery, he was honored with Nobel Prize in 2008 ("Harald Zur Hausen—Autobiography". Nobelprize.org.)

1980: Pediatric oncology as a specialty was virtually nonexistent in the India. Most children were treated by adult oncologists. The first dedicated pediatric cancer unit was started in Tata Memorial Hospital in 1985 (Advani SH, Agarwal R, Venugopal P, Saikia TK. Paediatric Oncology in India. Indian J Pediatr. 1987;54:843–5 Pub Med).

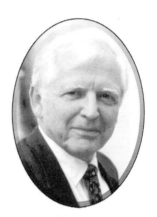

Harald Zur Hausen

2009: John A Boockvar: An American neurosurgeon, who performed the world's first intra-arterial delivery of the high-potency chemotherapeutic agent Avastin (bevacizumab) directly into a malignant brain tumor. He started a new era of "interventional neuro-oncology ("World's first delivery of intra-arterial Avastin directly into brain tumor". sciencedaily.com. Nov 17, 2009).

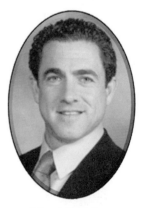

John A Boockvar

Father's figures of cancer pathology: Giovanni Battista Morgagni, Marie-Francois Xavier Bichat, Johannes Muller and Rudolf Ludwig Karl Virchow were known as father figure of cancer pathology. They were the first to describe microscopically the appearance of malignant tumors, the tumor stroma, the pathways of metastases and the association of inflammation and cancer (Neoplastic Diseases. Philadelphia, PA: WB Saunders Company; 1919).

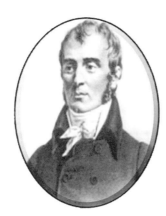

Giovanni Battista Morgagni
(1682–1771: From Padua)

Marie-Francois Xavier Bichat
(1771–1802: From France)

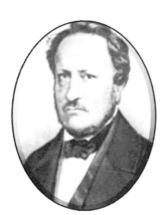

Johannes Muller
(1801–1858)

***History of Radiotherapy**
1869: The 'cathode rays' were discovered by Hittorf.

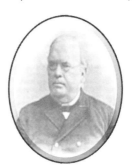

Hittorf

1895: Roentgen made the first X-ray photo.
1896: Voigt in Germany irradiated the first patient with a cancer of the throat
1939: Cyclotron was invented.
1940: Betatron was invented.
1948: Cobalt-60 unit was invented.
1953: Brachytherapy and linear accelerator was invented.

***History of Chemotherapy**
*460 to 370 BC: Hippocrates' remedy was a mixture of momordica elaterium, cucumber, honeycomb and water in juice was used for treatment of cancer.
*100AD: Dioscurides of Anazarous used terebinth oil, frankincense, hedge mustard and honey in plasters for hidden cancers.
*100AD: Leonides of Alexandria used ass's milk, opium, pork fat, fresh butter and rose oil in plasters for cancer treatment.
*200AD: Galen of Pergamum used an ointment consisting of calcined shells of whelk, purple shell fish, oysters, sea urchin, crab, sour wine, honey, pork fat for external cancers.
*1900: German chemist Paul Ehrlich coined the term "chemotherapy".

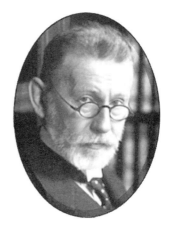

Paul Ehrlich

*1910: George Clowes of Roswell Park Memorial Institute in New York, developed the first transplantable tumor systems in rodents.

*1946: Gustaf Lindskog: He was a thoracic surgeon, who administered nitrogen mustard to a patient with non-Hodgkin's lymphoma having severe airway obstruction. Marked regression was observed in this and other lymphoma patients. The use of nitrogen mustard for lymphomas spread rapidly throughout the United States after the publication of this article.

*1948: Farber showed the antifolate activity of methotrexate in childhood leukemia.

*1949: Farber, Heinle and Welch tested folic acid in leukemia and they came to the conclusion that it actually accelerated leukemia cell growth (Farber S, Incurable cancers. Blood, 1949; 4:160–7).

*1950: Penicillin was initially thought to have antitumor properties that were never confirmed. But later on another antibiotic, actinomycin D was studied for antitumor properties and which is commonly used in pediatric tumors (Pinkel D. Actinomycin D in childhood cancer; a preliminary report. Pediatrics, 1959;23:342-7).

*1968: Dr Min Chiu Li: He was a pioneer chemotherapist who developed new curative chemotherapy for metastatic choriocarcinoma and testicular cancer.

*20th century: The use of chemotherapy for the treatment of cancer began (Cancer Res 2008; 68, 21:8643-53).

Despite all these inventions and modalities of management, the morbidity and mortality related with pediatric malignancies is challenge to forthcoming pediatricians and pediatric oncosurgeons. The important massage by this "History of Pediatric Oncology" chapter is to relieve pain of child and his family due to malignancy.

SUGGESTED READING

1. Advani SH, Agarwal R, Venugopal P, Saikia TK. Paediatric oncology in India. Indian J Pediatr.1987;54:843-5.
2. Antman K, Chang Y. Kaposi's sarcoma. New Engl J Med. 2000;342-14:1027-38.
3. Campbell De Morgan's 'Observations on cancer'- John M Grange, John L Stanford, Cynthia A Stanford SRN. Journal of the Royal Society of Medicine. 2002;95:296-9.
4. Conspiracy of Cells: One Woman's Immortal Legacy and the Medical Scandal it Caused. ISBN 978-0-88706-099-1.
5. Dobson J Percivall Pott in Annals of the Royal College of Surgeons of England. Vol. 50, 1972.pp.54-65.
6. Epstein MA, Achong BG, Barr YM. Virus particles in cultured lymphoblast from Burkitt's lymphoma. Lancet, 1964;1(7335):702-3.
7. Kass AM, Kass EH. Perfecting the World: The life and times of Dr Thomas Hodgkin, 1798–1866, Harcourt Brace Jovanovich 1988.
8. Lee RE, Young RH, Castleman B. James Homer Wright: A biography. Am J Surg Pathol. 2002;26(1):88-96.
9. Marilyn Yalom. "A history of the breast". New York: Alfred A Knopf. 1997. ISBN 0-679-43459-3.
10. Miller, Denis R. A tribute to Sidney Farber – the Father of Modern Chemotherapy. British Journal of Hematology 134. July 2006.
11. Opera Omnia. Vol XI, XII. Kuhn CG (editor). Leipzig, Germany; 1826. p. 139-41.
12. Pinkel D. Actinomycin D in childhood cancer; a preliminary report. Pediatrics, 1959;23:342-7.
13. Pioneer in X-ray Therapy. Science, New Series, 125(3236):18-9. January 1957. JSTOR 1752791.
14. Rutherford A. The Cell: Episode 1 the Hidden Kingdom. BBC4. August 2009.

Epidemiology of Childhood Cancer

Astha Tiwari, Sumantra Sarkar

INTRODUCTION

Cancer is an important cause of mortality in many of the economically developed nations of the world. Malignant diseases in developed countries cause 10% of all deaths in children below 15 years of age. In the developing world, childhood cancers are yet to be recognized as a major pediatric illness due to several other competing causes of death like diarrhea and respiratory illness. However, due to considerable reduction in infant and child mortality rates experienced in a few developing countries, it is now emerging as a distinct entity to be dealt upon.

Childhood cancers are unique in the sense that they arise from embryonic cells, respond to treatment rapidly. Unlike incidence pattern in adults, where cancer rates tend to increase rapidly with increasing age, in children two peaks are seen in early childhood and in adolescence. During the first year of life, embryonic tumors such as neuroblastoma, nephroblastoma (Wilms' tumor), retinoblastoma, rhabdomyosarcoma, hepatoblastoma, and medulloblastoma are most common. Embryonal tumors, acute leukemias, non-Hodgkin lymphomas, and gliomas peak in incidence from 2–5 years of age. As children age, bone malignancies, Hodgkin disease, gonadal germ cell malignancies (testicular and ovarian carcinomas) are more common.

RISK FACTORS

The etiology of cancer in children is poorly understood. Epidemiological studies have recognized that mechanism is multifactorial possibly resulting from potential interactions between genetic susceptibility traits and environmental exposures. The most notable genetic conditions that impart childhood cancer susceptibility are neurofibromatosis types 1 and 2, Down syndrome, Beckwith-Wiedemann syndrome, tuberous sclerosis, Von Hippel-Lindau disease, xeroderma pigmentosum, ataxia-telangiectasia, nevus basal cell carcinoma syndrome and Li-Fraumeni (P53) syndrome, etc. Viruses have been associated with certain pediatric cancers, such as polyomaviruses (BK, JC, SV40) associated with brain cancer and Epstein-Barr virus with non-Hodgkin lymphoma, but the etiologic importance remains unclear.

INCIDENCE OF CHILDHOOD CANCER

The incidence of childhood cancer in most populations in the world ranges from 75 to 150 per million children per year. Worldwide, the annual number of new cases of childhood cancer exceeds 200,000 and more than 80% of these are from the developing world. There is paucity of accurate vital statistics of childhood cancer in India. Children comprise approximately 40% of India's population. Annual incidences of cancer are about 75 to 80 per 10000 men and women respectively. Approximately, 5% of these are in pediatric age group as estimated by population based cancer registries. Approximately 40,000 new pediatric cancers are estimated to be diagnosed annually. The proportion of childhood cancers relative to all cancers reported by Indian cancer registries varied from 2.1 to 6.2%. However, the reported age of the standardized incidence rate for India, ranges from 38 to 124 per million children per year.

In India, though there being a higher proportion of childhood cancer relative to the developed world, it has not been a priority in healthcare. This is because of its contribution to overall childhood mortality. Only 2% of all deaths in this age (< 15 years) group are reported to be cancer-related deaths. Excluding neonatal deaths, infectious and parasitic diseases are the most common causes of death in children in India. Cancer contributes to less than 5% of the total cancer burden in India, with approximately 45,000 children diagnosed with cancer every year.

CANCER TYPES

Leukemias and lymphomas comprise nearly half of childhood cancers. Leukemia is the most common childhood cancer in India, frequency being 25 to 40%. Acute lymphoblastic leukemia (ALL) comprises 60 to 85% of all leukemias. The biology of ALL appears different in India, with a higher proportion of T-Cell ALL (20–50% as compared to 10–20% in the developed world, hypodiploidy and translocations t(1;19), t(9;22), and t(4;11), all of which contribute to a poorer prognosis of this leukemia. It has been proposed that T-Cell ALL predominates in economically disadvantaged areas.

In the developed world, CNS tumors are the second most common childhood cancer (22–25%) and lymphomas a distant third (10%). In contrast, in India lymphomas often exceed CNS tumors, particularly in males. Although the frequency data from AIIMS demonstrated a similar to developed country where leukemia is followed by brain tumor and lymphoma (Fig. 2.1). This may be explained due to better diagnostic facilities in developed countries due to availability of CT and MRI scanners. In India proportion of Hodgkin's disease exceeds non-Hodgkin's lymphoma (NHL), a pattern opposite to that seen in the developed world. In India, mixed cellularity is the most common Hodgkin's disease subtype, presents at a younger age, compared to the peak seen at ages 16 to 30 years in the developed world, where nodular sclerosis is most common. The high proportion of mixed cellularity in India is thought to be related to early childhood Ebstein-Barr virus exposure.

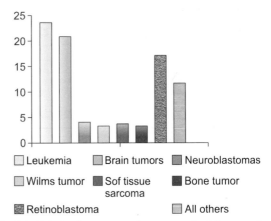

Fig. 2.1: Relative frequency of cancer under 15 years of age (population-based data) from AIIMS

VARIATION IN SEX

Cancer in childhood is more common among males than females. The male to female ratio is around 1.2:1. The male to female ratio for magnitude of childhood cancers ranges from 1.1 to 2.5 in different registries. Cancers like retinoblastoma, Wilms' tumor, osteosarcoma, and germ cell tumor show a slight female preponderance.

The reported incidence of childhood cancer in India in males (39–150 per million children per year) is higher than in females (23–97 per million children per year). Male preponderance is seen in Hodgkin's disease (HD). Gender bias in seeking healthcare, including treatment of cancer is one possible explanation. Childhood cancer risk among males is also higher as compared to females.

Relative frequency of cancer under 15 years of age (population-based data) from AIIMS	
Types	*Frequency (%)*
Leukemia	23.8
Brain tumors	21
Lymphomas	11.5
Neuroblastomas	4.1
Wilms tumor	3.3
Soft tissue sarcoma	3.8
Bone tumor	3.3
Retinoblastoma	17.2
All others	11.8

INCIDENCE TRENDS OF CHILDHOOD CANCERS

The incidence of childhood cancer is increasing by 1.1% every year in Europe, being different for individual cancer types. The incidence of CNS tumors is increasing by 1%. lymphomas by 0.9%, and leukemia by 0.6%. On the other hand the incidence of bone tumors, liver tumors, and retinoblastoma is unchanged.

The changing attributed by early suspicion, diagnostic facilities, lifestyle pattern may contribute to increasing trends. In India, the reported incidence of childhood cancer has increased over the last 25 years, but the increase is much larger in females (44–76%) than males (12–27%).

SURVIVAL RATE

Advances in treatment of childhood cancers have dramatically increased survival rate to around 70% in developed countries. Although this constitutes a remarkable medical achievement, the late morbidity in this growing survivor population has become area of concern. The highest survival in India is seen for Wilms' tumor and Hodgkins' disease where approximately two-third of the children survive for five years or more. The prognosis for leukemia and CNS tumors is less satisfactory where approximate only 33% and 25% of the children survive at five years. This low survival may be related to late diagnosis, an advanced stage at presentation, and suboptimal chemotherapy regimens and incomplete treatment due to financial constraints.

CONCLUSION

The hallmark of success in pediatric oncology in developed country is multidisciplinary approach executed through combined modality team comprising of a pediatric surgeon, radiologist, diagnostic specialist and supportive care service. Curative therapy with chemotherapy, radiation, and/or surgery may adversely affect a child's development and result in serious long-term medical and psychosocial effects in both childhood and adulthood. Potential adverse late effects include subsequent malignancy, early mortality, infertility, reduced stature; systemic diseases, neurocognitive impairment, etc. needs special focus.

SUGGESTED READING

1. Arora RS, Eden TOB, Kapoor G. Epidemiology of childhood cancer in India. Indian Journal of Cancer. 2009;46(4):264-73.
2. Ghai OP, Paul VK, Bagga Arvind (Eds). Essential Pediatrics. 7th Edn. CBS Publishers, New Delhi. 2009.
3. Kliegman R, Stanton B, St Geme J, Schor N, Behrman R (Eds). Nelson Textbook of Pediatrics. 19th Edn. Saunders 2011 Philadelphia.
4. Parthasarathy A (Ed). IAP Textbook of Pediatrics. 5th Edition 2013. Jaypee Brothers Medical Publishers (P) Ltd. New Delhi.
5. Satyanarayana L, Asthana S. Childhood Cancer Risk Trends in India (1982-2000). Indian Pediatrics, 2007;44:939-41.

3 Immune Biology of Malignancy

Rakesh Mondal, Anirban Chatterjee

Nature can be explored on many levels; none is more or less profound, none is more or less correct, but they are different. Which one you choose depends upon inclination, talent, accident, but most of all, unfortunately, upon fashion" written as a "Preface to a Grammar of Biology" book.

Immunology comes in handy in explaining the defensive mechanisms of the body against the attack of infection. The inventions of human blood groups, transfusion achieve the immunology of transplantation. Immunologists realize that tumors can be induced by viruses. Again it was found that some cancers have evidence of microscopic immune reaction around the cancers. Cancer has been induced in animals by experimental therapeutics by injection of cancer cells in them. Lymphoreticular neoplasm is well-documented with congenital immunodeficiency, such as Wiskott-Aldrich syndrome, ataxia telangiectasia, common variable immunodeficiency syndrome and acquired immunodeficiency states, e.g. in transplant receiver, AIDS patient. Non-Hodgkin lymphoma commonly occurs with these conditions. Some autoimmune diseases have been associated with malignancy, e.g. systemic lupus erythematous is linked with Non-Hodgkin lymphoma, Hashimoto thyroiditis with thyroid lymphoma. The idea is that breakdown of immune system is directly related to immune disorders and cancer cell proliferation. Again there are subjective evidences of spontaneous regression of malignancy and degeneration of distant metastasis after surgical removal of primary cancer. All these point towards a role of immune system in pathology of immunohematopoietic cell malignancy as well as its treatment.

THE MECHANISM FOR PREVENTION OF NEOPLASIA

All nucleated cells of mature immunohematopoietic system and the differentiating immature precursor cell can produce cancer. These malignancies are classified by clinical examination as well as by histopathological and molecular study of the malignant cell. Human immune system consists of T cell, B cell, natural killer (NK) cell, monocyte, neutrophil, basophil and esonophil. Innate immunity against tumor development is present in host.

The information necessary to distinctively and precisely identify the different malignancies reside in a comparatively small gene locus. Cell mediated immunity (CMI) is chiefly responsible for destruction of cancer cells. Cytotoxic T cell, the monocyte-macrophage system and natural killer cell (NK cell) constitute the CMI. T-cell immune responses could be divided into those promoting cell mediated immunity (Th1) and those promoting humoral responses (Th 2). Cytotoxic T lymphocytes are released from spleen, are attached to tumor cell then undergo lysis. The monocyte-macrophage system secretes substances called cytokines, e.g. tumor necrosis factor and interferon. The NK cells are large granular cell having azurophilic cytotoxic granules similar to lymphocytes. They kill malignantly transformed cells as target cells express little or no HLA class I molecules. NK cells express receptors that inhibit killer cell function when self MHC class I molecules are present. NK cells bind with cellular activating receptors and their ligands to recognize cancer cell and remove them. Regulatory T cells can inhibit naturally developing immune reaction to cancers. Most of the IL-17 families of cytokines induce TH1 types of T cell responses that direct to cytotoxic T cell effector function. Because of antigenic or immunological stimulation, polyclonal normal lymphocytes transform into monoclonal neoplastic cells and lymphoproliferative disease (LPDs) or lymphoma develops. This transformation is a multistep process and the reason for change of a non-neoplastic condition into neoplastic stage is not exactly clear. The hypotheses of multistep process is established by abnormal clones which are sensitive to normal controllers of growth and differentiation. The proliferation of such clones are subclinical and additional genetic changes make it irreversible. At the same time, a group of lymphoid disorders are each at a dissimilar stage of clonal development. The disease is often multiclonal in character. A large quantity of cell division resulting from polyclonal proliferation leads to random chromosomal reorganizations which are incapable of controlling oncogenes that switch normal cells to an irreversible malignant process. This clonal sequence of development requires a long time to grow in immune-competent individuals and less than one year in extremely immunocompromised individuals.

Immune system is responsible for surveillance to stop growth of cancer cells. Due to "end organ failure" or immature T- and B-cell series, "Stem cell overdrive" can stimulate differentiation and working of a functionally disordered T- or B-cell precursor group. This leads to enhanced mitotic activity of B- and T-ancestor population, which produce enhanced-risk of neoplastic proliferation. This is perhaps the reason for a development of lymphoreticular malignancies in immunodeficiency states. Using experimental approaches, it has been found that immunologically important molecules such as IFN-γ, IL-12, or cells such as NK-cells are essential for useful cancer immunosurveillance. IFN-γ and lymphocyte dependent tumor suppressor mechanisms have overlapping functions. Cancers can be recognized and eliminated by natural tumor-specific immune

responses. This observation is backed by the finding that the immune system can definitely defend against the expansion of spontaneous and chemically induced tumors. The immunogenicity of a malignancy is dependent on the immunological environment where it grows and the immune system can sometimes build up natural reactivity against the antigens of the tumor. Cancer is often undetectable due to the various mechanisms by which it is destroyed by the immune system. Tumor develops when the tumor is not immunogenic as other tumor antigens and the tumor cells are not lost during the progress of development of the cell. Defects in presenting tumor antigens to immune system and the production of immunosuppressive molecule that activates immunosuppressive responses also help in tumor development. This is the rationale, due to which immunotherapy can be effective.

IMMUNOEDITING

The term immunoediting is more precise than immunosurveillance. Immunoediting highlights dual role of the immune system in the progression. If stimulated, T cells may distinguish powerful immunogenic antigens. T cell recognition leads to complete or partial elimination of immunogenic and metastatic parts of cancer cells. Immune system has host protective action as well as an action to assist to form tumor. Immunoediting is consisting of the three phases: Elimination, equilibrium, escapes (Es). After cellular alteration and the stoppage of intrinsic tumor suppressor means, a growing tumor is identified by the immune system. It is determined by the host protective actions of immunity in elimination phase or it retained in a dormant or equilibrium state, it is called equilibrium phase. In escape phase, it escapes tumor suppressor actions of immunity by either becoming non-immunogenic or through the elaboration of immunosuppressive molecules. The cancer immunoediting hypothesis holds that the immune system not only protects the host against tumor development but can also promote tumor development by selecting for tumor escape variants with reduced immunogenicity. The first phase is called Elimination, which is the same as cancer immunosurveillance, in which cells and molecules of the innate and adaptive immune systems recognize and destroy developing tumors, thus protecting the host against cancer. The second phase is Equilibrium, similar to the concepts of tumor dormancy or viral latency, which is a protracted period in which the tumor and immune system enter into a dynamic equilibrium of tumor destruction and tumor escape. The third phase is Escape, where tumor variants that emerge from an immune selection process of the equilibrium phase develop into clinically apparent tumors that grow in an unrestricted manner in the immunocompetent host. First, several studies have now shown that immunosuppressed transplant patients display a significantly higher susceptibility to the formation of a variety of different cancers of non-viral origin. Second, a positive correlation has been made between the presence and location of T cells—particularly CD 8 + T cells — in a tumor and the survival of patients with a variety of different cancers. Third, cancer patients often develop spontaneous immune responses to the tumors that they carry. These findings now strongly support the statement that immunosurveillance happens.

GENETICS OF IMMUNOMALIGNANCY

There are two chief groups of cancer related genes: (a) The first group consists of oncogenes and tumor suppressor genes. The oncogenes positively influence cell growth and tumor suppressor genes have a negative effect on cell growth. These genes influence tumor growth by control of cell division or by apoptosis.

In cancer cells, single allele mutated oncogenes in dominant fashion generate increased activity of the gene product (proto-oncogene). The normal function of tumor suppressor genes is to control abnormal cell growth and this function is lost in cancer. As a consequence of the diploid character of mammalian cells, both alleles have to be dormant in recessive pattern of cell multiplication.

(b) The second group of cancer genes, the caretakers, preserve the integrity of its genome. Absence of these genes increases the rate of mutations in all the genes, such as oncogenes and tumor suppressor genes. Point mutations and large deletions are the most important types of somatic lesions detected in tumor suppressor genes

at some point in tumor development. Point mutations within the coding region of tumor suppressor genes produce truncated protein or nonfunctional proteins. Heterozygosity in tumor DNA is regarded as a hallmark for the occurrence of a tumor suppressor gene at an exacting locus. Heterozygosity studies have been valuable in the positional cloning of many tumor suppressor genes. A different mechanism of tumor suppressor gene inactivation is gene silencing. This takes place in combination with hypermethylation of the promoter.

IMMUNE MEDIATORS OF IMMUNOMALIGNANCY

Immune systems are not able to attack cancer cell effectively. Malignant cells develop multiple behaviors to prevent immune surveillance. They are different from normal cell major histocompatibility complex antigens helping them to mask identification by T cells. They are incompetent in presenting against themselves antigens to the immune cell. They envelop themselves in a defensive shell of fibrin to reduce contact with surveillance immune systems. They generate a variety of soluble molecules which are of help in preventing the immune system to recognize the cancer cells. They also create defects in T cells so that they can avoid their activation and cytotoxic activity. Cancer treatment reduces the host immunity.

In cell-mediated immunity, it has been found that the immune system shows significant strong anticancer effect. Three categories of experimental measures have been taken by using the capacity of T cells to destroy cancer cells. These are as follows:

1. In three main ways, allogeneic T cells can be transfused. Allogeneic bone marrow transplantation, pure lymphocyte transfusions subsequent to bone marrow revival following allogeneic bone marrow transplantation, minitransplants—pure lymphocyte transfusions after that immunosuppressive without myeloablation.

   Adoptively transferred donor T cells increase in the cancer-developing host and identify the cancer cell as foreign due to minor histocompatibility dissimilarity and can produce remarkable anticancer effects. Because of the negligible dissimilarity between the cancer and the normal cells, which increase risk of graft-versus-host disease. This therapy is highly successful in hematologic malignancy.

2. Autologous T cells—T cells are taken out from the cancer-bearing host and processed through some technique in vitro, and administered back to that particular host. The two main category of autologous T cell management are (a) to produce cancer antigen–specific T cells and (b) increase to huge quantity over many weeks in vitro before transfusion to stimulate the cells by polyclonal stimulators.

3. Vaccination approach is by peptide, protein or recombinant vaccine. All vaccination procedures have engaged immunization against shared cancer antigens. Autologous cancer cell vaccines or autologous heat shock protein vaccines is exceptional which have unique antigens. The objective of cancer vaccines is to enhance T cell action. T cell identify intracellular mutant oncogenes as targets to destroy as something is dissimilar regarding malignant cells. The most important problem lies into receive the tumor-specific peptides accessible in an order to prime the T cells. Malignant cells do not expose own antigens to T cells as the initial antigen for the process of priming. Priming is done very well by antigen presenting dendritic cells. Vaccine adjuvant GM-CSF draw antigen presenting cells to a cancer antigen. A microscopic residual disease of follicular lymphoma has been suppressed by this process. The process produces tumor-specific T cells. Particular tumor antigens or growth, its membranes added with purified antigen-presenting cells and carried as a vaccine. Cancer cells are able to be transfected with genes, which draw antigen-presenting cells. Vaccines against lymphomas show minimal clinical success.

ANTICANCER ANTIBODIES AND CYTOKINES

The hybridoma techniques produce huge quantity of high affinity antibody directed at a tumor for treatment of cancer. The first study of a monoclonal antibody in malignancy was published in 1980 and established that many hurdles are needed to be overcome to make the approach successful. It is better to attack a molecule which is not disassociated or modulated by the tumor. A target, which is responsible for an essential action for the tumor cells should be important point than physiologically irrelevant target. Murine antibodies are not very effectual as it is not involved in human effectors mechanisms. Rituximab is humanized antibodies against the CD 20 molecule expressed on B cell lymphomas and become important tool for the oncologists. It can singly cause tumor regression mainly in B cell lymphoma and also to potentiate the effects of combination chemotherapy.

Antibodies to CD 52 are useful in chronic lymphoid leukemia. Antibodies can be conjugated with drugs and toxins and also with isotopes, photodynamic substance and other killing molecule. Ibritumomab tiuxetan with yttrium-90 is radioconjugates attacking CD 20 on lymphomas and it has been used successfully. But problems are antigenicity, instability and poor tumor penetration.

Cytokines are soluble glycoprotein. Cytokines are formed by hematopoietic cell like T cells, NK cells, mast cells, basophils, monocytes/macrophages, B cells, and some nonhematopoietic cell. Cytokines are concerned with the growth, development and establishment of immune system and having various biologic functions. Cytokines are pleiotropic that means they can act on many diverse cell types due to the expression of same receptors on multiple cell. The action of cytokines can be the target cell is the same (autocrine) or the target cell is in close proximity (paracrine) or the cytokine goes to the circulation to act remote (endocrine). The basis of name of cytokines either assumed targets or assumed functions. Those cytokines, which act primarily on leukocytes named interleukins (IL). Sometimes granulocyte colony-stimulating factor or G-CSF name is given due to originally have definite function retained the name. Chemokines are cytokines which control cell movement and trafficking. Chemokines act through G protein-coupled receptors and have a distinctive three-dimensional structure.

Cytokines are more than 70 different proteins and with various biologic function in humans: IFN family, IL-1 to 29 and the tumor necrosis factor (TNF) family which includes lymphotoxin, TNF-related apoptosis-inducing ligand (TRAIL), CD 40 ligand and the chemokine family. Among them only few like IFN-α-2a and IL-2 are in clinical therapy.

In vitro interferon antitumor action occurred by antagonizing with thymidine. IFN-α2a and 2b are the commercially available two recombinant types. Anticancer action of interferon is dose-related, and IFN is most effective. Interferon is not curative but can bring partial responses in follicular lymphoma, hairy cell leukemia. It is also used as adjuvant in follicular lymphoma with indecisive effects on survival. Adverse effects of IFN are fever, flu like syndrome, myelosuppression, depression and autoimmune disease.

Monoclonal antibody is essential component of diagnostic procedure of tumor immunology. Cancer specific antigens which are tumor marker found in circulation, in others body fluid, in specific tissue. ELISA and RIA methods detect the tumor markers by using monoclonal antibodies. In immunocytochemistry, tumor markers are detected by monoclonal antibody technique in cytological specimen and similarly when used in histological specimen are called immunohistochemistry. These are also attached with radioactive isotope and this method is known as radioimmunodetection (RID).

The monoclonal antibody technology invents numerous new leukocyte surface molecules. The First International Workshop on Leukocyte Differentiation Antigens was held in 1982 and since then a nomenclature for cell-surface molecules of human leukocytes had been started. Thereafter, leukocyte differentiation workshops develop the cluster of differentiation (CD) classification of leukocyte antigens. CD antigen characterize mostly for different subtypes of T and B cells. It applies to classification of malignancies like leukemia and lymphoma.

IMMUNOTHERAPY

At present immunotherapy has appeared as the latest mode of treatment in cancer. It is used as an adjuvant to standard therapeutic modalities, such as chemotherapy, radiotherapy and surgery.

Immunotherapy is defined as an approach that modifies the immunological relationship between host and tumor in such a way that it alters the host's immune response to tumor cell in a therapeutically beneficial way. Standard therapy like chemotherapy, radiotherapy, surgery directly eradicate cancer cells. Immunotherapy doesn't kill the malignant cell but boost and stimulate the normal host immune mechanisms, so that regression of cancer can start. The term 'Biological response modifier' are the substances, which originate from biological sources and are applied as immunogenic reagent. Immunomodulators in malignancy are the agents that alter the host response to malignant cells, improve host resistance and directly inhibit tumor growth.

Immunotherapeutic approaches can be stratified as follows:

a. *Cytomodulatory:* This is to amplify the tumor associated antigen or major HLA antigen on surface of malignant cell

b. *Active:* It is used for specific (vaccine) or non-specific (macrophage or NK cell) stimulation of innate immune system

c. *Passive:* This is mediated by exogenously formed antibodies

d. *Restorative:* Restitution of poor immune response, e.g. to inhibit suppressor T cell or to abrogate the suppressor macrophage.

Recombinant DNA technology is important for huge production of highly purified biological molecule such as cytokines, which has immune regulatory action.

After high-dose chemotherapy, colony stimulating factor (GM-CSF) or progenitor stimulating factor (G-CSF) is used for accelerating bone marrow expansion and also to boost the quantity of progenitor cell in blood so that high concentration of stem cells can be achieved by apheresis, which can be cryopreserved and utilized for autologus bone marrow transplant.

Interferons (IFN) have cytotoxic, immunmodulatory and antiproliferative properties. Immunomodulatory actions can be achieved by increased T cell cytotoxic action and NK cell activity. It modifies expression of HLA and tumor associated antigen. After randomized trial, IFN-α-2a has been approved for use in few types of low grade NHL lymphoma and hairy cell leukemia. IFN also increases efficiency of chemotherapeutic drugs like ara-c.

Interleukins are secreted by immune cells. The most used IL-2 is a T cell proliferative factor and is the most important factor for clonal expansion of lymphocyte. IL-2 has direct anti-tumor action and indirectly stimulates IFN and tumor necrosis factor. Cytotoxic action and cell proliferation can be induced by incubating lymphocyte harvested from cancer with IL-2 ex vivo. These are called lymphocyte activated killer cell. IL-2 therapy has numerous clinical side effects such as fever, chills, skin rash intravascular volume depletion, capillary leak syndrome, adult respiratory distress syndrome, hypotension, and impaired renal and liver function. Adoptive immunity is defined as transmission of immune reactive cell, which would be able to produce anti-malignant activity to the cancer bearing host. The main problem is the failure to recognize the specific cancer cell in host. Lymphocyte activated killer cell have specific aptitude to make out cancer cells. Monoclonal antibodies can attack tumor surface antigens and so it can be used to treat specific targeted cancer cells. For effective monoclonal treatment, the concentration of antigen in cancer cell should be several times more than that of normal cells. Monoclonal antibody therapy in T and B cell lymphoma has low efficiency. Monoclonal antibodies incorporated with toxin like ricin and used to treat cancer are called immunotoxin therapy. Similarly, when it integrates with radioactive isotope it is called radioimmunotherapy and combination with chemotherapeutic agent, called chemoimmunotherapy. These therapies are used for compartmental administration and is on clinical trial for intralesional therapy.

APOPTOSIS

Apoptosis is most important in regulating normal immune responses to antigen. Many human diseases have been demonstrated that are the effect of or that are associated with mutated apoptosis genes. Due to under expression of bcl-2 and bcl-10 protein, non-Hodgkin's lymphoma develops in human beings. Under expression of c-IAP2 may lead to development of low-grade MALT lymphoma in humans. Mutation of gene Fas and of Fas ligand can lead to development of lymphoproliferative disorders. There is a correlation of mutated genes in the apoptotic pathway with certain malignant diseases. Bone marrow forms lymphocytes. These lymphocytes are clonally increased in periphery after attaching with antigen. So cell death is necessary to sustain a constant lymphocytic pool. Cells in immune system have normal life span. Lymphocyte antigens and different signals are responsible for cell survival and apoptotic cell death. Metazoans have developed a genetic program that stimulates the programmed death of cells. This course is known as apoptosis. Interactive intra- and extracellular signals are required to control cell division in the core cell cycle system. So these signals adjust a core enzymatic mechanism that controls cell death and survival.

Two main pathways are important for apoptosis.

(a) In the extrinsic pathway (death induced apoptosis)–The super family "death receptor" and ligands belonging to TNF are essential for immune system. The largest "death receptors" family are the tumor necrosis factor receptor (TNF-R) family which includes TNF-R 1, TNF-R 2, Fas (CD 95), death receptor 3 (DR 3), death receptor 4 (TRAIL-R1), and death receptor 5 (DR 5, TRAIL-R 2).

Apoptosis is triggered by attachment of the tumor necrosis factor (TNF) receptor superfamily, e.g. CD95 (Fas) by its ligand (CD95L), or the binding of death receptors DR 4 and DR 5 by their ligand TRAIL (TNF-related apoptosis-inducing ligand). These bring on the association of FADD (Fas-associated death domain) and procaspase-8 to death domain component of the receptors. Caspase-8 is activated and it activates effector caspases-3 and-7, which then target cellular components for proteolysis including DNA, cytoskeletal proteins, and a variety of regulatory proteins. This leads to apoptosis.

(b) The intrinsic or stress induced pathway (involving p53 suppresor gene)—a group of lethal stimuli, including DNA damage, loss of adherence to the extracellular matrix (ECM), oncogene-induced proliferation, and growth factor deprivation produce stress on cell. The response is accomplished by energy source of cell-mitochondria. The genome of mitochondria is enclosed in two layers of membrane with cytochrome C which lies in between. Apoptosis is initiated by the release of cytochrome C and SMAC (second mitochondrial activator of caspases) from the mitochondrial intermembrane space to cytosol.

Pro caspases 9 in cytosol is activated to release caspases. The caspases responsible for activation of caspases 3 and caspases cascade make catalytic cleavage of cell substrate.

MALIGNANT DISORDER OF THE IMMUNE SYSTEM

Human immune system consists of T cell, B cell, natural killer (NK) cell, monocyte, neutrophil, basophil and esonophil. All nucleated cells of mature immunohemopoietic system may undergo neoplastic changes and cause cancer. The same is true for precursor cell. When malignancy involved all bone marrow and lymphoid cell types designed as in both localized solid tumor and disseminated leukemia type. Each of these has unique clinical spectrum in matter of age, localization clinical feature and cellular and molecular analyses of neoplastic cell. Immnusupressed state increases incidence of neoplastic disorder. An intact immune system plays strong "surveillance role" to protect against development of malignancy. Molecular defect and genetic damage results in DNA damage with malignant transformation.

NORMAL B CELL ONTOGENY

The normal stages B cell differentiations are characterized by expression of cell surface and cytoplasmic antigen.

B cell grouped as Pan B cell antigen—span ontogeny appear non resting B cell. It appear after activation at terminal state of differentiation. Pre-B cell differentiation takes place in prenatal-fetal liver and bone marrow; Adult-bone marrow; Pre B antigen cell surface antigen— CD 19 (the most reliable cell marker of B lineage in pre B cell, this is a glycoprotein of Ig gene super family), CD 34 (early stem marker also present in myeloid progenitor cells) CD 22 is B cell restricted antigen present in cytoplasm of earliest stage of B cell and it is then exported to the cell surface at mature resting B cell. After CD 19 and cytoplasmic CD 22, cell express CD 10 or common acute lymphocytic leukemia antigen (CALLA). Next pre B cell express pan B cell restricted antigen CD 20. Last stage characterized by the expression of the cytoplasmic Ig μ heavy chain without the expression of light chain. Pan B cell antigen CD 9, CD 24, CD 40, CD 45r, CD 72,

CD 73, CD 74, CD w78 are expressed during pre B cell development, these are decreased prior to plasma cell stage. Mature resting B cell express surface IgM or IgD, HLA-DR, CD 19, CD 20, CD 24 and CD 22 but not CD 10. Resting B cell also express CD 44 which is involved in lymphocytic reticulation and homing including the adhesion of lymphocyte to high endothelial venules. CD 21, CD 35 is two complement component receptor present in resting B cell. Following triggering with antigen or various polyclonal mitogens, the resting B cell is activated and subsequently proliferates. Within 24 hours of activation, they begin to lose surface IgD, CD 21, CD 22. The activation antigen includes CD 71, CD 54, CD 25, CD 5 and CD 23. Following activation B cell are competent to proliferate and subsequently secrete Ig. The terminal differentiation stage is also characterized by the appearance of several other antigens including CD 38, which is expressed on plasma cell.

NORMAL T CELL ONTOGENY

During embryonic and early postnatal life the bone marrow precursor cell migrate to thymus. Stage I of intrathymic differentiation express CD 2, CD 71, CD 38, CD 7. Stage II thymocyte are characterized by loss of CD 71 and acquisition of CD 1 and co-expression of CD 4, CD 8. These populations constitute 70% of the lymphocyte. In stage III with further maturation, the cell loses CD 1 and acquires mature T cell antigen CD 3, CD 5, CD 6. In addition, they express the T cell antigen receptor (TCR). When cells leave the thymus, they no longer express CD 38 and are segregated into cell expressing CD 4, CD 8. The latter constitute 60 to 70 per cent and 30 to 40 per cent of the peripheral blood T cell respectively. Peripheral T cell also expresses CD 25 (IL 25 receptor) and CD 26 followed by reappearance of CD 71, CD 70, CD 9, and CD 38.

Non-Hodgkin Lymphoma (NHL)

Low Grade NHL

These are follicular small cleaved and follicular mixed small cleaved and large-cell lymphoma. Immunological studies show presence of C 3 receptor, monoclonal surface immunoglobulin (Ig isotope μ ± δ or μ ± γ).

Virtually all cases express HLA-DR, CD 1, CD 19, CD 20, CD 21,CD 24, CD 10, CD 45 R.

Diffuse Small Lymphocytic Lymphoma

These tumors represent B cell chronic lymphocytic leukemia. The small lymphocytic lymphoma expresses HLA-DR, CD 19, CD 20, CD 21, CD 24, and CD 44.

Leukemia

Acute Leukemia

Immunophenotypically, the ALL can be classified into B cell and T cell leukemia (Table 3.1).

B cell lineage ALL divided in six subgroups on basis of expression of HLA DR, CD 19, CD 10, CD 20, cytoplasmic immunoglobulin and surface immunoglobulin. This classification based on the stage of differentiation with group 1 representing the least differentiated blast and group 6 the most differentiated blasts (Table 3.2).

Table 3.2: Classification of B lineage acute lymphoblastic leukemia

Group	HLA-DR	CD 19	CD 10	CD 20	Cytoplasmic μ	Surface membrane IG
I	+	–	–	–	–	–
II	+	+	–	–	–	–
III	+	+	+	–	–	–
IV	+	+	+	+	–	–
V	+	+	+	+	+	–
VI	+	+	+	+	–	+

T cell lineage ALL are generally classified according to the stages of thymocyte maturation:

i. Stage 1—early thymocytes express CD 7, CD 2, CD 5, CD 38, and CD 71.and acquire surface expression of CD 1, CD 4, and CD 8.

ii. Stage II—medullary lymphocyte loses CD 71, express CD 3 and CD 4 CD 8. The cytoplasmic CD 3 is reliable marker for the early thymocyte.

In B cell lineage ALL, the various immunophenotypes have demonstrated to have some significance. A few recent studies suggest that patient with early T cell phenotype respond poorly to treatment.

Table 3.1: Monoclonal antibodies useful in the study of ALL

Lymphoid-B

CD group	Antibodies	Reactivity
CD 19	B4, Leu12	B lymphocyte
CD 20	B 1, Leu 16	
CD 22	Leu 14, SHC 11	
CD 21	B2, CR 2	
CD 10	CALLA, J 5	Immature B cell

Lymphoid-T

CD group	Antibodies	Reactivity
CD 1	T 6, leu 6	Thymocytes
CD 2	T 11, leu 5b	T cell, subset of NK cell
CD 3	T 3, leu4	
CD 4	Leu 9, 3A1, WT1	T lymphocyte,
CD 5	Leu1, T1	small subset of B cell

SUGGESTED READING

1. Dunn GP, Old LJ, Schreiber RD. The three Es of cancer immunoediting. Annu Rev Immunol. 2004;22:329-60.
2. Jones A. Hormonal therapy and Immunotherapy for cancer. Medicine International. 1998;430-3.
3. Old LJ. Immunotherapy for cancer. Sci Am 1996;275: 136-43.
4. Robert D. Schreiber Cancer Vaccines 2004 opening address: The molecular and cellular basis of cancer immunosurveillance and immunoediting; Cancer Immunity, 2005;5(1).
5. Stein H, Hummel M, Marafioti T, et al. Molecular biology of Hodgkin's disease. Cancer Surv. 1997;30:107-23.

4 Cytogenetics in Pediatric Cancers

Anup Kumar Roy, Anjan Das, Rakesh Mondal

INTRODUCTION

It has been recognized for quite some time now that genetic factors contribute to the development of a number of human cancers. These factors may be particularly important in the etiology of pediatric malignancies because, in most cases, these young patients have been minimally exposed to environmental mutagens and carcinogens. For example, certain hereditary disorders, such as neurofibromatosis and immunodeficiency, predispose the host to specific childhood cancers. Likewise, certain constitutional chromosomal abnormalities, chromosomal breakage syndromes and defects in DNA repair are associated with increased risk for cancer in these children. There are solid tumors like retinoblastoma and Wilm's tumor, which occur in a hereditary form. Over the past decades great strides have been made towards elucidating the cytogenetic mechanisms involved in carcinogenesis.

Genetic factors play an important role in the development of some pediatric cancers. These factors are more predominant in the pediatric age group because environmental exposures have been minimal. Several pediatric solid tumors, including retinoblastoma and Wilms' tumor, are hereditary. Specific constitutional chromosome abnormalities have been found in these patients which may explain tumorigenesis in some of them. Molecular genetic studies have provided insight into the events occurring at the DNA level in these gene regions. The role of genetics in other sporadic pediatric malignancies are elucidated today as specific chromosome abnormalities are being discovered in the malignant cells of these karyotypically normal individuals now. Certain hereditary disorders, such as neurofibromatosis

and immunodeficiency, predispose the host to specific childhood cancers. Likewise, certain constitutional chromosome abnormalities, chromosomal breakage syndromes and DNA repair defects are associated with an increased risk for cancer in children. Technical advances in cytogenetics have made it possible to define specific constitutional and acquired chromosome abnormalities that are associated with specific cancers, thus implicating certain gene regions as being involved in the process of malignant transformation. The rapidly progressing field of molecular genetics is providing further insight into the events occurring at the DNA level in these gene region.

BASIC GENETICS

Between 2 to 5% of all liveborn infants have genetic disorders or congenital malformations. Many diseases in adult life also have a considerable genetic predisposition, including cancer or diabetes.

Classification of Genetic Disorders
A. Traditional modes of inheritance
　I. Mendelian (Single Gene) disorders
　　i. Autosomal dominant (AD)
　　ii. Autosomal recessive (AR)
　　iii. X-linked recessive (XLR)
　　iv. X-linked dominant (XLD
　II. Chromosomal disorders
　　i. Numerical abnormalities
　　ii. Structural abnormalities
　III. Multifactorial disorders
B. Non-traditional modes of inheritance
　I. Mosaicism
　II. Genomic imprinting
　III. Uniparental disomy (UPD)
　IV. Inheritance of unstable mutations
　V. Cytoplasmic/mitochondrial inheritance

Chromosomal Disorders

The autosomes are divided in 7 groups according to the position of centromere.

Group A – Chromosome Pairs 1, 2, 3
Group B – Chromosome Pairs 4, 5
Group C – Chromosome Pairs 6, 7, 8, 9, 10, 11, 12
Group D – Chromosome Pairs 13, 14, 15
Group E – Chromosome Pairs 16, 17, 18
Group F – Chromosome Pairs 19, 20
Group G – Chromosome Pairs 21, 22

Each chromosome has a short arm designated as 'p' and a long arm 'q', the arms are joined together at a constriction called centromere 'c'. The types of chromosomes are metacentric (centromere in the middle), submetacentric (centromere towards short arm) and acrocentric (with secondary constriction and satellites). The majority of chromosomal disorders have a low risk of recurrence in the family. 4.5% of stillbirths and 0.6% of live borns have chromosomal abnormalities—numerical or structural. These abnormalities have a close relationship to development of neoplasia.

Numerical Abnormalities

A cell with exact multiple of the haploid number, e.g. 46, 69 is referred to as 'euploid'. Euploid cells with more than the normal diploid number of 46 is called 'polyploid'. Cells deviating from euploid number is 'aneuploid'. The presence of one additional chromosome to the normal homologous pair is called 'trisomy'. A chromosomal number one less than the diploid number is called 'monosomy'. An individual with two or more cell lines are called 'mosaic'.

Structural Abnormalities

Translocation: The transfer of all or part of a chromosome to another non-homologous chromosome, usually through a reciprocal event during meiosis. It can be:
Balanced: In which a full complement of genetic material is present. There is risk of offspring inheriting an unbalanced form in next generation.
Unbalanced: Here, due to deletion or duplication, full complement of genetic material is not present. This may result in spontaneous abortions or multiple physical/mental defects.
Robertsonian: This is translocation of 2 aerocentric chromosomes, in which, the small fragment formed by 2 short armed is usually lost.

Deletion: This is loss of portion of a chromosome, either terminal (5p-) or middle portion, i.e. interstitial (11p-)
Fragile site: Constriction sites other than centromere is known as fragile site which shows a tendency to break, e.g. Fragile X syndrome.
Duplication: It is presence of two copies of a segment of chromosome. It arises by unequal crossing over during meiosis.
Inversion: This is reverse joining of portion of a chromosome. This can be pericentric (on either side of centromere, involving both arms) or paracentric (on one side of centromere, in one arm only) e.g. 9q.
Ring chromosome: Both arms joining at terminal portion with loss of fragments to give a ring-like appearance, e.g. ring chromosome 18.
Contiguous gene syndrome: This involves microdeletion or microduplication resulting in involvement of genes that are adjacent to each other on a chromosome.

Somatic Cell Mutation

Some cancers can be inherited as simple Mendelian traits, with clear patterns of transmission. But though most cancers involve quite substantial changes in the genetic material, such mutations are somatic and there is no risk to further generations.

Mosaicism

Mosaicism is presence of two or more genetically different cell lines. Phenotype expression in mosaicism depends on dosage-affect relationship. It occurs as a postzygotic event and can be:

Chromosomal Mechanism

It has been recognized in cultured lymphocytes of patients with aneuploidy, e.g. Down syndrome, Turner syndrome, Diploid/Triploid phenotype, Pallister-Killian (12p isochromosome) syndrome, hypomelanosis of Ito.

Single Gene Mosaicism

Isomatic mosaicism for single gene mutation, e.g. Maccune-Albright syndrome.

Germline Mosaicism

Presence of mosaicism in germ cells, e.g. found in DMD, chronic granulomatous disease.

Genomic Imprinting

This means that the level of expression of the genes depends on the parent of origion. The genes are modified during gametogenesis and as a result are activated or inactivated. Deletion in chromosome 15q 11 or 13 region results in Prader-Willi syndrome, if inherited from father and in Angelman's syndrome, it inherited from mother. Other examples include Beckwith-Wiedeman syndrome and transient neonatal diabetes mellitus.

Uniparental Disomy

An individual may inherit both homologous chromosomes from only one of his parents. Thus a father with hemophilia can have an affected son and a child with cystic fibrosis may be born to a couple in which only the mother was carrier.

Unstable Mutation

Also known as Triplet Nucleotide Repeats. Fragile X mutations consists of an increase in the size of region in fragile X mental retardation (FMR-I) gene. This region contains a long CGG trinucleotide repeat sequence. In normal persons there are between 10–15 copies of this repeat and this is inherited in stable fashion. A small increase between 50–200 makes this sequence unstable, a condition known as premutation. A man carrying premutation is a 'normal transmitting male'. If this reaches a critical size of greater than 200 CGG triplets, it becomes a full mutation. Unstable mutations also reported in myotonic dystrophy, Huntigton's chorea and Kennedy's disease.

Mutations

A mutation may be defined as a detectable and heritable change in genetic material that is not caused by genetic recombination, a permanent change in the DNA. Mutations that affect germ cells are transmitted to the progeny giving rise to inherited diseases. Somatic cell mutations, though do not cause hereditary diseases, but are very important in the genesis of cancers and congenital malformations. Based on the extent of genetic changes, mutations have been classified into three categories.

Genome Mutation

This involves loss or gain of whole chromosomes, giving rise to monosomy or trisomy, i.e. numerical changes.

Chromosome Mutation

This results from rearrangement of genetic material and gives rise to structural changes in the chromosome.

These two mutations are transmitted only infrequently, because most are incompatible with survival. The vast majority of mutations associated with hereditary diseases are submicroscopic gene mutation. These may result in partial or complete deletion, substitution or insertion of a gene or more often a single nucleotide base. Mutation involving a single nucleotide base is termed a point mutation.

Point Mutation within Coding Sequences

There are different types:

Silent mutation: Mutation results in a different codon but the amino acid coded is the same as that of the original codon.

Missense mutation: Mutation results in coding of a new amino acid in place of the original resulting in production of an abnormal protein. If the substituted amino acid causes little change in the function of the protein, the mutation is called a conservative missense mutation. But, if the normal amino acid is replaced by a totally different one, it is called a non-conservative missense mutation, e.g. sickle mutation. The nucleotide triplet GAG codes for glutamic acid in β-globin chain of normal hemoglobin. In sickle cell anemia, this triplet is changed to GTG, which codes for valine, resulting in abnormal hemoglobin.

Nonsense mutation: Mutation results in introduction of a stop codon causing premature termination of protein synthesis resulting in a truncated protein. In β-globin, a pint mutation affecting the codon for glutamine (CAG) creates a stop codon UAG, if U substitutes C. This leads to premature termination of β-globin gene translation, resulting in β°-thalassemia.

Frame-shift mutation: Mutation causing single-base insertion or deletion resulting in a shift of the translational reading frame which leads to production of a completely different sequence of amino acids. Singe base deletion at ABO locus leading to frame-shift mutation in A allele can lead to O allele.

Point Mutation with Non-coding Sequences

Mutations in promoter region and introns can result in abnormal production, i.e. in excess or less. Mutation in exon/intron boundary may lead to differently spliced mRNA.

Polymorphisms

Some germline mutations occur in frequency of more than 1% in general population, which mostly have no relevance in health or disease. These are called polymorphisms and they may help in the process of evolution.

Protective Mutation

Uncommonly, mutations may be protective. HIV uses a chemokine receptor CCR5, to enter cells. A deletion in the CCR5 gene can protect from HIV infection.

Mutagens

Mutations may be generated spontaneously by rare errors that occur during DNA replications. More frequently mutations are produced by exposure to certain agents called mutagens, like high energy radiation (e.g. X-ray, U-V rays, γ-rays), certain viral infections (E-B virus, Herpes simplex, HPV, Coxsackie B) and certain chemicals (arsenic, asbestos, benzene, cadmium, ethylene oxide), etc.

Gain-of-function Mutation

This can result in an increase in the ability of a protein molecule to perform one or more normal functions or in overexpression of a gene product. Most frequently they produce autosomal dominant disorders as in achondroplasia or Charcot-Marie-Tooth disease, type-IA.

Loss-of-function Mutation

They are frequently observed in autosomal recessive disorders in which loss of 50% enzyme activity in the heterozygote continued to allow for normal function. They can have a dominant negative effect when the abnormal protein product activity interferes with the function of the normal protein product. Loss-of-function mutations can result in conditions in which 50% of the gene product is insufficient for normal function. This is termed as haploinsufficiency.

Genetic disorders are far more common than widely appreciated. The lifetime frequency of genetic diseases is estimated to be 670 per 1000. Included in this figure are not only the "classic" genetic disorders, but also cancer, diabetes or cardiovascular diseases.

A neoplasm is defined as an abnormal mass of tissue, the growth of which exceeds and is uncoordinated with that of the normal tissue and persists in the same excessive manner after cessation of the stimuli which evoked the change. The persistence of growth, even after withdrawal of the inciting stimulus, results from heritable genetic alterations that are passed down to the progeny of the tumor cells. These genetic changes allow excessive and unregulated proliferation that becomes autonomous. The entire population of cells within a tumor arises from a single cell, that has incurred genetic change, and hence the growth is said to be clonal. Certain anatomic features suggest the benign nature of a growth, while others point towards a malignant potential. Differentiation refers to the extent to which neoplastic cells resemble comparable normal cells, both morphologically and functionally. Lack of differentiations is called anaplasia. Anaplasia is marked by several morphologic changes. Both the cells and the nuclei characteristically display variation in size and shape, which is called pleomorphism. The nuclei contain an abundance of DNA and are extremely dark-staining, i.e. hyperchromatic. The nuclei are disproportionately large, and the nucleus to cytoplasm ratio may approach 1:1, instead of normal 1:4 to 1:6. Undifferentiated tumors usually possess large numbers of mitoses, reflecting the higher proliferative activity. Thus, malignant cells show atypical, bizarre mitotic figures, sometimes producing tripolar, quadripolar or multipolar spindles. The orientation of anaplastic cells is markedly disturbed, i.e. there is loss of normal polarity. Another important feature of anaplasia is the formation of tumor giant cell, some possessing a single huge polymorphic nucleus and other having two or more nuclei. Some anaplastic growths have scanty vascular stroma, and there are large central areas of ischemic necrosis. Dysplasia means disordered growth, which is mainly encountered in epithelia, and is characterized by constellation of changes that include a loss in the uniformity of individual cells as well as their architectural orientation.

GENETIC PREDISPOSITION TO CANCER

For a large number of cancer types, there exist not only environmental influences, but also genetic predispositions. Lung cancer is related to cigarette smoking, yet mortality from lung cancer has been shown to be four times greater among non-smoking relatives of lung cancer patients than among non-smoking relatives of smoker controls. Genetic predisposition to cancer have been divided into three categories:

Autosomal Dominant Inherited Cancer Syndromes

There are several well-defined cancers in which inheritance of a single mutant gene greatly increases the risk of developing a tumor. Usually, this is a point mutation occurring in a single allele of a tumor suppressor gene. The defect in the second allele occurs in the somatic cells, as a consequence of chromosome deletion. This is the classic two-mutation hypothesis of Knudson. Childhood retinoblastoma is the most striking example in this category. Approximately 40% of retinoblastomas are hereditary. Carriers of a mutant of RB tumor suppressor gene have a 10,000-fold increased risk of developing the tumor. The D group chromosome involved in all cases is chromosome 13, and the band common to all the deletions is 13q14. These data suggest that the retinoblastoma gene is located within this chromosomal band. Gene dosage studies have demonstrated that the locus for the enzyme esterase D is also located in band I 3q 14, and is closely linked to the retinoblastoma gene 13. Thus, there is a biochemical marker for small deletions of this region of chromosome 13. Most of the patients with this specific chromosomal deletion have other phenotypic abnormalities in addition to retinoblastoma. Although there is no classical phenotype, developmental delay, microcephaly, microphthalmia, and skeletal and genitourinary malformations have been reported. There is also an increased risk for the development of a second primary malignancy, usually an osteogenic sarcoma, both within and outside the field of radiation therapy. Again, individuals who inherit the autosomal dominant mutation of adenomatous polyposis coli (APC) tumor suppressor gene, have innumerable polypoid adenomatous growth of colon, virtually 100% of which are fated to develop a carcinoma later. Other examples in this category are Li-Fraumeni syndrome resulting from germline mutation of p53 gene, multiple endocrine neoplasia (MEN-1 and 2), hereditary nonpolyposis colonic cancer. Both incomplete penetrance and variable expressivity occur here like other autosomal dominant conditions. Neurofibromatosis has been linked to NF-1 and NF-2 genes. Deletion in short arm of chromosome 11 is associated with Wilms' tumor.

Common Features of Hereditary Cancers

a. High incidence of same or related tumors among family members
b. Bilateral involvement of organs
c. Multiple primary malignant neoplasms
d. Early age of onset with minimal exposure to environmental carcinogens
e. Autosomal dominant inheritance pattern.

Defective DNA Repair Syndromes

These conditions generally have an autosomal recessive pattern of inheritance. They are characterized by defects in DNA repair and resultant DNA instability. Included in this group are xeroderma pigmentosum, ataxia-telangiectasia and bloom syndrome. Hereditary non-polypoid colon cancer (HNPCC), although an autosomal dominant condition, may be included in this category. This is caused by inactivation of a DNA mismatch repair gene.

Familial Cancers

Virtually all the common types of cancers that occur sporadically have also been reported to occur in familial forms, without any clearly defined pattern of transmission. Examples included carcinomas of colon, breast, ovary, brain and melanoma. Two breast cancer susceptibility genes, namely BRCA-1 and BRCA-2 have been identified. Mutation of p16INK4A tumor suppressor gene has been linked to familial melanomas.

Molecular Basis of Cancer (Flow chart 4.1)

There are some fundamental points regarding the molecular basis of cancers and carcinogenesis. The most important are listed below:

Flow chart 4.1: Schematic diagram showing oncogenesis

Nonlethal genetic damage: This lies at the heart of carcinogenesis. Such damage may be inherited through germline or may be acquired by external agents, e.g. chemicals, radiation or viruses. Some mutations may even be spontaneous, without any detectable insults.

Clonal expression of a single precursor cell: Tumors are mostly monoclonal. The most commonly used method to determine tumor clonality involves the analysis of methylation pattern adjacent to the highly polymorphic locus of human androgen receptor gene. For neoplasms with a specific translocation, as in myeloid leukemias, the presence of translocation can be used to assess clonality. Immunoglobulin receptor and T-cell receptor gene rearrangements act as markers of clonality in B- and T-cell lymphomas, respectively.

Regulatory genes: There are four classes of normal regularity genes—the growth-promoting protooncogenes, the growth-inhibiting tumor suppressor genes,

programmed cell death regulating apoptosis genes and those involved in DNA repair—the DNA repair genes. Mutant alleles of protoancogenes are considered dominant because they transform cells despite the presence of a normal counterpart. In contrast, both normal alleles of the tumor suppressor genes have to be damaged for transformation to occur. So, this family of genes is referred to as recessive oncogenes. But, due to haploinsufficiency some tumor suppressor genes may lose their suppressor activity when a single allele is lost or inactivated.

Mutator phenotype: DNA repair genes affect cell proliferation or survival indirectly by influencing the ability of the organism to repair non-lethal damage in other genes, including proto-oncogenes, tumor suppressor genes and apoptosis genes. A disability in the DNA repair genes can predispose to mutations in the genome and hence to neoplastic transformations. Such propensity to mutations is called mutator phenotype. Both alleles of DNA repair genes must be inactivated to induce such genomic instability.

Tumor progression: Carcinogenesis is a multistep process, at both phenotypic and genetic levels. The phenotypic attributes of a malignant neoplasm, like excessive growth, local invasiveness, distant metastasis, etc. are acquired in a stepwise fashion, a phenomenon called tumor progression.

Essential Alterations for Malignant Transformation

Till date, hundreds of cancer-associated genes have been discovered. Some, such as p53, are commonly mutated. Others, such c-abl, are affected only in certain leukemias. There are certain fundamental changes in the cell physiology that together determine malignant phenotype.

Self-sufficiency in growth signals: Neoplasms have the capacity to proliferate with external stimuli, usually as a consequence of an oncogene activation.

Inability to sense growth-inhibitory signals: Tumors may not respond to signals from growth-inhibitory molecules like transforming growth factor-β (TFG-β) or CDK inhibitors Cip/Kip and INK4/ARF families.

Evasion of apoptosis: Tumors may be resistant to programmed cell death, as a consequence of inactivation of p53 or other genes.

Defects in DNA repair: Tumors may fail to repair DNA damage caused by carcinogens or unregulated cellular proliferation.

Limitless replicative potential: Malignant cells have unrestricted proliferative capacity, associated with telomere length and function.

Sustained angiogenesis: The vascular supply and angiogenesis are induced by various factors, the most important being vascular endothelial growth factor (VEGF).

Ability to invade and metastasize: This depends on processes that are intrinsic to the cell or are initiated by signals from surrounding tissue.

The orderly progression of cells through the various phases of cell cylce ($G_1 \rightarrow S \rightarrow G_2 \rightarrow M$) is orchestrated by cyclins, cyclin-dependent kinases (CDKs) and by their inhibitors. There are two check-points at G1/S and G2/M transitions. The S phase is the point of no return in cell cycle, and before a cell makes the final commitment to replicate, G1/S checkpoint checks for DNA damage. If DNA damage is present, DNA repair machinery are put in motion. If the damage is not repairable, apoptotic pathways are activated to kill the cell. The G2/M checkpoint monitors the completion of DNA replication and checks whether the cell can safely initiate mitosis and separate sister chromotids. Defects in G2/M checkpoints give rise to chromosomal abnormalities. These checkpoint defect is a major cause of genetic instability in cancer cells. Cell-cycle arrest in both of the checkpoints are mainly mediated by p53, which induces cell cycle inhibitor p21.

Specific chromosomal abnormalities have been identified in most leukemias and lymphomas. Two types of chromosomal rearrangements can activate protooncogenes—translocation and inversion. Translocations are much more common. In lymphoid tumors, specific translocations result in overexpression of protooncogenes by removing them from their regulatory elements. In many hematopoietic neoplasms, the translocations allow normally unrelated sequences from two different chromosomes to recombine and form hybrid genes that encode growth-promoting chimeric proteins. The Philadelphia chromosome, characteristic of CML and subset of ALL, provides the prototypic example of an oncogene formed by fusion of two separate genes. In these cases, a reciprocal translocation between chromosomes 9 and 22 relocates a truncated portion of protooncogene c-ABL (from chromosome 9) to BCR (Breakpoint Cluster Region) on chromosome 22. The hybrid fusion gene BCR-ABL encodes a chimeric protein that has constitutive tyrosine kinase activity leading to activation of multiple pathways. Overexpression of a protooncogene caused by translocation is best exemplified by Burkitt's lymphoma. All such tumors carry one three translocations, each involving chromosome 8q24, where MYC gene has been mapped, as well as one of the three Ig gene-carrying chromosomes. The MYC-containing segment of chromosome 8 is translocated to chromosome 14q band 32 placing it close to Ig heavy-chain (IgH) gene. Transcription factors are often the partners of gene fusion. For instance, the MLL gene on 11q23 is known to be involved in 25 different translocations with different partner genes (Table 4.1). The MLL gene is affected in childhood ALL and ANLL. The Ewing Sarcoma gene (EWS) at 22q12 was first described in t(11;22)(q24;12) reciprocal translocation, but may be found in other types of sarcomas as well.

Reduplication and amplification of DNA sequences may also activate protooncogenes leading to overexpression. Such amplification may produce several

Table 4.1: Translocations and oncogenes

Childhood malignancy	Translocation	Genes
Acute leukemias (ALL & ANLL)	(4;11)(q21;q23) (6;11)(q27;q23)	AF4 4q21 MLL 11q23 AF6 6q27 MLL 11q23
T-cell ALL	(8;14)(q24;q11) (10;14)(q24;q11)	C-MYC 8q24 TCR-α 14q11 HOX11 10q24 TCR-α 14q11
Burkitt lymphoma	(8;14)(q24;q32)	C-MYC 8q24 IgH 14q32
Follicular lymphoma	(14;18)(q32;q21)	IgH 14q32 BCL-2 18q21
Chronic myeloid leukemia	(9;22)(q43;q11)	ABL 9q34 BCR 22q11
Ewing sarcoma	(11;22)(q24;q12)	FC-1 11q24 EWS 22q12

hundred copies of the protooncogene in the tumor cell. Two patterns are seen—multiple small, chromosome-like structures called double minutes (dms) and homogeneous staining regions (HSR). The latter derive from the assembly of amplified genes into new chromosomes. In about 30% cases of neuroblastomas, there is amplification of N-MYC genes, present both dms and HSR. Other examples are breast carcinoma (ERB-B2), small cell lung cancer (C-MYC, L-MYC, N-MYC) and squamous cell carcinoma (CYCLIN-D1).

SUGGESTED READING

1. Arthur CD. Genetics and Cytogenetics of Pediatric Cancers; Cancer, 1986;58:534-40.
2. Barr FG. Molicular genetics and pathogenism of stabdomyosarcoma, J Pediatr Hematol Oncol. 1997;19:483-65.
3. Kramarira E, Stiller CA. The international classification of childhood cancer. Int J Cancer. 1966;68:759-91.
4. Xia SJ, Pressey JG, Barr F6. Molecular pathogenesis of abdomyosarcoma, Cancer Biol Ther. 2002;1:97-104.

5

Flow Cytometric Immunophenotyping in the Diagnosis of Acute Leukemias

Arnab Chattopadhyay

INTRODUCTION

Flow cytometric immunophenotyping (FCI) first appeared in clinical laboratories in the 1980s, in the wake of the AIDS epidemic. Initially utilized to assess CD 4, T cells, the technique was soon applied to lymphoid and eventually myeloid neoplasms. Since initiation of application of the technology to clinical practice, there has been tremendous improvements in flow cytometry instrumentation and availability of an expanded range of antibodies and fluorochromes. This has led to more accurate phenotyping of cells, leading to enhanced identification of abnormal populations, even when present in a small proportion of cells analyzed. The 2001 World Health Organization (WHO) classification of hematological neoplasms has led to refinement of the criteria used to identify distinct disease entities and has been widely adopted. This classification endorses a multiparametric approach to diagnosis with identification of morphologic, phenotypic, and genotypic features that are characteristic of each disease entity. As such, FCI has become an indispensable tool for the diagnosis, classification, staging, and monitoring of hematological neoplasms. Although the diseases where flow cytometry is helpful in diagnosis is well-known, a practical problem is that the diagnosis is often not known until after flow cytometry is done. As such, description of the signs and symptoms that would prompt the clinician to ask for flow cytomerty in the first place is potentially more useful than diagnosis-based indications for flow cytometry. But this issue largely remained unaddressed till recently.

FLOW CYTOMETRY IMMUNOPHENOTYPING (FCI) GUIDELINE

In 2006, consensus recommendations for flow cytometric testing based on clinical presentations were formulated in an international conference at Bethesda, USA. Accordingly, FCI is indicated in the following clinical conditions:

- Cytopenias, especially bicytopenia and pancytopenia
- Elevated leukocyte count, including lymphocytosis, monocytosis, and eosinophilia
- Atypical cells or blasts in the peripheral blood, bone marrow, or body fluids
- Plasmacytosis, or monoclonal gammopathy (in adult)
- Organomegaly and tissue masses including but not limited to lymphadenopathy, and skin, mucosa, and bone infiltrates.

It should be remembered that just because a patient with a hematopoietic neoplasm may have one of these signs or symptoms does not mean that flow cytometry is indicated in any patient with these signs or symptoms. Flow cytometry is not a screening test. For many signs and symptoms like anemia and thrombocytopenia, flow cytometry is indicated only after an appropriate work-up to exclude non-neoplastic causes of disease. In some circumstances (e.g. identification of blasts in blood or marrow), flow cytometry is appropriately used as a frontline test. In contrast, the Bethesda group agreed that flow cytometry was generally not indicated in the following situations:

- Mature neutrophilia
- Polyclonal hypergammaglobulinemia

- Polycythemia
- Thrombocytosis
- Basophilia.

Although thrombocytosis, polycythemia and granulocytic leukocytoses are common presentations of some hematopoietic neoplasms (chronic myeloproliferative neoplasms), these diseases lack characteristic flow cytometric findings so that immunophenotyping is not indicated. For atypical cells in blood, marrow or fluids, flow cytometry has an increased sensitivity and specificity compared to morphology and therefore helps to confirm the presence of blasts suspected by morphology, classify leukemias, or may demonstrate that an atypical population is reactive. In addition, the consensus group agreed that flow cytometry is a useful tool for staging a previously diagnosed hematolymphoid neoplasm, detection of minimal residual disease (MRD), documenting relapse or progression, and diagnosing an intercurrent hematologic malignancy, such as therapy-related myelodysplastic syndrome (MDS).

FCI evaluates individual cells in suspension for the presence or absence of specific antigens (phenotype). The phenotypic information thus obtained can be used to assess following aspects of the hematological malignancies:

- Identification of cells from different lineages and determination of whether they are mature or immature
- Detection of abnormal cells through identification of antigen expression that differs significantly from normal
- Detailed documentation of the phenotype of abnormal cell populations (i.e. the presence or absence of antigens, intensity of fluorescence for an antibody in comparison to the normal counterparts)
- Arrive at a definitive diagnosis from the information available; if that is not possible, a list of differential diagnosis should be developed with suggestion of additional studies that might be of diagnostic value such as immunohistochemistry, cytogenetics, fluorescent in situ hybridization (FISH), and molecular studies
- Provision of immunophenotypic information that might be of additional prognostic value, including

the identification of targets for potential directed therapy:

PROCEDURE

Immunophenotypic analysis may be performed on a variety of specimens including, and not limited to:

- Peripheral blood
- Bone marrow aspirates
- Bone marrow biopsies
- Lymphoid tissue biopsies
- Serosal fluids
- Spinal fluid
- Skin
- Mucosa (endoscopic biopsies)
- Fine needle aspirates.

Peripheral blood and bone marrow aspirates are the specimens most commonly used and processed. In general, the specimens should be transported to the flow cytometry laboratory, processed, and stained for analysis immediately after collection. Any available clinical or diagnostic information pertinent to the specimen should accompany it, if possible. All specimens should be maintained at room temperature (16°C–28°C). Using sodium heparin as anticoagulant for blood and bone marrow aspirates, the specimens may be stored for up to 72 hours while with ethylenediamine tetra-acetate (EDTA), the storage time appears to be ~ (12–24) hours due to depletion of myeloid cells under these conditions. Other anticoagulants are generally not recommended for FCI.

USES

Acute leukemia can present with blasts in the peripheral blood, bone marrow, body fluids, or infiltration into the extramedullary sites. FCI can assist in the identification of abnormal cells, their distinction from immature cells normally present in the marrow, and determination of lineage in order to differentiate between acute myeloid and lymphoblastic leukemias (AML & ALL), and occasionally can aid in further classification.

Blasts often differ from more mature cells by expressing markers of immaturity and lacking antigens expressed by more mature cells. For example, myeloblasts can be

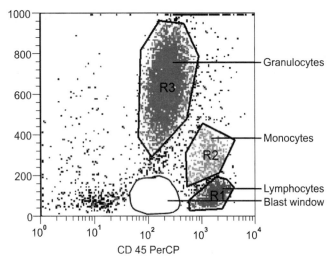

Fig. 5.1: CD 45 vs Side scatter histogram from a normal peripheral blood *(For color version, see Plate 1)*

distinguished from maturing myeloid cells if they display low orthogonal (side) light scatter, markers of immaturity such as CD 34 and CD 117, and lack markers of maturation such as CD 11b, CD 15, and CD 16. Immature B-lymphoid cells can be distinguished from mature B-lymphoid cells if they express CD 34 and TdT, and lack surface immunoglobulin and CD 20. Immature T-lymphoid cells can be distinguished from mature T-lymphoid cells if they express CD 34, TdT, or CD1a, or lack surface expression of CD 3. A plot of CD45 versus orthogonal (side) light scatter is very useful in identifying blasts by their low side light scatter and weak intensity expression of CD 45. This representation can help to distinguish blasts from lymphocytes (bright CD 45), erythroid precursors (essentially negative CD 45), neutrophilic precursors and eosinophils (higher side light scatter), and monocytes (higher side light scatter and brighter CD 45) (Fig. 5.1). However, basophils usually fall within the blast region in this plot due to loss of granules during processing.

Through the analysis of many thousands of cells, flow cytometric studies can determine the precise percentage of the total cells analyzed that demonstrate phenotypic features of immature cells. However, the percentage of immature cells determined by flow cytometry often differs from the blast count determined by manual differential counting performed on aspirate smears. Despite inaccuracies inherent in manual differential counting, this method is still used in the current classification

schemes and therefore remains the gold standard for determining blast percentage. However, flow cytometric analysis can certainly assist in identifying neoplastic cells that might, otherwise, be overlooked because of atypical morphological features or less than optimal smears.

Neoplastic blasts often have an abnormal phenotype that permits their distinction from normal immature cells. Phenotypic abnormalities include expression of markers not normally present on cells of that lineage, such as myeloid markers on lymphoblasts or lymphoid markers on myeloblasts, and deviations from the well-coordinated gain or loss of antigens seen with normal maturation. For example, although ALL may closely resemble one stage of B cell maturation, such as precursor B cells, the phenotype may contain some feature unexpected for that stage of maturation, such as surface CD 20 expression. However, a subset of nonneoplastic immature myeloid and monocytic cells may demonstrate an unusual phenotype following growth factor stimulation or regeneration, such as low-level expression of CD 56 and possible CD 5.

Reliable distinction between AML and ALL is important for the selection of appropriate therapy. AML usually express antigens characteristic of neutrophilic or monocytic differentiation such as CD 13, CD 15, CD 33, CD 64, CD 117, and myeloperoxidase. In ALL, CD 19 has the highest sensitivity and specificity for the B-lineage and cytoplasmic CD 3 for the T-lineage. Cytoplasmic CD 22 is also a sensitive and specific B-lineage marker. Although CD 79a was proposed as a specific marker of B-lineage, subsequent studies have demonstrated staining of some cases of precursor T-cell ALL and AML.

Leukemic blasts may aberrantly express antigens for another lineage. Lymphoid antigens frequently expressed in AML include CD 7, CD 56, CD 2, and CD 19. ALL frequently demonstrates expression of one or more myeloid antigens, which does not appear to have any independent prognostic significance, and should not be used to diagnose biphenotypic leukemia.

Determination of lineage can be difficult if the leukemic blasts express antigens from more than one cell line or demonstrate very few lineage-associated antigens. Approximately 5% of acute leukemias were found to have lineage heterogeneity, either biphenotypic leukemia (expression of antigens from more than one lineage by a single population of blasts) or bilineal leukemia (2 populations of blasts of different lineages). To assist in standardization, a scoring system was proposed that gave weight to phenotypic findings in the assignment of lineage. For example, cytoplasmic expression of CD 3 is a strong indicator of T cell lineage, whereas CD 7 is frequently expressed in AML and therefore carries less weight for the assignment of a T-cell lineage. However, this scoring scheme does not include all the markers used in the current clinical practice and does not address the weighting of partial expression or intensity of expression of antigens. Therefore, when faced with a blastic malignancy expressing antigens from more than one lineage, the leukemic cells should be thoroughly characterized using a multiparametric approach including morphology, cytochemical staining, FCI, and cytogenetic analysis. Neoplasms with recurrent cytogenetic abnormalities recognized in the WHO classification are more easily categorized. For the remaining neoplasms, the information should be weighed up and, where possible, a diagnosis of AML or ALL favored. A similar multiparmetric approach can be taken to the characterization of patients expressing very few antigens, in an attempt to minimize the number of patients falling in the acute undifferentiated leukemia category.

The identification of recurrent genetic abnormalities has assumed priority in the classification of AML. However, FCI studies remain of value in its distinction from ALL. In addition, flow cytometric studies are also of value in the identification of megakaryocytic differentiation with expression of CD 41, CD 61, and pure erythroid leukemia with expression of CD 235a (Glycophorin A) or CD 36 in the absence of CD 64, myeloperoxidase, and other myeloid-associated antigens. Although flow cytometric studies can also evaluate for monocytic differentiation, cytochemical stains remain part of the current WHO classification scheme. Flow cytometric evaluation for CD 14 lacks sensitivity for the detection of monocytic differentiation. However, it has been suggested that the sensitivity of the flow cytometric assay can be improved by evaluation of other monocyte-associated antigens such as co-expression of CD 36 and CD 64 bright and intermediate CD 15 plus bright CD 33.

Some phenotypes in AML are associated with presence of recurrent genetic abnormalities. But these FCI results lack specificity and sensitivity required for the detection of the genotypic abnormalities. FCI of AML is also of value in patients being considered for gemtuzumab ozogamycin therapy by demonstrating expression of target antigen CD 33.

FCI is important for the distinction between ALL and AML, identification of B cell or T cell lineage, and assessing response to treatment, including the identification of early responders and the detection of MRD. Some phenotypes in ALL are associated with the presence of prognostically significant cytogenetic and molecular abnormalities. But they also lack in either sensitivity or specificity and cannot be used as a suitable surrogate tool for detection of these subtypes of ALL.

LIMITATION

In the past 10 years, clinical flow cytometry has evolved from a technique primarily used to characterize large populations of abnormal cells to one that can routinely evaluate small populations of cells for subtle aberrancies in antigen expression. Adoption of these more sophisticated techniques has reinforced the need for optimization of flow cytometric procedures and for interpretation by individuals who are familiar with all aspects of the testing that may affect the quality of the data. In addition, it is important that interpreters of flow cytometric data have a thorough knowledge of the phenotypes of diverse normal cell populations, can recognize deviations from normal, and are able to discuss the potential clinical significance of the flow cytometric findings.

SUGGESTED READING

1. Bene MC, Castoldi G, Knapp W, et al. Proposals for the immunological classification of acute leukemias: European Group for the Immunological Characterization Leukemias (EGIL). Leukemia. 1995;9:1783-6.
2. Bhargava P, et al. CD79a is heterogeneously expressed in neoplastic and normal myeloid precursors and megakaryocytes in an antibody clone-dependent manner. Am J Clin Pathol. 2007;128:306-13.
3. Craig FE, Foon KA. Flow cytometric immunophenotyping for hematologic neoplasms. Blood 2008;111: 3941-67.

4. Davis BH, Foucar K, et al. US-Canadian consensus recommendations on the immunophenotypic analysis of hematologic neoplasia by flow cytometry: data reporting. Cytometry 1997;30:245-8.

5. Davis BH, Holden JT, Bene MC, et al. 2006 Bethesda International consensus recommendations on the flow cytometric immunophenotypic analysis of hematolymphoid neoplasis: medical indications. Cytomerty B Clin Cytom. 2007;72B: S5-13.

6. Digiuseppe JA. Acute lymphoblstic leukemia: diagnosis and detection of minimal residual disease following therapy. Clin Lab Med. 2007;27:533-49.

7. Dunphy CH, Orton SO, Mantell J. Relative contributions of enzyme cytochemistry and flow cytometric immunophenotyping to the evaluation of acute myeloid leukemias with a monocytic component and of flow cytometric immunophenotyping to the evaluation of absolute monocytoses. Am J Clin Pathol. 2004;122:865-74.

8. Jaffe ES, Harris NL, Stein H, Vardiman J. Tumours of haematopoietic and lymphoid tissues. World Health Organization Classification of Tumours. Lyon, France: IARC Press; 2001.

9. Mckenna RW, Washington LT, et al. Immunophenotypic analysis of hematogones (B-lymphocyte precursors) in 662 consecutive bone marrow specimens by 4-color flow cytomerty. Blood. 2001;98:2498-2507.

10. Stelzer GT, Marti G, et al. 1997 US-Canadian consensus recommendations on the immunophenotypic analysis of hematologic neoplasia by flow cytometry: standarization and validation of laboratory procedures. Cytometry. 1997;30:214-30.

11. Wood B. 9-colour and 10-colour flow cytometry in the clinical laboratory. Arch Pathol Lab Med. 2006;130:680-90.

12. Wood BL. Myeloid malignancies: myelodysplastic syndromes, myeloproliferative disorders, and acute myeloid leukemia. Clin Lab Med. 2007;27:551-75.

APPENDIX

I. **Basic antibody panel in use in (Institute of Hematology and Transfusion Medicine) IHTM for the diagnosis of acute leukemia:**

B-lineage: CD 19, CD 20, CD 10, cytoplasmic CD 22

T-lineage: CD 4, CD 5, CD 7, cytoplasmic CD 3 (cCD 3)

Myelomonocytic lineage: CD 13, CD 33, CD 117, cytoplasmic MPO

Non-lineage specific: CD 34, HLADR

II. **Phenotypic changes during normal myeloid differentiation:**

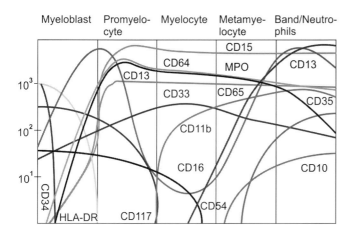

III. **Phenotypic changes during normal differentiation of the monocytic lineage:**

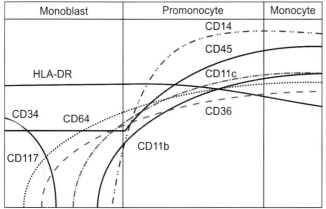

IV. **Phenotypic changes during normal B-lineage maturation:**

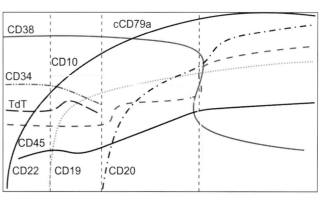

The figures in the Appendix showing phenotypic changes during maturation of normal hematopoietic cells have been kindly provided by Prof Maria Arroz, Lisbon, Portugal and Prof Alberto Orfao, Salamanca, Spain.

(For color version of these graphs, see Plate 1)

6

Chemotherapy in Pediatric Oncology

Rakesh Mondal, Suhas Ganguly

INTRODUCTION

Childhood malignancies and their treatment seem to occupy more and more of our pediatric practice in city hospitals with the explosive advancement of newer diagnostic and treatment modalities. While fundamental principles of cancer treatment are still enormously important but certain nuances of pediatric cancer care make it one of its kind in the clan. The most commonly used modality in the treatment of childhood malignancies is chemotherapy, often using a combination of anti-cancer drugs. Here we describe the pharmacological properties of the leading anticancer drugs with a review of their therapeutic applications in some common childhood neoplasms. It is needless to say that elaboration of treatments of individual diseases is given separately.

GENERAL PRINCIPLES OF CANCER CHEMOTHERAPY

Cancer chemotherapy aims at striking neoplastic cells with a lethal cytotoxic effect that arrests progression of tumors. The mechanisms of action differ considerably depending on the different classes these agents belong to. However, the attack is generally targeted at the metabolic pathways resulting in production of the building blocks for DNA or RNA synthesis. The high replication rate of the malignant cells confers them with an increased susceptibility to the damages caused by these drugs. This also explains some of the toxic effects like iatrogenic myelosuppression, dermatitis, mucositis and hepatitis resulting from increased susceptibility of these rapidly proliferating tissues compared to their slowly growing counterparts.

A. Treatment Strategies

1. **Goal of treatment:** The goal of chemotherapy is long-term disease free survival or palliation depending on the diagnosis and biological milieu of the subject. Both of these require destruction of as many neoplastic cells as possible, often using adjunct modalities like surgery and radiation for such "debulking."

2. **Tumor susceptibility and the growth cycle:** Both cell cycle specific and cell cycle non-specific drugs are in use. The former group targets only the replicating cells (Fig. 6.1). The latter group, though more toxic, destroys tumors with low percentage of replicating cells. Some cell cycle specific drugs are antimetabolites, bleomycin peptides, antibiotics, vinka alkaloids and etoposide. Alkylating agents, cisplatin, some antibiotics and nitrosoureas, on the other hand, are cell cycle non-specific.

B. Problems Associated with Chemotherapy

A. Resistance

Drug resistance can be primary or secondary. Some tumors, for example a melanoma, are resistant to most chemotherapeutic agents to start with. Some tumor types acquire resistance to standard drugs by mutating. A variety of mechanisms is responsible for development of

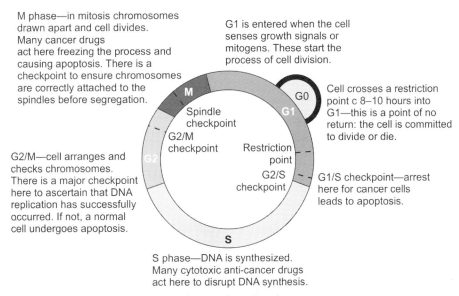

M phase—in mitosis chromosomes drawn apart and cell divides. Many cancer drugs act here freezing the process and causing apoptosis. There is a checkpoint to ensure chromosomes are correctly attached to the spindles before segregation.

G1 is entered when the cell senses growth signals or mitogens. These start the process of cell division.

Cell crosses a restriction point c 8–10 hours into G1—this is a point of no return: the cell is committed to divide or die.

G2/M—cell arranges and checks chromosomes. There is a major checkpoint here to ascertain that DNA replication has successfully occurred. If not, a normal cell undergoes apoptosis.

G1/S checkpoint—arrest here for cancer cells leads to apoptosis.

S phase—DNA is synthesized. Many cytotoxic anti-cancer drugs act here to disrupt DNA synthesis.

Fig. 6.1: The cell cycle

drug resistance. The detailed discussion of that, however, is beyond the scope of this concise book.

B. Toxicity

Therapies targeted at the neoplastic cells eventually also kill normal cells in sizeable numbers. This gives rise to the chemotherapy induced adverse effects. The rapidly proliferating cells like bone marrow, gastrointestinal mucosa, and buccal mucosa are particularly susceptible to such damage. Some toxic effects can be ameliorated by different techniques like perfusing the tumor locally (for example, a sarcoma in the arm) or by removing some of the patient's own marrow prior to chemotherapy and then reimplanting it, or by promoting hydration and intensive diuresis to prevent bladder toxicities. Again, with the availability of human granulocyte colony stimulating factor, the neutropenia consequential to chemotherapy can be partially reversed.

C. Treatment Induced Neoplasms

This is a unique aspect of cancer chemotherapy. Since most antineoplastic agents are mutagens second tumors (e.g. leukemias) can arise long time after the first tumor was treated. Treatment induced neoplasms are particularly important in case of treatment with alkylating agents.

Classification of Anti-cancer Drugs

A. **Antimetabolites:**
1. Capecitabine
2. Cladribine
3. Cytarabine
4. Fludarabine
5. 5-Fluorouracil
6. Gemcitabine
7. 6-Mercaptopurine
8. Methotrexate
9. 6-Thioguanine.
B. **Antibiotics:**
1. Bleomycin
2. Dactinomycin
3. Daunorubicin
4. Doxorubicin
5. Epirubicin
6. Idarubicin.
C. **Alkylating agents:**
1. Busalfan
2. Carmustine
3. Chlorambucil
4. Cyclophosphamide
5. Dacarbazine

6. Ifosfamide
7. Lomustine
8. Mechlorethamine
9. Melphalan
10. Streptazocin
11. Temozilamide.
D. **Microtubule inhibitors:**
1. Docetaxel
2. Paclitaxel
3. Vinblastine
4. Vincristine
5. Vinorelbine.
E. **Steroid hormones and their antagonists:**
1. Aminoglutethimide
2. Anastrozole
3. Bicalutamide
4. Estrogens
5. Exemestane
6. Flutamide
7. Goserelin
8. Letrozole
9. Leuprolide
10. Megestrol acetate
11. Nilutamide
12. Prednisone
13. Tamoxifen
14. Toremifene.
F. **Monoclonal antibodies:**
1. Bevacizumab
2. Cetuximab
3. Rituximab
4. Trastuzumab.
G. **Others:**
1. Asparaginase
2. Cisplatin
3. Carboplatin
4. Etoposide
5. Gefinitib
6. Imatinib
7. Interferons
8. Irinotecan
9. Oxaliplatin
10. Procarbazine
11. Tropotecan.

ANTINEOPLASTIC AGENTS USED IN PEDIATRIC ONCOLOGY

Not all the above drugs belonging to the different classes are used in pediatric practice. In the part of the article that follows, we will restrict ourselves to the commonly used drugs in treatment of different pediatric cancers.

A. Methotrexate

Methotrexate, an antimetabolite, plays key role in a variety of reactions involving "one carbon metabolisms."
Mechanism of action: Methotrexate inhibits the enzyme dihydrofolate reductase (DHFR) and thus acts as a folic acid antagonist.
Resistance: Nonproliferating cells are relatively resistant to methotrexate probably due to deficiency of the enzyme DHFR. Apart from this several other mechanisms of resistance like amplification of DHFR producing genes, decreased affinity of the enzymes to MTX and reduced drug influx from impaired transport have been identified.
Pharmacokinetics: Poorly absorbed from GIT and does not cross blood brain barrier. Hence, intrathecal administration is required to attain therapeutic concentration sufficient to destroy neoplastic cells in the CNS. High concentration of drug has been reported in liver, kidney and ascitic and pleural fluids.

Excretion of the drug including its 7-OH metabolite occurs chiefly through urine. This makes it important to keep the patient adequately hydrated and urine alkaline to prevent adverse renal events. A small proportion of the drug, however, undergoes enterohepatic circulation and is excreted in stool.
Route of administration: IV, IM or intrathecal.
Adverse effects: Myelosuppression, stomatitis, dermatitis and hepatitis are the predominant adverse effects. With long-term administration osteopenia and fractures are also reported. Central nervous system and renal toxicities are usually consequences of use in increased dosage. Intrathecal administration can lead to arachnoiditis, leukoencephalopathy and leukomyelopathy. Children who are maintained on methotrexate rarely develop pulmonary manifestations like cough, dyspnea, cyanosis

and bilateral radiologic infiltrates which disappear on withdrawing the medication.

Therapeutic use:
1. Acute lymphoblastic leukemia
2. Non-Hodgkin lymphoma
3. Osteosarcoma
4. Hodgkin lymphoma
5. Neuroblastoma.

B. 6-Mercaptopurine

6-MP is a thiol analogue of hypoxanthine and is one of the first purine derivatives acting against neoplastic cells.

Mechanism of action: The mechanism of action of 6-MP can be described in the following three steps:
1. **Nuclotide formation:** After penetrating the cell 6-MP gets converted into 6-MP ribose phosphate (better known as 6-thionic acid or TIMP).
2. **Inhibition of purine synthesis:** A number of metabolic pathways that get affected by TIMP is interrupted at several steps resulting in inhibition of purine synthesis.
3. **Incorporation into nucleic acids:** TIMP is converted to TGMP, which after phosphorylation and diphosphorylation, gets incorporated into DNA giving rise to non-functional nucleic acids, i.e. DNA and RNA.

Resistance: The following pharmacological mechanisms of resistance have been reported from different biological models:
1. An inability to transform 6-MP into TIMP due to congenital deficiency of HGPRT—the salvage pathway enzyme (e.g. in Lesch Nyhan Syndrome).
2. An increased dephosphorylation.
3. Increased metabolism of the drug to thiouric acid or other metabolites.

Pharmacokinetics: Oral absorption is erratic. Allopurinol, a xanthine oxidase inhibitor, frequently used on patients receiving chemotherapy, results in increased drug accumulation and hence toxicities. So, dose may need to be adjusted. Metabolites are excreted through kidney.

Route of administration: Oral.

Adverse effects: Myelosuppression, hepatitis and mucositis are the main adverse effects. Other minor adverse effects include nausea, vomiting and diarrhea.

Therapeutic use:
Acute leukemia (during the maintenance phase).

C. Cytarabine (Ara-C):

Cytarabine is an analogue of 2'-deoxycytidine in which the natural ribose residue is replaced by D-arabinose. Ara-C acts as a pyrimidine antagonist.

Mechanism of action: After entry to cell through a carrier mediated process the drug gets phosphorylated to form the nucleotide are-CTP and becomes cytotoxic. It gets incorporated into the DNA and inhibits chain elongation. This drug is specific for the S-phase of the cell cycle.

Resistance: Four mechanisms of resistance have been described:
1. A defect in the transport process.
2. A change in the phosphorylating enzyme deoxycytidine kinase.
3. Increased pool of the natural dCTP nucleotide
4. Increased deamination of the drug to Ara-U

Pharmacokinetics: Since it is converted into a non-cytotoxic metabolite Ara-U by intestinal enzymes, it is not effective orally. Though the drug does not cross the blood brain barrier, intrathecal injections can be effective in the treatment of meningeal leukemia. Ara-C is extensively metabolized to Ara-U by oxidative deamination. Both Ara-C and Ara-U are excreted in urine.

Route of administration: IV and intrathecal.

Adverse effects: Nausea, vomiting, myelosuppression are the main side effects. Intrathecal administration is sometimes associated with arachnoiditis, leukoencephalopathy and leukomyelopathy.

Therapeutic use:
1. Acute lymphoblastic leukemia
2. Acute myeloblastic leukemia
3. Non-Hodgkin lymphoma
4. Hodgkin lymphoma.

D. Cyclophosphamide

This is an alkylating agent with a broad range of clinical effects including use in some non-neoplastic diseases like nephrotic syndrome.

Mechanism of action: Cyclophosphamide is first converted to phosphoramide mustard and acrolein by cytochrome P450 system. The reaction between phosphoramide mustard and DNA is said to be the cytotoxic step. Alkylates guanine and inhibits DNA synthesis.

Resistance: Three mechanisms have been reported:
1. Increased DNA repair.
2. Decreased drug permeability.
3. Reaction of the drug with thiols like glutathione.

Route of administration: Oral/IV.

Pharmacokinetics: Good oral absorption. Excretion is both via stool and urine. Since action requires hepatic transformation, the drug is less effective in children with hepatic dysfunction.

Adverse effects: The most prominent side-effects of the drug are diarrhea, vomiting, alopecia, myelosuppression and hemorrhagic cystitis. The latter is attributed to acrolein and can be prevented by adequate hydration of the patient and IV injection of MESNA (Sodium 2-mercaptoethane sulphonate). Other adverse events include bladder cancer, pulmonary fibrosis, inappropriate ADH secretion and anaphylaxis. Effects on germ cells leading to testicular atrophy and amenorrhea have been also noted.

Therapeutic uses:
1. Acute lymphoblastic leukemia
2. Acute myeloblastic leukemia
3. Non-Hodgkin lymphoma
4. Hodgkin lymphoma
5. Soft tissue sarcoma
6. Ewing's sarcoma.

E. Ifosfamide

This drug is similar to cyclophosphamide in most of its properties, and belongs to the same genre.

Mechanism of action: Alkylates guanine inhibits DNA synthesis.

Pharmacokinetics: Same as cyclophosphamide.

Adverse effects: Same as cyclophosphamide.

Therapeutic uses:
1. Non-Hodgkin lymphoma
2. Wilms tumor

3. Rhabdomyosarcoma
4. Ewing's sarcoma.

E. Doxorubicin and Daunorubicin

Both doxorubicin and daunorubicin are anthracycline antibiotics, and doxorubicin is the product obtained after hydroxylation of daunorubicin. Doxorubicin is one of the most widely used anti-cancer agents.

Mechanism of action: The anthracyclines have three major actions which lead to antineoplastic effects. All the three are maximal in the S and G2 phase of the cell cycle:
1. **Intercalation into DNA:** This leads to local uncoiling due to nonspecific insertion of the drug between the sugar-phosphate moieties and thus causes interruption of DNA and RNA synthesis.
2. **Binding to the cell membranes:** This results in impaired cellular transport consequential to activation of phosphatidylinositol.
3. **Generation of oxygen radicals:** Free radical induced cellular damage.

Pharmacokinetics: The anthracyclines are considerably protein bound and have large volume of distribution. They do not penetrate blood brain barrier or testes. The major route of excretion is through bile, which necessitates reduction of dose in children with impaired hepatic function. However, renal excretion is not so high as to require dose adjustment. Poor oral absorption makes it mandatory for the drug to be given IV. Local extravasations, however, has been associated with tissue necrosis.

Route of administration: IV

Adverse effects: Cardiomyopathy, red urine, myelosuppression, radiation dermatitis and arrhythmia are the main side-effects.

Therapeutic use:
1. Acute lymphoblastic leukemia
2. Acute myeloblastic leukemia
3. Ewing's sarcoma
4. Osteosarcoma
5. Hodgkin lymphoma
6. Non-Hodgkin lymphoma
7. Neuroblastoma.

F. Dactinomycin

Dactinomycin, also known as actinomycin D, is the first antimicrobial to be successfully used in cancer chemotherapy.

Mechanism of action: Three mechanisms of action have been identified:

1. Intercalation into the minor grooves between guanine-cytosine analogues forming a stable Dactinomycin-DNA complex. This complex interferes with DNA dependent RNA polymerase.
2. Hinders DNA synthesis at high doses.
3. Cause single strand breaks, possibly by effect on topoisomerase II and free radical induced damage.

Resistance: Resistance is mainly due to increased efflux of the drug from the cell.

Pharmacokinetics: Widely distributed in body but does not enter CSF. The drug is mostly excreted unchanged in bile.

Route of administration: IV

Adverse effects: Nausea, vomiting, tissue necrosis on extravasation and myelosuppression are the main adverse effects. Stomatitis and alopecia are also not infrequent. Dactinomycin is a radiosensitizer.

Therapeutic use:

1. Wilms tumor
2. Rhabdomyosarcoma
3. Ewing's sarcoma.

G. Bleomycin

Bleomycin is a mixture of different copper chelating glycopeptides and acts mainly in the G2 phase of the cell cycle.

Mechanism of action: A DNA-Bleomycin-Fe 2^+ complex undergoes oxidation to bleomycin-Fe 3^+ giving rise to birth of one hydroxyl free radical in the process. This free radical causes DNA strand breakage and chromosomal aberrations.

Resistance: No specific mechanism of resistance has been yet identified but increased efflux of the drug from the cell and DNA repair mechanisms are two plausible conjectures that are in vogue at present.

Pharmacokinetics: The bleomycin inactivating enzyme, a hydrolase occurs in less concentration in organs like skin compared to liver and spleen. This makes toxicity on the former organ more likely. The drug is excreted almost unchanged in urine and requires dose reduction in patients with reduced GFR.

Route of administration: IV, IM, SC and intracavitary.

Adverse effects: Nausea, vomiting, stomatitis, Raynaud's phenomenon, pulmonary fibrosis and dermatitis are the common side effects of therapy.

Therapeutic uses:

1. Hodgkin disease
2. Non-Hodgkin lymphoma
3. Germ cell tumors.

H. Vincristine

Vincristine (VX) and Vinblastine (VBL) are related compounds derived from periwinkle compound *vinca rosea*. Therefore, they are referred to as vinka alkaloids.

Mechanism of action: Both VX and VBL are cell cycle specific and they prevent formation of microtubules. They bind with the protein tubulin in a GTP dependent fashion and prevent its polymerization to form the microtubules. The paracrystalline aggregates comprising of the drug and the tubulin dimers results in dysfunctional tubules and frozen metaphase. Thus cell proliferation is impaired.

Resistance: Resistance is due to increased efflux of the drugs from the cells and may be also due to altered structure of the microtubules.

Pharmacokinetics: Vinca alkaloids are concentrated and metabolized in the liver. They are excreted in bile and stool. Dose must be adjusted in children with impaired liver function. Intravenous injection of these agents leads to very rapid destruction of cells and consequent hyperuricemia. Xanthine oxidase inhibitors need to be administered with these agents.

Route of admininstration: Intravenous only.

Adverse effects: Constipation, ileus, local cellulitis, jaw pain, SIADH, seizures, ptosis, minimal myelo-suppression, peripheral neuropathy, local cellulitis at sites of extravasation.

Therapeutic use:

1. Acute lymphoblastic leukemia
2. Non-Hodgkin lymphoma
3. Hodgkin disease
4. Wilms' tumor
5. Ewing's sarcoma

6. Neuroblastoma
7. Rhabdomyosarcoma.

I. Decarbazine

It is an important chemotherapeutic agent used for treating children with cancer.

Mechanism of action: Alkylating agents which form methyldiazonium ions that attack neucleophilic groups in DNA. It also inhibits DNA, RNA and protein synthesis by cross-linking DNA strands.

Pharmacokinetics: Distributes to the liver. CSF penetration is poor. Protein binding is minimal. N demethylated in the liver by microsomal enzymes. Half-life is maximum. It is excreted mainly by tubular secretion through urine.

Uses: It is used in pediatric solid tumors, i.e. neuroblastoma, Hodgkin diseases. It is administered parenterally as IV infusion. Its use is monitored by periodic check up of CBC and liver function tests.

Adverse reactions: It includes myelosuppression, leukopenia, vomiting, hepatocellular dysfunction, etc.

J. Vinblastine

It is a vinca-alkaloid group of chemotherapeutic agents

Mechanism of action: It binds to microtubular protein of the spindle causing metaphase arrest.

Pharmacokinetics: It is rapidly distributed into body tissue but have poor penetration into CSF. Protein binding is 75%. It is extensively metabolized by liver and mainly extracted through bile.

Uses: It is used in Hodgkin disease, histiocytosis, germ cell tumors, etc.

Its use is monitored by CBC, uric acid, liver function tests, etc.

It is administered as short push or IV infusion.

Adverse reactions: It includes skin rash, vomiting, hypersensitivity, myelosuppression, leukopenia, and peripheral neuropathy.

K. Etoposide

It is a topoisomerase inhibitor which is used in pediatric cancer.

Mechanism of action: It inhibits mitotic activity. It also inhibits DNA type II topoisomerase producing single and double strand DNA breaks.

Pharmacokinetics: It has variable bioavailability penetratetes CSF poorly. It is 90% protein bound and metabolized mainly in liver. It is excreted in urine either as unchanged drug or its metabolites.

Uses: It is used in germ cell tumor, Hodgkin disease, leukemia, neuroblastoma, Ewing's sarcoma, Wilms' tumor, brain tumors, etc. It is used as 100 mg/m^2/day IV infusion. CBC and platelet counts, liver function tests, renal function tests should be monitored during its use.

Adverse reaction: It can cause vomiting, rash, urticaria, myelosuppression, etc. Its special adverse reaction includes peripheral neuropathy hypersensitivity, reaction, etc.

L. Asparaginase

Mechanism of action: Indirect DNA-interacting agents.

Pharmacokinetics: Poorly absorbed from GIT and does not cross blood brain barrier. High concentration of drug has been reported in liver, kidney and ascitic and pleural fluids.

Route of administration: IV, IM or SC.

Adverse effects: Protein synthesis defect, clotting factors abnormalities, glucose metabolism defect, hypersensitivity, CNS dysfunction, pancreatitis, hepatic dysfunction, myelosuppression, stomatitis, are the predominant adverse effects.

Therapeutic use:
1. Acute lymphoblastic leukemia
2. Non-Hodgkin lymphoma.

M. Cisplatin

Mechanism of action: It is hypothesized that in the intracellular environment, the positively charged species generated from cisplatin is an efficient bifunctional interactor with DNA, forming Pt-based cross-links. Cisplatin requires administration with adequate hydration, including forced diuresis with mannitol to prevent kidney damage.

Pharmacokinetics: Poorly absorbed from GIT and does not cross blood-brain barrier. High concentration of drug has been reported in liver, kidney and ascitic and pleural fluids.

Route of administration: IV infusion.

Adverse effects: Hypomagnesemia, hypocalcemia, tetany, neurotoxicity with stocking and glove sensorimotor neuropathy, hearing loss. Cisplatin is intensely emetogenic, requiring prophylactic antiemetics. Myelosuppression is less evident than with other alkylating agents. Renal toxicities are usually very significant side-effects.

Therapeutic use:

1. Neuroblastoma.
2. Nephroblastoma.
3. Rhabdomyosarcoma.

SUGGESTED READING

1. Berg SL, Grisell DL, DeLaney TF, et al. "Principles of treatment of pediatric solid tumors". Pediats Clin North Am. 1991;38:249-67.
2. Chabner BA, Longo DL (Eds). Cancer chemotherapy and biotherapy: principles and practice, 3rd ed. Philadelphia, Lippincott Williams & Wilkins, 2001.
3. Mondal R, Nandi M, Chandra PK. Neurofibromatosis, pathological fracture and hypervitaminosis-D. Indian Pediatr. 2010;47:881-2.
4. Mondal R, Nandi M, Tiwari A, Chakravorti S. Diabetic ketoacidosis with L-asparaginase therapy. Indian Pediatr. 2011;48:735-6.
5. Roden DM, George AL. The genetic basis of variability in drug responses. Nat Rev Drug Discovery. 2002;1:37.
6. Sausville E, et al. Signal transduction-directed cancer treatments. Annu Rev Pharmacol Toxicol. 2003;43:199.

7

Acute Lymphoblastic Leukemia

Supratim Datta, Kalpana Datta

Acute Lymphoblastic Leukemia (ALL) is the most common malignancy in children below 15 years of age comprising about 30% of all pediatric cancer patients. In United States, about 3000 new cases of childhood leukemia are found annually of which 80% are ALL. In India, no such community based data is available. Because of the improvement of the multiagent chemotherapy, the survival of ALL patients has improved dramatically in the past 40 years and 80% of patients with ALL are long-term relapse free survivors.

The disease has a peak incidence in between 2–6 years of age, excepting the T cell ALL, which is common in adolescent boys. Overall, the ALL is more common in boys.

ETIOLOGY

In a vast majority of cases, etiology is not known. There are several **Genetic syndromes** and **Environmental factors**, which are associated with increased incidence of ALL.

Genetic syndromes: Few genetic syndromes, which are associated with increased incidence of ALL, are:

- Down's syndrome
- Bloom syndrome
- Fanconi syndrome
- Diamond-Blackfan syndrome
- Ataxia telangiectasia
- Klinefelter syndrome
- Turner syndrome, etc.

Environmental factors: Of the environmental factors, ionizing radiation has been proved as an established factor.

Certain anticancer drugs can give rise to ALL. These are alkylating agents, nitrosourea and epipodophyllotoxin. EB-virus has been associated with B cell ALL.

CLASSIFICATION

ALL is characterized by clonal proliferation of lymphoid precursors, whereby lymphoblasts replace the normal marrow elements. Classification of ALL is based on characteristics of these lymphoblasts. Therefore, the classifications of ALL depend on morphology, cytochemistry, immunophenotype, chromosomal and molecular genetic aberrations of these blast cells.

Morphologic Classification

A classification system based on morphology has been devised by French-American-British (FAB) co-operative working group and is popularly known as FAB classification. According to this, the ALL is divided into three subtypes- L1, L2, L3.

The L1 type is the most common one and found in 85% cases of ALL. L1 cells have scanty cytoplasm. L2 is found in 15% cases of ALL and blast cells here are pleomorphic with more abundant cytoplasm. L3 morphology is found in only 1–2% cases and prominent cytoplasmic vacuoles are found here. L3 subtype is nearly always associated with mature B cell immunophenotype.

With the current multiagent intensive chemotherapy the prognosis between L1 and L2 morphology does not differ.

CYTOCHEMICAL CHARACTERISTICS

Lymphoblasts

- React positively with Periodic acid-Schiff (PAS) stain which stains cytoplasmic glycogen
- TDT (Terminal deoxynucleotidyl transferase) activity may be found in T & B cell lymphoblast. Prognostically not significant
- Lymphoblasts are myeloperoxidase, specific and non-specific enolase and Sudan black negative. On the contrary myeloblasts are myeloperoxidase positive in 75% of cases.

Immunophenotype of ALL

Identification of immunophenotype helps in precise categorization of leukemia than morphological classification with better predict ability of prognostic outcomes and in difficult situation helps to differentiate leukemic blast cells from normal lymphoid precursors. It also helps in detection of minimal residual disease (MRD) which is useful in prognostication and more intensive therapy in the induction phase.

Immunophenotyping is based on presence of some maturation specific antigen present on the cell surface and cytoplasm of lymphoblasts. Based on reactivity with monoclonal antibody flow cytometry technique can be used to categorize the following immunophenotypes in ALL:

1. B cell-progenitor ALL 85%.
2. B cell ALL (mature B cell ALL) 1%.
3. T cell ALL (mature T cell ALL) 14%.

B Cell-progenitor ALL (CD9+, CD19+, CD20+)

This is differentiated from mature B cell ALL by the surface Ig. B cell-progenitor ALL has again 3 subjects depending on various cell surface markers and cytoplasmic Ig (CIg). These subsets include:

Pro-B ALL: 3–4% of ALL patients. These cells are CD10+ and CIg. This subset occurs mainly in infancy.
Early pre-B ALL (60–70% of patients). CD10+ but lacks CIg. This is also referred to as common ALL.
Pre-B ALL (20–30%): Both CD10+, CIg positive.

Mature B cell-ALL: Surface Ig positive and associated with L3 morphology.
Mature T cell-ALL: Commonly found in boys of older age group, associated with mediastinal mass, high leukocyte count and bad prognosis.

CLINICAL FEATURES

ALL is primarily a disease manifestation due to infiltration of bone marrow by leukemic blast cells. The disease may present acutely with life-threatening hemorrhage, infection or severe anemia or insidiously. Many times the disease is diagnosed incidentally on routine blood examination in an asymptomatic child.

Usual Features

The cardinal features of ALL are pallor, fever (due to infection or malignancy) and bleeding manifestations (due to thrombocytopenia). The average duration of illness is 2–4 weeks at the time of presentation. Many times the disease presents like acute viral febrile illness and in due course the pallor, bleeding manifestations and other features of ALL appear. The important clinical signs are enlargement of liver and spleen (30–50% cases) often >4 cm below the costal margins. Generalized lymphadenopathy is found. Anemia, purpuric spots and tenderness of bones are the other usual signs (Fig. 7.1).

Other Features

CNS: Less than 5% of patients with ALL have CNS symptoms at the time of diagnosis. CNS symptoms could be features of raised ICT (like headache, vomiting, papilledema and lethargy), seizures and neck rigidity. Rarely cranial nerve palsies, specially 7th cranial nerve palsy may be found. Other rare manifestations may be hypothalamic involvement (excessive weight gain), cerebellar involvement, multifocal leucoencephalopathy. Spinal cord compression has been found.
Bones and joints: Many patients with ALL present with bone pain and joint pain or swelling and may be confused with Juvenile idiopathic arthritis (JIA) or acute rheumatic fever. Bone pain may be due to leukemic

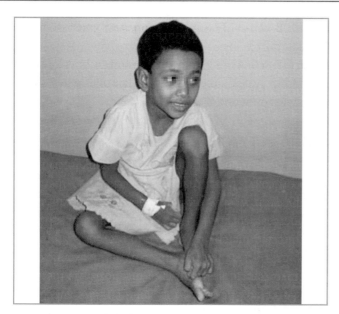

Fig. 7.1: A sick looking child with acute lymphoblastic leukemia having pallor and wasting

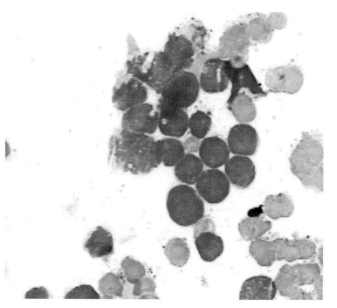

Fig. 7.2: Bone marrow slide of acute lymphoblastic leukemia *(For color version, see Plate 2)*

infiltration of periosteum or expansion of marrow cavity by blast cells (Fig. 7.2). Sometimes the child may present with pathological or vertebral compression.

Thoracic: ALL may present with mediastinal mass with life-threatening compression of tracheobronchial tree and cardiovascular complication. This mediastinal mass is nearly always associated with T cell leukemia. Pleural effusion is another pulmonary feature, which may need urgent intervention. Pericardial effusion may lead to cardiac tamponade. Cardiomyopathy is usually induced by chemotherapy.

Testes: Painless enlargement of one or both testes.

Kidneys: Both the kidneys maybe enlarged due to leukemic infiltration.

Priapism: Due to elevated leukocyte count giving rise to leukostasis in dorsal veins.

Gastrointestinal: Acute abdomen due to perforation of small bowel rarely found mainly in relapsed ALL.

Ocular: Leukemia can affect all the structures of eyes.

Skin: Skin infiltration may be found in congenital leukemia.

DIAGNOSIS

Diagnosis is mainly done by examination by:
1. Peripheral blood.
2. Bone marrow.

Differential Diagnosis

The following conditions are to be differentiated from ALL in some situations:

1. **Infectious mononucleosis:** Atypical lymphocytes in peripheral blood may be indistinguishable from blast cells. Sometimes monospot test and PCR technique for EBV may be helpful to differentiate.
2. **ITP:** It will be prudent to do a bone marrow examination before giving corticosteroid in a patient with ITP to rule out acute leukemia.
3. **Aplastic anemia:** Bone marrow biopsy may be needed to differentiate it from ALL.
4. **JIA:** As there is no confirmatory test for JIA, bone marrow examination is mandatory to exclude ALL before giving corticosteroid in JIA.
5. **Neuroblastoma, rhabdomyosarcoma, and Ewing's tumor** with extensive marrow involvement are to be considered in the differential diagnosis.
6. **Myelodysplasia and myeloproliferative disorders** rarely terminate in ALL.

CLINICAL AND BIOLOGICAL FACTORS PREDICTING OUTCOME

There are certain risk factors in ALL children which when present indicate increased chance of relapse and bad prognosis. The dramatic improvement in event free survival (EPS) in ALL children in last 40 years is mainly because of identification of these risk factors and categorizing ALL children into standard (low) risk group and high-risk group. Risk adapted therapy (high-risk group ALL needing intensive multiagent chemotherapy) has drastically improved the remission of ALL patients (>95% remission) and at the same time less side effects of therapy and more EFS (>80% EFS). The following clinical and biological factors indicate outcome in ALL:

Age: Prognosis favorable in between 1–9 years.

Sex: Female sex has favorable prognosis.

WBC count (at presentation): <50,000/mm^3 favorable. >50,000 unfavorable.

Genotype: Hyperdiploidy (>50 chromosomes), T cell (12:21) or TEL/AML1 fusion carry good prognosis. Whereas hypodiploidy (<45chromosomes), t(9:22) or BCR/ABL fusion, t(4:11) or MLL/AF 4 fusion indicate bad prognosis.

Immunophenotype: Common ALL indicate good prognosis and Pro-B, T cell ALL predict bad prognosis.

Early response to induction therapy: Recently detection of MRD (Minimal Residual Disease) in bone marrow during the first month of therapy either by flow cytometry or by molecular genetics have been shown to have a prognostic significance. Good responders mean MRD even in early months of therapy. Poor responders (MRD in early months)need intensification of therapy.

MANAGEMENT

The management of leukemia is entirely a team effort that needs pediatric oncologist, radiation oncologist, trained nurses, psychologist, nutritionist and social workers. Improved survival has been documented following improved supportive care and modern chemotherapeutic agents.

The strategy of the treatment is systemic combination chemotherapy together with CNS prophylaxis. There are several regimens for the treatment like the BFM protocol, UK protocol, MCP 841 protocol. The choice of therapy is based on estimated clinical risk of relapse, prognostic expected outcome and subtypes of ALL.

The treatment is based on following components. Outlines of therapy given below:

Induction: This is aimed to rapidly destroy blast cells and minimize leukemia burden. Currently 3 drugs are used for induction remission: Vincristine, prednisolone and L-asparaginase. Addition of anthracycline has been shown to be of benefit in ALL children > 10 years of age.

Several studies have shown total oral dexamethasone (6 mg/m^2) instead of oral prednisolone decreases the bone marrow or CNS relapse. Dexamethasone penetrates blood brain barrier better.

Induction phase usually lasts from 4–6 weeks, complete remission means <5% blast cells in bone marrow plus no evidence of extramedullary leukemia.

CNS Directed Therapy: Most children have subclinical CNS involvement at the time of diagnosis. As the brain and spinal cord are not penetrated by anti-leukemic drugs CNS directed therapy is required to prevent CNS relapse and increase survival rate. Whether intrathecal triple therapy with weekly methotrexate (MTx), cytarabine, glucocorticoid is better than single weekly MTx therapy is still not clear. Along with intrathecal therapy intermittent high-dose MTx and 6 MP is given as consolidation therapy.

Experts also recommend low-dose (1800 CGY) cranial irradiation with intrathecal MTx.

Re-induction: With drugs comparable to be used in induction and consolidation have got proven value in preventing risk of relapse.

Intensification (Consolidation) Phase: A period of intensified treatment administered shortly after remission induction to prevent drug resistance usually to those with high-risk cases. Commonly used agents are high-dose MTx, L-asparaginase, epipodophyllotoxin, cytarabine the resultant prolonged granulocytopenia may need supportive therapy with broad spectrum antibiotics and blood products.

Continuation Phase: With weekly oral MTx and daily oral 6 MP, oral corticosteroid, vincristine and IT therapy is given. This phase is continued for 2–3 years.

Stem Cell Transplantation (SCT)

Autologous SCT is not helpful in childhood ALL. Although allogeneic SCT has been tried in high-risk ALL in first remission, its role is still unknown.

Future Therapy

New genomic techniques and targeted therapy with biological like imatinib, desatinib, etc. may be helpful in future.

Relapse

With current therapy > 90% patients with ALL will achieve remission and > 80% cases will have > 5 years event free survival. Relapse occurs in about 20% cases. Common sites of relapse are: Bone marrow, CNS, testes, ovaries, etc. (Fig. 7.3).

Prognosis in relapse cases depend on many factors, such as site of relapse, (medullary relapse has bad prognosis as compared to isolated CNS or testicular relapse), longer initial remission had favorable prognosis. T cell ALL and older age (>10 years) had bad prognosis.

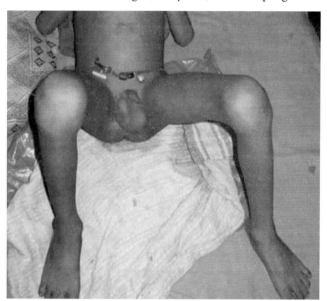

Fig. 7.3: Clinical photograph of testicular relapse of acute lymphoblastic leukemia

Medullary Relapse

It is treated with intensive chemotherapy and allogenic SCT. Long-term survival is 25–60%.

Isolated CNS Relapse

It is treated with cranial irradiation and intensive systemic chemotherapy. Long-term survival is 45–70%.

Isolated Testicular Relapse

Testiculars radiation and intensive systemic chemotherapy are used in this condition.

SUGGESTED READING

1. Behrmann RE, Kliegman RM, Jenson HB. Nelson text book of pediatrics. 17th edition; Philadelphia; WB Saunders.
2. Choudhury VP. In Recent advances in hematology. Jaypee Brothers, New Delhi. 2004.
3. Mondal R, Nandi M, Tiwari A, Chakravorti S. Diabetic ketoacidosis with L-asparaginase therapy. Indian Pedtr. 2011;48(9):735-6.
4. Nathan and Oski's Hematology of infancy and childhood; Sixth edition; 2003;1335-56.
5. Parotid gland enlargement as a presenting manifestation of acute lymphoblastic leukemia. JK Science. 2005;7(3):167-8.
6. Pediatric Oncology. The Pediatric Clinic of North America. 1997;44;4 P831-46.
7. Pediatric Oncology. The pediatric Clinic of North America. 2008;55;1;101-86.
8. Philip Pizzo A. Principles and Practices of Pediatric Oncology; 4th edition; Lippincott William and Wilkins; Philadelphia; USA, 2002.

8 Hodgkin's Disease

Anirban Chatterjee

In 1832, Thomas Hodgkin first discovered a morbid condition of 'Absorbent' gland and spleen. Later it is recognized as malignant disorder, lymphoma, which is called Hodgkin's disease. Hodgkin's lymphoma clinically presents as lymph node enlargement and spread of the disease from one lymph node group to another and systemic symptoms appear with advanced disease. Pathological hallmark of the disease is Reed-Sternberg cells (RS cells). Disease is associated with defective cellular immunity. In the early stages, the cure rate is approximately 93%. Advanced stages of the disease have a significantly worse prognosis. Hodgkin's lymphoma can be cured by radiation.

EPIDEMIOLOGY

Hodgkin's lymphoma is responsible for less than 1% of all cancers in world. In developing countries, highest incidence is in younger age group.

Its incidence is stable or slightly decreasing at present.

Age

Hodgkin's disease has bimodal age curve. A peak is in 10–35 years and another peak later in life (55 years).

Hodgkin's lymphoma shows a three form of age incidence curve in epidemiologic studies. It develops in three different age groups, childhood (≤14 years) young adulthood (15–35 years age) and older adult (55–74 years of age) and the peak varies within different ethnic group. It occurs rarely below five-year.

Sex

It is more common in males and mostly below ten years of age. Exception is the nodular sclerosis, where females are more common.

In developing countries, the most cases showed that presence of Epstein-Barr virus in the Reed-Sternberg cells. Rarely, Hodgkin's disease is familial. The incidence of Hodgkin's lymphoma upsurges in HIV infection.

CLINICAL FEATURES

Hodgkin's lymphoma present with the following symptoms:
- **Lymph nodes:** The painless enlargement of one or more lymph nodes is the most frequent symptom of Hodgkin lymphoma. On palpation the lymph nodes are rubbery and swollen. The cervical and supraclavicular lymph node enlargements are most common presenting symptom (80–90%). Inguinal and axillary lymphanedopathy are occasional. The lymph nodes of mediastinum are involved in two-third cases and these are revealed on a chest X-ray and rapidly disappear with therapy. Rarely, involved nodes are characteristically painful after alcohol ingestion in youth.
- Splenomegaly, which is rarely massive in 30% of Hodgkin's lymphoma. The size of the spleen usually varies during the course of treatment
- Hepatomegaly is present in about five percent of cases

- **Systemic symptoms:** About one-third (⅓) of Hodgkin disease present with systemic symptom, systemic symptoms are low-grade fever; night sweats; unexplained weight loss of at least 10% of the total body mass in last six months or less, itchy skin (pruritus) because of eosinophilia in the blood; or fatigue (lassitude). Systemic symptoms fever, night sweats, and weight loss are regarded as B symptoms; which indicate that stage of the disease is, for example, 1B rather than 1A
- **Cyclical fever:** A cyclical high-grade fever occurs in Hodgkin disease. It is known as the Pel-Ebstein fever. There is controversy about whether P-E fever truly exists
- **Extranodal disease:** On depending of extent of involvement of node, disease may present with airway obstruction pleural or pericardial effusion, hepatocellular dysfunction, bone marrow infiltration.

Autoimmune disorder like Nephrotic syndrome is well-known and rare presentation. Other autoimmune disorder, autoimmune hemolytic anemia, immune thrombocytopenia and autoimmune neutropenia are also reported.

Concomitant tuberculosis, fungal infection and varicella-zoster infection are common due to impaired cellular immunity and immunosuppressive treatment (Fig. 8.1).

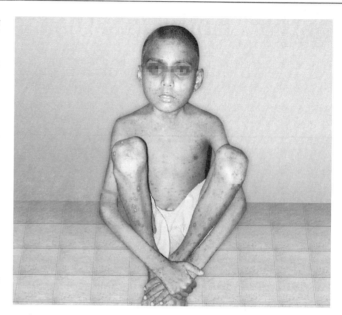

Fig. 8.1: Clinical photograph of a child with Hodgkin's disease developed disseminated chickenpox

DIAGNOSIS

Excision biopsy of lymph node with microscopic examination is done to confirm diagnosis. Complete blood count, chest skiagram, liver function test, renal function test are performed to evaluate function of major organs and to judge safety of chemotherapy. Positron emission tomography (PET) is necessary to identify small lesion, which is not able to detect on CT-scan. Gallium scans are also useful sometimes as for a PET-scan. Useful but not essential tests are cell-surface marker phenotypic analysis and gene rearrangement analysis (Fig. 8.2).

PATHOLOGY

The shape of lymph node is maintained as cancer cell, usually do not invade the capsuler of nodes. In general,

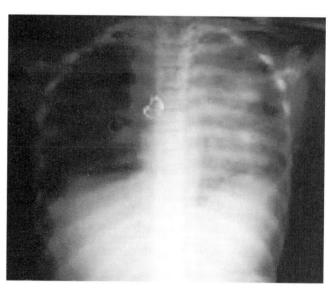

Fig. 8.2: X-ray of chest showing mediastinal mass in a case of Hodgkin's disease

the cut surface is white-grey and uniform. Nodular sclerosis may show a nodular appearance.

Microscopy

Microscopic examination of the lymph node biopsy shows total or partial destruction of the lymph node by diffused large cancer cells known as Reed-Sternberg cells (typical and variants) and mix with a reactive cell infiltrate, consist of different proportion of lymphocytes, histiocytes, eosinophils, and plasma cells. Isolated RS cells separated by micro-dissection technique showed that B cell type monoclonal immunoglobulin (Ig) gene rearrangement in 98% of cases and T-cell type monoclonal T-cell receptor gene rearrangement in 2% of cases.

The Reed-Sternberg cell is large cell with multiple or multilobulate nuclei is regarded as hallmark of Hodgkin disease and shows an unusual CD45–, CD30+, CD15+/– immunophenotype. The Epstein-Barr virus genome present in the Reed-Sternberg cells in 50% to 97% of cases. EBV infection induces expression of latent membrane antigen (LMP) 1 that makes hindrance of the apoptosis for RS cells.

Classic Reed-Sternberg cells consist of large size, ample, amphophilic, thinly granular/homogeneous cytoplasm; two mirror-image nuclei (owl eyes) each with prominent eosinophilic nucleolus and a thick nuclear membrane, in which chromatin is spread at peripheral region.

Variants of RS Cell

Hodgkin's cell is atypical mononuclear cell, which is similar but mononucleated variant of RS cell. Lacunar RSC consists of a single nucleus, and cytoplasm pull around the nucleus, forming a vacant space ("lacunae").

Pleomorphic RSC contains many uneven nuclei.

"Popcorn" RSC (lympho-histiocytic variant) is a small cell, with lobulated nucleus, small nucleoli.

"Mummy" RSC contains a dense nucleus, no nucleolus and basophilic cytoplasm.

HD invasion to adjacent lymph node in arranged manner and spread to bloodstream for distant metastasis. Cytokines are increases in blood and HD culture tissue. Systemic symptoms are due to cytokine. Interleukin 1or 2 causes fever, weight loss is due to tumor necrosis factor, transforming growth factors causes suppression of immunity and help to grow RS cell.

Genotype

Classic HL shows mutation in VG (variable region of Ig heavy chain gene).

Crippled B cell due to defect in immunoglobulin gene regulatory elements that is down-regulation of transcription factors. Nodular lymphocytic predominance shows normal gene transcription and Ig production and no crippled B cell.

Cell Cycle Analysis

The typical features of Reed-Sternberg cells and classical Hodgkin's lymphoma is greatly positive for proliferation markers. Abortive mitotic cycles, which form multinucleation and cell death in mitosis are characteristic of these cells. They have high expression of G(1)-phase cyclins in classical Hodgkin's lymphoma and this is the explanation of the high percentage of cells staining for proliferation markers.

The correlation between increased p27 and p53 expression status and higher expression levels of G2/M cyclins indicates that the impairment of the growth inhibitory activity of the p27 and p53 tumor suppressor pathway usually promote the proliferation of Hodgkin's and Reed-Sternberg cells.

PATHOLOGICAL CLASSIFICATION OF HD

There are four pathologic subtype of Classical Hodgkin's lymphoma (Table 8.1). These subclassification is based upon Reed-Sternberg cell morphology and reactive cell infiltrate in the lymph node disease specimen.

Non-classical nodular lymphocyte predominant Hodgkin's lymphoma (NLPHL) is not a form of classic Hodgkin's lymphoma. Because of NLPHL composed of RSC variants of large popcorn-shaped RSC, which express B lymphocyte markers such as CD 20 and negative of CD 15 and CD 30. For this reason, this is an atypical form of B cell lymphoma. NLPHL can transform into diffuse large B cell lymphoma (Table 8.2).

STAGING

Staging HD is essential to determine the region of the body invaded. These require diagnostic histology of HD, a physical examination, blood tests, chest X-ray, computed tomography (CT) scans or magnetic resonance

Table 8.1: Classification of HD (WHO)

Family	Name	Description
Classical	Nodular sclerosing	This is the most common variety. It consists of large tumor nodules which is organized by numerous classic RS, often pleomorphic RS cells with lacunar RS cells and merely few reactive lymphocytes Differential: Diffuse large cell lymphoma
Classical	Mixed-cellularity subtype	This is a common subtype and consists of numerous classic RS cells and numerous reactive cells which are lymphocytes, histiocytes, eosinophils, and plasma cells
Classical	Lymphocyte-rich	Is a rare subtype
Classical	Lymphocyte depleted	Is a rare subtype
Non classical	Lymphocyte predominant	Uncommon subtype

Table 8.2: Immunophenotyping of HD

Hodgkin lymphoma immunophenotyping	CHL (95%) NS,MC,LR,LD	NPL-HL (5%)
CD 30	+	–
CD 15	+/–	–
EMA	–	+
CD 45	–	+
CD 20, 79	+/– in 25%	On 100%
CD 3	+ in 20%	–
Dendritic cell background	Poor CD 21 Polyclonal T	Strong CD 21 Polyclonal B

imaging (MRI) scans of the chest, abdomen and pelvis, and a bone marrow biopsy. At present, positron emission tomography (PET) scan is used in place of the gallium scan for staging.

At present time lymphangiograms or laparotomies are very rarely necessary, as due to improvements in imaging with the CT-scan and PET-scan. The Ann Arbor staging classification scheme is commonly used and on the basis of staging, the classifications are:

Stage I—involvement of a single lymph node region (I) or single extralymphatic site (Ie)

Stage II—involvement of two or more lymph node regions on the same side of the diaphragm (II) or of one lymph node region and a contiguous extralymphatic site (IIe)

Stage III—involvement of lymph node regions on both sides of the diaphragm, which may include the spleen (IIIs) and/or limited contiguous extralymphatic organ or site (IIIe, IIIes);

III₁: with splenic hilar, celiac, portal nodes; III₂: with para-aortic, iliac, mesenteric nodes

Stage IV—disseminated involvement of one or more extralymphatic organs.

'A' add to the stage when absence of systemic symptoms

'B' add to the stage when presence of systemic symptoms.

X. Bulky disease (>1/3 widening of mediastinum >10 cm maximum dimension of nodal mass)

E. Involvement of a single, localized, extranodal site.

PROGNOSIS

The unfavorable prognostic factors recognized in the international study are:

a. Stage IV disease
b. Hemoglobin <10.5 g/dL
c. Lymphocyte count <600/μL or <8%
d. Male sex
e. Albumin <4.0 g/dL
f. White blood count $\geq$15,000/μL

These can correctly predict the success rate of standard treatment of local or advanced stage Hodgkin's lymphoma. Freedom from progression (FFP) at 5 years are precisely correlated with these factors. The 5-year FFP without any factors is 84%, when each factor adds, it lowers the 5-year FFP rate by 7%.

Other important poor prognostic factors, which are reported by study are mixed-cellularity or lymphocyte-depleted histologies, large number of involved nodal sites, the presence of B symptoms, high erythrocyte sedimentation rate, and widening of the mediastinal widening is more than one third, the size of nodal mass more than 10 cm in any dimension.

INTERVENTION

The current treatment can cure more than 90% of new onset Hodgkin's disease (Table 8.3).

Table 8.3: Treatment of HD

Stages	Treatment of choice	Cure rate
IA and IB	Involved field reduceddose radiation therapy + combination chemotherapy (3–4 cycles)	90%
IIA and IIB	Combination chemotherapy with reduced dose field irradiation to involved areas	80 to 90%.
IIIA, IIIB and IV	Combination chemotherapy alone or combination chemotherapy and low dose radiation for bulky disease or more extensive fields or residual disease after chemotherapy	< 50%

Radiation therapy   80–90% RC
mantle field
para-aortic field
pelvic field
Combination chemotherapy
ABVD   80% RC
BEACOPP   90% RC

Therapy of early stage disease (IA or IIA) is radiation or chemotherapy. Age, sex, bulk and the histological subtype of the disease determine the choice of therapy. Combination chemotherapy alone is the treatment for advance stage of disease (III, IVA, or IVB). Large thoracic mass are commonly treated by combined chemotherapy and radiation therapy at any stage of the disease.

Majority Hodgkin's disease in pediatric age group is treated with combination chemotherapy with or without low dose (1,500–2,500 cGy) field radiation for primary treatment. Radiation therapy for HD should be providing at institute with Modern megavoltage equipment that comprise linear accelerators of six mega voltage energy and planned simulators. In prepubescent child, low dose involved field radiation with chemotherapy. The standard treatment for older adolescents and young adult with nonbulley, localized and good prognosis disease can be high dose, extended field radiation along with transposition of ovaries to midline and midline pelvic block to protect ovarian function. Testicular shield or sperm banking in male patient. As standard radiation dose (3,600–4,000 cGy) treatment causes severe skeletal and dermatological abnormalities in prepubescent children and also correlated with high incidence of subsequent breast cancer in teenage females. Complications of this therapy are sterility, cardiopulmonary toxicity and second malignancies. Radiation therapy can cause solid tumors, such as sarcomas and breast cancer. The detrimental effect of low-dose mantle radiation therapy is thyroid dysfunction and/or thyroid nodules, thyroid cancer.

Multi-agent regimen for Hodghin's should be non-cross-resistant chemotherapeutics. Each drug must kill the cancer cells independently. Every drug in multidrug regimen should have different target point to kill cancer cell so that resistance could not be approached and there are no similar toxicities in multiagent drugs so that full dose can be given.

Regimens of combination chemotherapy for Hodgkin's disease in pediatrics are cyclophosphamide, vincristine, prednisone and procarbazine (COPD) or adriamycin/doxorubicin, vinblastine, bleomycin and dacarbazine or etoposide (ABVD or ABVE). COPP/ABVP is hybrid regimens which are also frequently used (Table 8.4).

The ABVD chemotherapy regimen is the gold standard therapy for Hodgkin's disease at present. In the 1970s the four drugs regimen grow up in Italy. The ABVD treatment is typically six to eight months duration, sometimes longer duration treatments may be needed.

The other mode of treatment is BEACOPP which is used predominantly in Europe. BEACOPP regimen has 10–15% higher cure rate than standard ABVD in metastatic disease. This regimen is not well-accepted in US physicians probably due to higher incidence of secondary leukemia. BEACOPP is costly due to simultaneous use of GCSF to boost production of white blood cells.

The delayed harmful effects of treatment are cardiovascular disease and second malignancies like acute leukemias, lymphomas, and solid tumors in the field of radiation therapy. For this reason, treatment of early stage disease is shortened chemotherapy and field radiation therapy. Clinical research strategies are exploring reduction of the duration of chemotherapy and dose and volume of radiation therapy in an attempt to reduce late morbidity and mortality of treatment while maintaining high cure rates.

Table 8.4: Chemotherapy regimen in Hodgkin disease

Name	Drugs	Dosage route	Days
COPD	Cyclophosphamide	600 mg/m^2	1, 8
	Vincristine (Oncovin)	1.4 mg/m^2 IV	1, 8
	Procarbazine	100 mg/m^2 P.O	1–15
	Prednisone	40 mg/m^2 PO	1–15
ABVD	Doxorubicin	25 mg/m^2 IV	1, 15
	Bleomycin	10U/m^2 IV	1,15
	Vinblastine	6 mg/m^2	1, 15
	Dacarbazine	375 mg/m^2	1, 15

*Repeat cycle 28 days

The secondary malignancy like acute leukemia, depends on the type of treatment, such as dual mode treatment with some chemotherapeutic regimens and irradiation is correlated with enhanced risk than single modality of treatment. Radiation therapy alone can cause much less incidence of secondary acute leukemia than chemotherapy.

Chemotherapy has a dose response curve; a higher dose increases the risk of secondary leukemia. Newer combined chemotherapy regimens will be less-risk of malignancy than previous combinations that consist of alkylating agents, such as mechlorethamine and procarbazine. It also maintains fertility in males, as it is less gonadotoxic.

Usually chemotherapy and radiation therapy are used in massive mediastinal disease, which means more than one third of the maximum intrathoracic diameter and invasive disease affecting the pericardium or chest wall in the stage I or stage II disease.

Monitoring of mediastinal disease commonly done by chest X-ray, chest computed tomography (CT) scan, magnetic resonance imaging (MRI), 67-gallium single photon emission computed tomography (SPECT) imaging, and positron emission tomography (PET) scanning. progressive/relapse pediatric Hodgkin's disease. There are three groups of treatment failure.

Relapse of HD

Majority of relapse are found in the first 3 years and may be as long as 10 years of preliminary diagrams. The final outcome of different salvage therapy is limited in pediatrics.

Definitions

1. Primary progressive HD—never complete remission (CR) occur.
2. Early relapse—within one year of CR.
3. Late relapse—after one year of CR.

The poor prognostic factors are presence of B symptoms and extranodal disease at the time of relapse/progression.

Relapse after initial chemotherapy is found in Stage I or II disease 10 to 15% and Stage III or IV disease 30 to 50%. Sites of relapse following different chemotherapy regimen is described in the Table 8.5.

The diagnosis of progressive or relapse of disease is done by CT-scan of chest/abdomen and pelvis (Diagnostic accuracy 56%), PET-scan (Diagnostic accuracy 92%), biopsy and clinical analysis.

Prognostic Factors for Salvage Therapy

- Age <30 years
  - Disease status at relapse untreated refractory
  - Stage I or II at relapse
  - No B symptoms at relapse, Stage I–III at original diagnosis
  - Nodal only relapse, disease extent at relapse.

There are Conventional Dose Salvage Therapy

- Several regimens (ESHAP, DHAP, ICE, ASHAP, VIM-D, CAPE/PALE, ABDIC)
- Commonly used: ESHAP, ICE.

High Dose Chemotherapy with Autologous Stem Cell Transplantation

The definite indication for treatment with high dose chemotherapy/hematopoietic stem cell transplantation (HDC/HSCT) for relapse of Hodgkin's lymphoma after primary chemotherapy are relapse <1 year after completion of primary chemotherapy, relapse B symptom, relapse extranodal site and, relapse previously irradiated site.

Most significant factors for autologous transplantation are:

a. Serum albumin <4
b. HB <10.5 g
c. Age >45
d. Lymphocytopenia.

Table 8.5: Sites of relapse

Regimen	Nodal sites	Sites of prior disease	Remarks
MOPP chemotherapy	75% central axial nodes and left SC area the most common nodal site	92%	New nodal sites tended to be adjacent to prior sites
			13% previously irradiated nodes
ABVD ±XRT	71%	—	Previously uninvolved nodal regions or extranodal sites like lung and live
XRT	—	—	

Ten years event-free survival:

0–1 factors—38%

2–3 factors—23%

>4 factors—7%

SUGGESTED READING

1. Bayle-Weisgerber C, Lemercier N, Teillet F, et al. Hodgkin's disease in children: results of therapy in a mixed group of 178 clinically and pathologically staged patients over 13 years. Cancer. 1984;54:215-22.

2. Biggar RJ, Jaffe ES, Goedert JJ, Chaturvedi A, Pfeiffer R, Engels EA. "Hodgkin lymphoma and Immunodeficiency in persons with HIV/AIDS". Blood. 2006;108:3786–91.

3. Donaldson SS, Whitaker SJ, Plowman PN, et al. Stage I–II pediatric Hodgkin's disease: long-term follow-up demonstrates equivalent survival rates following different management schemes. J of Clin Onco. 1990;8:1128-37.

4. Gehan EA, Sullivan MP, Fuller LM, et al.: The intergroup Hodgkin's disease in children: A study of stages I and II. Cancer. 1990;65:1429-37.

5. Gupta RK, Gospodarowicz MK, Andrew Lister T. Clinical Evaluation and Staging of Hodgkin's Disease. Hodgkin's Disease. 1999;230-1.

6. Hasenclever D, Diehl V. "A Prognostic Score for Advanced Hodgkin's Disease". New Engl J of Medi. 1998;339:1506-14.

7. Kaldor JM, Day NE, Clarke EA, et al. Leukemia following Hodgkin's disease. New Engl J of Med. 1990;322:7-13.

8. Longo DL, Glatstein E, Duffey PL, et al. Alternating MOPP and ABVD chemotherapy plus mantle-field radiation therapy in patients with massive mediastinal Hodgkin's disease. J of Clin Oncol. 1997;15:3338-46.

9. Schellong G. The balance between cure and late effects in childhood Hodgkin's lymphoma: the experience of the German-Austrian Study Group since 1978. German-Austrian Pediatric Hodgkin's Disease Study Group. Annals of Oncology. 1996;7(Suppl 4):67-72.

10. Shah AB, Hudson MM, Poquette CA, et al. Long-term follow-up of patients treated with primary radiotherapy for supradiaphragmatic Hodgkin's disease at St. Jude Children's Research Hospital. Int J of Rad Oncol Biol Phys. 1999;44:867-77.

11. Stein RS, Morgan D (2003). Handbook of cancer Chemotherapy. Sixth edition. Lippincott Williams & Wilkins, 493, Table 21.2: "Hodgkin's Disease: Incidence of stages and results of therapy." ISBN 0-7817-3629-3.

12. Zinzani PL, Zompatori M, Bendandi M, et al. Monitoring bulky mediastinal disease with gallium-67, CT-scan and magnetic resonance imaging in Hodgkin's disease and high-grade non-Hodgkin's lymphoma. Leukemia and Lymphoma. 1996;22:131-5.

9 Non-Hodgkin's Lymphoma in Children

Prantar Chakrabarti

Lymphoma [Hodgkin and non-Hodgkin (NHL)] is the third most common childhood malignancy, and NHL accounts for approximately 7% of cancers in children younger than 20 years.

Although there is no sharp age peak, NHL occurs most commonly in the second decade of life, and occurs less frequently in children younger than 3 years. The incidence of NHL is increasing worldwide. The incidence of NHL is higher in Caucasians than in African-Americans, and NHL is more common in males than in females. Immunodeficiency, both congenital and acquired (HIV infection or post-transplant), increases the risk of NHL. Epstein-Barr virus (EBV) is associated with most cases of NHL seen in the immunodeficient population.

CLASSIFICATION AND CLINICAL PRESENTATION

- Burkitt and Burkitt-like lymphoma/leukemia
- Diffuse large B cell lymphoma (DLBCL)
- Lymphoblastic lymphoma
- Anaplastic large cell lymphoma
- Lymphoproliferative disease associated with immunodeficiency in children
- Rare non-Hodgkin lymphoma occurring in children.

In children, NHL is distinct from the more common forms of lymphoma observed in adults. While lymphomas in adults are more commonly of low or intermediate grade, almost all NHLs that occur in children are high grade. Classification of NHL in childhood and adolescence has historically been based on clinical behavior and response to treatment. A study by the Children's Cancer Group (CCG) demonstrated that the outcome for lymphoblastic NHL was superior with longer leukemia-like therapy consisting of induction, consolidation, and maintenance, while non-lymphoblastic NHL (Burkitt and large cell) had superior outcome with short, intensive, pulsed therapy.

The World Health Organization (WHO) has classified NHL on the basis of the following:

A. Phenotype [i.e. B-lineage, T-lineage, or natural killer (NK) cell lineage].
B. Differentiation (i.e. precursor versus mature/peripheral).

On the basis of clinical response to treatment, NHL of childhood and adolescence currently falls into three therapeutically relevant categories:

1. B cell NHL (Burkitt and Burkitt-like lymphoma/leukemia and DLBCL).
2. Lymphoblastic lymphoma (primarily precursor T-cell lymphoma and, less frequently, precursor B-cell lymphoma).
3. Anaplastic large cell lymphoma (T cell or null cell lymphomas).

NHL associated with immunodeficiency generally has a mature B cell phenotype and is more often of large cell than Burkitt histology. Post-transplant lymphoproliferative diseases (PTLDs) are classified according to standard NHL nomenclature as (1) early lesions, (2) polymorphic, and (3) monomorphic.

Other types of lymphomas are more commonly seen in adults and occur rarely in children.

Each type of childhood NHL is associated with distinctive molecular biological characteristics, which are outlined in Table 9.1. The Revised European-American Lymphoma Classification (REAL) and the WHO classification are the most current NHL classifications utilized and are shown below. The Working Formulation is also listed for reference. The WHO Classification applies the principles of the REAL Classification and focuses on the specific type of lymphoma for therapy purposes.

BURKITT AND BURKITT-LIKE LYMPHOMA/ LEUKEMIA

Burkitt and Burkitt-like lymphoma/leukemia accounts for about 50% of childhood NHL and exhibits consistent, aggressive clinical behavior. The malignant cells show a mature B cell phenotype and are negative for the enzyme terminal deoxynucleotidyl transferase (TdT). These malignant cells usually express surface immunoglobulin, most bearing surface IgM with either kappa or lambda light chains. A variety of additional B-cell markers (e.g. CD 20, CD 22) are usually present, and almost all childhood Burkitt/Burkitt-like lymphoma/leukemia express CALLA (CD 10). About 25% contain Epstein-Barr virus (EBV) genomes. Burkitt lymphoma/leukemia expresses a characteristic chromosomal translocation, usually t (8;14) and more rarely t (8;22) or t (2;8). Each of these translocations juxtaposes the c-*myc* gene to immunoglobulin locus regulatory elements, resulting in the inappropriate expression of c-*myc*, the gene involved in cellular proliferation. Pediatric Burkitt lymphoma patients whose tumors also contain cytogenetic abnormalities of 13 q and 22 q have a markedly poor survival on current chemotherapy protocols.

The distinction between Burkitt and Burkitt-like lymphoma/leukemia is controversial. Burkitt lymphoma consists of uniform, small, noncleaved cells (Fig. 9.1), whereas Burkitt-like lymphoma is a highly disputed diagnosis among pathologists owing to features that are

Table 9.1: Major histopathological categories of non-Hodgkin lymphoma in children and adolescents*

Category WHO classification/ updated REAL	Category (working formulation)	Immuno-phenotype	Clinical presentation	Chromosome translocation	Genes affected
Burkitt and Burkitt-like lymphomas	Malignant lymphoma small noncleaved cell	Mature B cell	Intra-abdominal (sporadic), head and neck (non-jaw, sporadic), jaw (endemic)	t (8;14) (q24 q32), t (2;8) (p11;q24), t (8;22) (q24; q11)	C-MYC, IGH, IGK, IGL
Diffuse large B cell lymphoma	Malignant lymphoma large cell	Mature B cell; maybe CD 30 +	Nodal, abdomen, bone, primary CNS, mediastinal	No consistent cytogenetic abnormality identified.	
Lymphoblastic lymphoma, precursor T cell/leukemia, or precursor B cell lymphoma	Lymphoblastic convoluted and non-convoluted	Pre-T cell Pre-B cell	Mediastinal, bone marrow Skin, bone	MTS1/ p16 ink 4 a deletion TAL1 t (1;14) (p34; q11), t (11;14) (p13;q11)	TAL1, TCRAO, RHOMB1, HOX11
Anaplastic large cell lymphoma, systemic	Malignant lymphoma immunoblastic or malignant lymphoma large	CD 30 + (Ki-1+) T cell or null cell	Variable, but systemic symptoms often prominent	T (2;5) (p23; q35)	ALK, NMP
Anaplastic large cell lymphoma, cutaneous		CD 30 + (Ki-usually) T cell	Skin only; single or multiple lesions	Lacks t (2;5)	

*Adapted from Percy et al.[22]

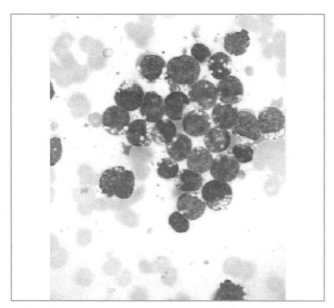

Fig. 9.1: Microphotograph showing lymphoblast proliferation suggestive of Burkitt's lymphoma *(For color version, see Plate 2)*

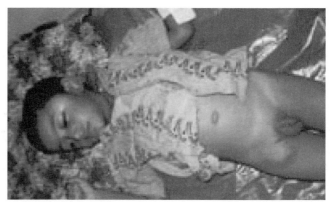

Fig. 9.2: Clinical photograph of a sick child with multiple lymph node enlargement and organomegaly in NHL

consistent with diffuse large B cell lymphoma (DLBCL). Cytogenetic evidence of c-*myc* rearrangement is the gold standard for diagnosis of Burkitt lymphoma. For cases in which cytogenetic analysis is not available, the WHO has recommended that the Burkitt-like diagnosis be reserved for lymphoma resembling Burkitt lymphoma or with more pleomorphism, large cells, and a proliferation fraction [i.e. Ki-67 (+) of at least 99%]. Despite the histologic differences, Burkitt and Burkitt-like lymphoma/leukemia are clinically very aggressive and are treated with very aggressive regimens.

The two most common primary sites of disease are the abdomen and head and neck region (Fig. 9.2). Other sites of involvement include testes, bone, peripheral lymph nodes, skin, bone marrow, and central nervous system (CNS).

DIFFUSE LARGE B CELL LYMPHOMA

DLBCL is a mature B-cell neoplasm that represents 10% to 20% of pediatric NHL. DLBCL occurs more frequently during the second decade of life than during the first. While classification systems have described morphologic variants (e.g. immunoblastic, centroblastic) of DLBCL, the WHO classification system for hematological malignancies does not recommend morphologic sub- classification. Pediatric

DLBCL may present clinically similar to Burkitt or Burkitt-like lymphoma, though it is more often localized and less often involves the bone marrow or CNS.

Non-mediastinal DLBCL in children and adolescents differs biologically from DLBCL in adults. Pediatric DLBCL belongs primarily to the germinal center B-cell type. Unlike adult DLBCL of the germinal center B-cell type, in which the t (14;18) translocation involving the immunoglobulin heavy-chain gene and the *BCL 2* gene is commonly observed, pediatric DLBCL rarely demonstrates the t (14;18) translocation. Outcomes for children with DLBCL are more favorable than those observed in adults, with overall 5-year event-free survival (EFS) rates of approximately 90% in children.

About 20% of pediatric DLBCL presents as primary mediastinal disease [primary mediastinal B cell lymphoma (PMBCL)]. This presentation is more common in older children and adolescents and is associated with an inferior outcome compared with other pediatric DLBCL. PMBCL is associated with distinctive chromosomal aberrations. PMBCL also has a distinctive gene expression profile in comparison with other DLBCL, suggesting a close relationship of PMBCL with Hodgkin lymphoma.

LYMPHOBLASTIC LYMPHOMA

Lymphoblastic lymphoma makes up approximately 20% of childhood NHL. Lymphoblastic lymphomas are usually positive for TdT, with more than 75% having a T cell immunophenotype and the remainder having a precursor B cell phenotype. Chromosomal abnormalities are not well-characterized in patients with lymphoblastic lymphoma.

Nearly 75% of patients with lymphoblastic lymphoma have an anterior mediastinal mass and may present with symptoms of dyspnea, wheezing, stridor, dysphagia, or swelling of the head and neck. Pleural effusions may be present, and the involvement of lymph nodes, usually above the diaphragm, may be a prominent feature. There may also be involvement of bone, skin, bone marrow, CNS, abdominal organs (but rarely bowel), and occasionally other sites such as lymphoid tissue of Waldeyer ring and testes. Abdominal involvement is rare compared with Burkitt lymphoma. Localized lymphoblastic lymphoma may occur in lymph nodes, bone, and subcutaneous tissue (Fig. 9.3). Lymphoblastic lymphoma within the mediastinum is not considered localized disease.

Involvement of the bone marrow may lead to confusion as to whether the patient has lymphoma with bone marrow involvement or leukemia with extramedullary disease. Traditionally, patients with more than 25% marrow blasts are considered to have leukemia, and those with fewer than 25% marrow blasts are considered to have lymphoma. It is not yet clear whether these arbitrary definitions are biologically distinct or relevant for treatment design.

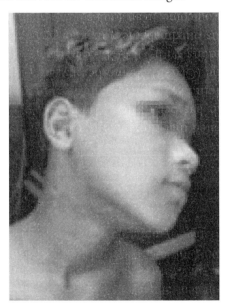

Fig. 9.3: Clinical photograph showing cervical lymphadenopathy in localized lymphoblastic type of NHL

ANAPLASTIC LARGE CELL LYMPHOMA

Anaplastic large cell lymphoma (ALCL) accounts for approximately 10% of childhood NHL. While the predominant immunophenotype of ALCL is mature T cell, null-cell disease (i.e. no T cell, B cell, or NK cell surface antigen expression) does occur. More than 90% of ALCL cases are CD 30-positive and have the translocation t (2;5) (p23;q35) leading to the expression of the fusion protein NPM/ALK, though variant *ALK* translocations have been reported. Clinically, ALCL has a broad range of presentations, including involvement of lymph nodes and a variety of extranodal sites, particularly skin and bone and, less often, gastrointestinal tract, lung, pleura, and muscle. Involvement of the CNS and bone marrow is uncommon. However, in a retrospective subset analysis, there was evidence that submicroscopic bone marrow and peripheral blood involvement, detected by reverse transcriptase-polymerase chain reaction (RT-PCR) from *NPM-ALK*, were found in approximately 50% of patients and correlated with clinical stage; marrow involvement detected by PCR was associated with a 50% cumulative incidence of relapse. ALCL is often associated with systemic symptoms (e.g. fever, weight loss) and a prolonged waxing and waning course, making diagnosis difficult and often delayed. There is a subgroup of ALCL with leukemic peripheral blood involvement. These patients usually exhibit significant respiratory distress with diffuse lung infiltrates or pleural effusions and have hepatosplenomegaly. Most of these cases have an aberrant T cell immunophenotype with frequent expression of myeloid antigens. Patients in this ALCL subgroup may require more aggressive therapy. Patients with ALCL may present with signs and symptoms consistent with hemophagocytic lymphohistiocytosis (HLH), but have mediastinal or other adenopathy that, when biopsied, is diagnostic of ALCL.

LYMPHOPROLIFERATIVE DISEASE ASSOCIATED WITH IMMUNODEFICIENCY IN CHILDREN

The incidence of lymphoproliferative disease or lymphoma is 100-fold higher in immunocompromised children than in the general population. The cause of such immune deficiencies may be a genetically inherited defect, secondary to HIV infection, or iatrogenic following transplantation [solid organ transplantation or allogeneic hematopoietic stem cell transplantation (HSCT)]. EBV is associated with most of these tumors, but some tumors are not associated with any infectious agent.

NHL associated with HIV is usually aggressive, with most cases occurring in extralymphatic sites. HIV-associated NHL can be broadly grouped into three subcategories: systemic (nodal and extranodal), primary CNS lymphoma (PCNSL), and body cavity–based lymphoma, also referred to as primary effusion lymphoma (PEL). Approximately, 80% of all NHL in HIV patients is considered to be systemic. PEL, a unique lymphomatous effusion associated with the *human herpesvirus-8* (*HHV 8*) gene or Kaposi sarcoma herpesvirus is primarily observed in adults infected with HIV but has been reported in HIV-infected children. Highly active antiretroviral therapy has decreased the incidence of NHL in HIV-positive individuals. Most childhood HIV-related NHL is of mature B cell phenotype but with a spectrum including PEL, PCSNL, mucosa-associated lymphoid tissue (MALT), Burkitt lymphoma, and diffuse large cell lymphoma. Most NHL in children with HIV present with fever, weight loss, and symptoms related to extranodal disease, such as abdominal pain or CNS symptoms.

NHL observed in primary immunodeficiency usually shows a mature B cell phenotype and large cell histology. Mature T cell and anaplastic large cell lymphoma have been observed. Children with primary immunodeficiency and NHL are more likely to have disseminated disease and present with symptoms related to extranodal disease, particularly the gastrointestinal tract and CNS.

Post-transplant lymphoproliferative disease (PTLD) represents a spectrum of clinically and morphologically heterogeneous lymphoid proliferations. Essentially all PTLD following HSCT is associated with EBV, but EBV-negative PTLD can be seen following solid organ transplant. The WHO has classified PTLD into three subtypes: early lesions, polymorphic PTLD, and monomorphic PTLD. Not all PTLD is B cell phenotype. EBV lymphoproliferative disease post-transplant may manifest as isolated hepatitis, lymphoid interstitial pneumonitis, meningoencephalitis, or an infectious mononucleosis-like syndrome. The definition of PTLD is frequently limited to lymphomatous lesions (localized or diffuse), which are often extranodal (frequently in the allograft). Although less common, PTLD may present as a rapidly progressive, disseminated disease that clinically resembles septic shock, which almost always results in death despite therapy.

RARE NON-HODGKIN LYMPHOMA OCCURRING IN CHILDREN

Mature T cell and NK cell NHL are much less common in children than in adults. Mature B cell lymphomas such as small lymphocytic, MALT, mantle cell lymphoma, myeloma, or follicular cell lymphoma are also rarely seen in children. It is unclear whether these histologies observed in children are the same diseases as those seen in adults. For example, follicular lymphoma observed in children express *bcl-2* only in a small number of cases. However, other diseases appear to reflect the disease observed in adult patients. For example, MALT lymphomas observed in pediatric patients usually present as localized disease and are associated with *H. pylori* and require no more than local therapy of surgery and/or radiation therapy to cure.

Other types of NHL may be rare in adults and are exceedingly rare in pediatric patients, such as primary cutaneous and primary CNS lymphomas. Reports suggest that the outcome of pediatric patients with primary CNS lymphoma may be superior to that of adults with primary CNS lymphoma and long-term survival can be achieved without cranial irradiation. One report showed that most of the children had diffuse large B cell lymphoma or ALCL. Results of this study showed that therapy with high-dose intravenous methotrexate and cytosine arabinoside was most successful and that intrathecal chemotherapy may be needed only when malignant cells are present in the cerebral spinal fluid.

Staging

The most widely used staging scheme for childhood non-Hodgkin lymphoma (NHL) is that of the St. Jude Children's Research Hospital (Murphy Staging).

Stage I childhood NHL: A single tumor or nodal area is involved, excluding the abdomen and mediastinum.

Stage II childhood NHL: Disease extent is limited to a single tumor with regional node involvement, two or more tumors or nodal areas involved on one side of the diaphragm, or a primary gastrointestinal tract tumor (completely resected) with or without regional node involvement.

Stage III childhood NHL: Tumors or involved lymph node areas occur on both sides of the diaphragm. Stage III NHL also includes any primary intrathoracic (mediastinal, pleural, or thymic) disease, extensive primary intra-abdominal disease, or any paraspinal or epidural tumors.

Stage IV childhood NHL: Tumors involve bone marrow and/or central nervous system (CNS) disease regardless of other sites of involvement.

Bone marrow involvement has been defined as ≥5% malignant cells in an, otherwise, normal bone marrow with normal peripheral blood counts and smears. Patients with lymphoblastic lymphoma with more than 25% malignant cells in the bone marrow are usually considered to have leukemia and may be appropriately treated on leukemia clinical trials.

CNS disease in lymphoblastic lymphoma is defined by criteria similar to that used for acute lymphoblastic leukemia [i.e., white blood cell count of at least 5/μL and malignant cells in the cerebrospinal fluid (CSF)]. For any other NHL, the definition of CNS disease is any malignant cell present in the CSF regardless of cell count. The Berlin-Frankfurt-Munster (BFM) Group analyzed the prevalence, clinical pattern, and outcome of CNS involvement in NHL in over 2,500 patients. Overall, CNS involvement was diagnosed in 6% of patients. Involvement by cell type was as follows:

- Burkitt lymphoma/leukemia: 8.8%
- Precursor B cell lymphoblastic lymphoma: 5.4%
- Anaplastic large cell lymphoma: 3.3%
- T cell lymphoblastic lymphoma: 3.7%
- Diffuse large B cell lymphoma: 2.6%
- Primary mediastinal large B cell lymphoma: 0%.

The probability of event-free survival (EFS) at 6 years for CNS-positive patients was 64% compared with 86% for CNS-negative patients. Presence of CNS involvement did not impact outcome for T cell lymphoblastic lymphoma patients, but had significant negative impact on patients with Burkitt lymphoma/leukemia.

As with histologic classification, there exist several different staging schemes for childhood NHL; none is perfect. For example, in the French Society of Pediatric Oncology and most recent international French-American-British study for B-lineage NHL, Group A is completely resected stage I and II disease; Group C is disease with leukemic disease (>25% marrow involvement) and/or CNS disease; and Group B consists of all other patients. For B-lineage NHL, the Berlin-Frankfurt-Munster group treats according to four risk groups: R 1 is completely resected disease; R 2 is unresected disease or stage III disease with lactate dehydrogenase (LDH) less than 500 u/L; R 3 is stage III and LDH concentrations of 500 to 1,000 u/L or leukemic disease (>25% marrow disease) with LDH levels higher than 1,000 u/L; and R 4 is stage III/IV disease or leukemic disease with LDH levels higher than 1,000 u/L and/or CNS involvement. In general, treatment for childhood NHL depends on localized versus disseminated disease. Localized disease is usually defined as stage I or II disease, while stage III or IV disease is generally considered disseminated.

Treatment Options: Overview (Table 9.2)

Children and adolescents with NHL should be referred to medical centers that have a multidisciplinary team of cancer specialists with experience treating the cancers that occur during childhood and adolescence.

NHL in children is generally considered to be widely disseminated from the outset, even when apparently localized; as a result, combination chemotherapy is recommended for most patients. There are two potentially life-threatening clinical situations that are often seen in children with NHL: (1) superior vena cava syndrome (or mediastinal tumor with airway obstruction), most often seen in lymphoblastic lymphoma (Figs 9.5 and 9.6); and (2) tumor lysis syndrome, most often seen in lymphoblastic and Burkitt or Burkitt-like NHL. These

Table 9.2: Results of recent multicenter studies on childhood NHL

Study	Period	No. of patients (Age in year)	pEFs at 3-5 years*	Stages (St. Jude staging system) No. of patients/pEFs I	II	III	IV	Comments
Lymphoblastic lymphoma								
CCG-502	10/83–03/90	281 (0.5–19)	NG	–	I+II 28/84%	219/70%	34/46%	Randomized trial Modified LSA$_2$-L$_2$ vs ADCOPM EFS 74% vs 64%
POG 8704	05/87–01/92	180 (1–21)	NG	NE	NE	NG	NG	Randomized trial 20 weekly L-Asp vs no 4-year pCCR 78 vs 64%
NHL-BFM 90-LBL	04/90–03/95	105 (0.5–18)	90%	2/100%	2/100%	82/90%	19/95%	T-LBL only
NHL-BFM 95-LBL	0495–03/01	198 (0–18)	80%		I+II 22/95%	123/79%	53/77%	Omission of pre-emptive cranial irradiation
SFOP-LMT 96	02/97–12/03	83 (ng)	87%	NG	NG	NG	NG	T-LBL only, BFM-backbone, early intensi- fication day 8
B-NHL								
POG total	10/86–11/91	133 (0–21)	NG	NE	NE	NE	59/79%	
B-ALL 74/65%								
CCG-hybrid	12/91–12/93	42 (0–21)	77%	NE	NE	82%	60% incl B-ALL	
SFOP/LMB 89	07/89–06/96	561 (0–17)	91%	31/93%	88/99%	278/91%	62/87%,	
B-ALL 102/87%								
NHL-BFM 90	04/990–03/95	413 (1–19)	98%	49/97%	115/98%	169/88%	24/73%,	
B-ALL 56/74%								
NHL-BFM 95	04/96–03/01	505 (0–18)	89%	53/98%	119/98%	221/87%	33/81% B-ALL 79/77%	Randomized trial HD-MTX intravenously over 24 hours vs 4 hours
FAB/LMB-96								
Anaplastic large cell lymphoma								
SFQP-HM 89/91	08/88–02/997	82 (1–17)	66%	–	I?II 23/94%	–	III/IV	
NHL-BFM-90	04/90–03/95	82 (0.8–17)	76%	8/100%	20/79%	55/74%	59/55%	
UKCCSG	06/90–05/96	72 (0–17)	59%		I/II 15/62%		6/50%	
AIEOP	01/93–10/97	34 (4–15)	65%	0/–	10/60%	17/65%	III/IV	
POG-8704-APO	12/94–04/100	86 (0–21)	72%	NE	NE	NG	57/58% 7/71% NG	

*Total group.

Abbreviations: pEFS Kaplan-Meier estimate of event-free survival; NG, not given; ADCOMP, L-asparaginase, daunorubicin, cyclophosphamide, vincristine, methotrexate, prednisone; L-asp, L-asparaginase; pCCR, probability of continuous complete remission; NE, not eligible; T LBL, T-cell lymphoblastic lymphoma; B-ALL, B-cell acute lymphoblastic leukemia; HD-MTX, high-dose methotrexate

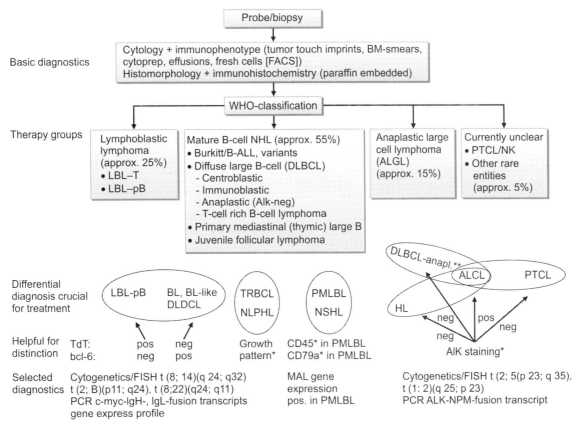

Fig. 9.4: Diagnostic work-up, classification, and stratification of childhood non-Hodgkin lymphoma (NHL) subtype into treatment groups

*Growth pattern diffuse into T cell—rich B cell lymphoma (TCRB), nodular, or nodular and diffuse in NLPH. An overlap between TCRB and NLPHL cannot be excluded at present.
**Rare cases of DLBCL (with immunoblast/plasmoblast-like cytology) express full-length Alk and can have t(2;17) (p23; q230 (Alk-clathrin) translocation (Gascoyne RD 2003).
Abbreviations: TRBCL, T cell rich B cell lymphoma; PMLBL, primary mediastinal (thymic) large B cell lymphoma; HL, Hodgkin lymphoma; NLPHL, nodular lymphocyte predominant Hodgkin lymphoma; NSHL, nodular sclerosis type Hodgkin lymphoma; PTCL/NK, peripheral T-cell/natural killer-cell lymphoma; FISH, fluorescence in situ hybridization; PCR, polymerase chain reaction.

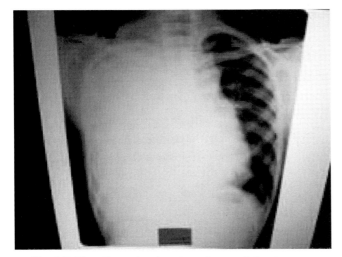

Fig. 9.5: Chest X-ray showing thoracic mass following non-Hodgkin lymphoma with superior vena caval syndrome

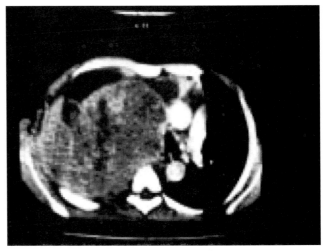

Fig. 9.6: CT scan chest showing thoracic mass following non-Hodgkin lymphoma with superior vena caval syndrome

emergent situations should be anticipated in children with NHL and addressed immediately.

Bone marrow aspirate and biopsy should always be performed early in the work-up of these patients (Figs 9.4 and 9.7). If a pleural effusion is present, a cytologic diagnosis is frequently possible using thoracentesis. In those children who present with peripheral adenopathy, a lymph node biopsy under local anesthesia and in an upright position may be possible. In situations in which the above diagnostic procedures are not fruitful, consideration of a computed tomography–guided core needle biopsy should be contemplated. Mediastinoscopy, anterior mediastinotomy or thoracoscopy are the procedures of choice when other diagnostic modalities fail to establish the diagnosis. A formal thoracotomy is rarely if ever indicated for the diagnosis or treatment of childhood lymphoma. Occasionally, it will not be possible to perform a diagnostic operative procedure because of the risk of general anesthesia or heavy sedation. In these situations, preoperative treatment with steroids or localized radiation therapy should be considered. Since preoperative treatment may affect the ability to obtain an accurate tissue diagnosis, a diagnostic biopsy should be obtained as soon as the risk of general anesthesia or heavy sedation is thought to be alleviated.

Tumor lysis syndrome results from rapid breakdown of malignant cells resulting in a number of metabolic abnormalities, most notably hyperuricemia, hyperkalemia, and hyperphosphatemia. Hydration and allopurinol or rasburicase (urate oxidase) are essential components of therapy in all but patients with the most limited disease. An initial prephase consisting of low-dose cyclophosphamide and vincristine does not obviate the need for allopurinol or rasburicase and hydration.

Children with limited disease have an excellent prognosis when treated with chemotherapy. Radiation is not used as frontline therapy for children. Radiation therapy can serve an ancillary role (i.e. as emergency treatment) for involvement of the nervous system, or when there is a severe mass effect, as in superior vena caval compression or airway obstruction.

Prognosis

With current treatments, about 80% of children and adolescents with NHL will survive at least 5 years, though

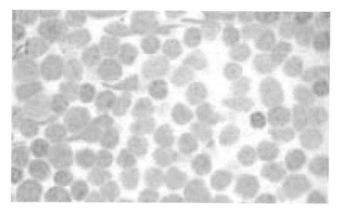

Fig. 9.7: Microphotograph of biopsy taken from enlarged lymph node of NHL *(For color version, see Plate 2)*

outcome is variable depending on a number of factors. The most important prognostic determinant, given optimal therapy, is the extent of disease at diagnosis as determined by pretreatment staging. Patients with localized disease (i.e. single extra-abdominal/extrathoracic tumor or totally resected intra-abdominal tumor) have an excellent prognosis (a 5-year survival rate of approximately 90%), regardless of histology. Patients with NHL arising in bone have an excellent prognosis regardless of histology, and testicular disease does not affect prognosis. Unlike adults, children and adolescents with non-lymphoblastic NHL involving the mediastinum have an inferior outcome, as compared with other sites of disease. Patients with intrathoracic or extensive intra-abdominal disease and patients with bone marrow or central nervous system involvement at diagnosis require intensive therapy. These intensive therapies have improved the outcome for patients with disseminated or advanced-stage disease.

Localized Non-Hodgkin Lymphoma in Children and Adolescents

Standard Treatment Options

Stage I and II patients with grossly resected (>90%) disease regardless of histology have an excellent prognosis, with 90% or better disease-free survival (DFS). A Children's Cancer Group (CCG) study demonstrated that pulsed chemotherapy with cyclophosphamide, vincristine, methotrexate, and prednisone (COMP) administered for 6 months for localized non-lymphoblastic non-Hodgkin lymphoma (NHL) was equivalent to 18 months of therapy with radiation to sites of disease and that it produced more than 85% DFS and more than 90% overall survival. Patients with lymphoblastic lymphoma had a much inferior outcome. A Pediatric Oncology Group (POG) study tested 9 weeks of short, pulsed chemotherapy with cyclophosphamide, doxorubicin, vincristine, and prednisone (CHOP), with or without radiation to involved sites and with or without 24 weeks of maintenance chemotherapy. The results showed no benefit of radiation or maintenance chemotherapy, but the DFS for nonlymphoblastic lymphoma was for localized B-NHL, defined as risk group R1 (completely resected disease), the Berlin-Frankfurt-Munster (BFM) group has used a 5-day cytoreduction phase followed by two cycles of multiagent chemotherapy (BFM-90). In the most recent BFM study (BFM-95), it was shown that reducing the dose of methotrexate did not affect the results for localized disease. The French Society of Pediatric Oncology (SFOP) has treated all completely resected stage I and abdominal stage II (Group A) with two cycles of multiagent chemotherapy (LMB-89).

For localized lymphoblastic lymphoma (grossly resected, i.e. >90% stage I/II disease), about 60% of patients can achieve long-term DFS with short, pulsed chemotherapy. However, using a leukemia approach with induction, consolidation, and maintenance for a total of 24 months, the BFM group (BFM-90/95) has shown more than 90% DFS for localized lymphoblastic lymphoma.

For localized anaplastic large cell lymphoma (ALCL) (grossly resected, i.e. >90% stage I/II disease), the best results have come from using pulsed chemotherapy similar to B-NHL therapy. The SFOP group added methotrexate to the first two cycles following cytoreduction and added four more cycles of pulsed multiagent chemotherapy (HM-89/91). With an additional cycle of chemotherapy, the BFM group had shown results similar to those obtained with the BFM-90 regimen for B-NHL. Primary cutaneous ALCL presents a particular problem. The diagnosis can be difficult to distinguish from more benign diseases such as lymphoid papulosis. Many cutaneous ALCL are ALK-negative and may be treated successfully with surgical resection and/or local radiotherapy without systemic chemotherapy. There are reports of surgery alone being curative for ALK-positive cutaneous ALCL, but extensive staging and vigilant follow-up is required.

Large cell lymphoma

Both diffuse large B cell lymphoma (DLBCL) and anaplastic large cell lymphoma (ALCL), vincristine, doxorubicin, cyclophosphamide, prednisone, mercaptopurine, and methotrexate.

DLBCL and Burkitt lymphoma

NHL-BFM-90 (B-NHL): Dexamethasone, cyclophospha-mide, methotrexate, cytarabine, prednisolone (IT), ifosfamide, etoposide, doxorubicin.
LMB-89: Cyclophosphamide, vincristine, doxorubicin, prednisone.

Lymphoblastic lymphoma

NHL-BFM-90/95 (Lymphoblastic)

Anaplastic large cell lymphoma

HM89/91: Vincristine, cyclophosphamide, prednisone, methotrexate, doxorubicin, etoposide (vinblastine and bleomycin HM91).
NHL-BFM-90 (ALCL): Dexamethasone, cyclophos-phamide, methotrexate, cytarabine, prednisolone (IT), ifosfamide, etoposide, doxorubicin.

Disseminated Childhood B cell Non-Hodgkin Lymphoma

Patients with disseminated mature B-lineage NHL (Burkitt or Burkitt-like lymphoma and diffuse large B cell lymphoma [DLBCL]) have 80 to 90% long-term survival. For the Berlin-Frankfurt-Munster (BFM) group, disseminated mature B-lineage NHL is defined as: R 2- unresected disease or stage III disease with lactate deyhdrogenase (LDH) levels lower than 500 u/L; R 3- stage III disease and LDH concentrations between 500 u/L and 1,000 u/L or leukemic disease (>25% marrow disease) with LDH levels lower than 1,000 u/L; R 4-stage III/IV disease or leukemic disease with LDH levels higher than 1,000 u/L and/or central nervous system (CNS) involvement. The R 2 group receives five cycles of intensive chemotherapy and has a disease-free survival (DFS) of more than 90%. The R 3 group receives six cycles of intensive chemotherapy and has about 85% DFS. The R 4 group receives seven cycles of intensive chemotherapy with approximately 80% DFS. For the French Society of Pediatric Oncology (FAB/LMB), Group B consists of all patients with unresected disease but excludes those with leukemic (>25% marrow involvement) and/or CNS involvement, while Group C patients have leukemic and/or marrow involvement. FAB/LMB 96 study identified response to prophase reduction as the most significant prognostic factor with poor responders (i.e. less than 20% resolution of disease), having an EFS of 30%. As opposed to mature B-lineage NHL seen in adults, there is no difference in outcome based on histology with current therapy in pediatric trials. This improvement has developed through the use of short, intensive, pulsed chemotherapy with aggressive CNS-directed chemotherapy without cranial radiation. The use of high-dose methotrexate (>5 g/m^2), cytarabine, and etoposide have appeared to be helpful. Even patients with CNS involvement can achieve a DFS of approximately 75% with current intensive therapy. Intrathecal methotrexate should be used in all patients, but prophylactic cranial radiation is not necessary.

Involvement of the bone marrow may lead to confusion as to whether the patient has lymphoma or leukemia. Traditionally, patients with more than 25% marrow blasts are classified as having mature B cell leukemia, and those with fewer than 25% marrow blasts are classified as having lymphoma. Patients with Burkitt leukemia should be treated with protocols designed for Burkitt lymphoma. Testicular disease at diagnosis does not seem to confer poor prognosis. Poor prognostic factors include high levels of LDH, primary mediastinal disease, and age of more than 15 years, though this appears to mainly involve females with DLBCL. It appears that secondary cytogenetic abnormalities, other than c-*myc* rearrangement, are associated with an inferior outcome. Treating children with B-NHL with short, intensive, pulsed multiagent chemotherapy has markedly improved results, particularly in patients with extensive disease. All patients should be considered for entry into a clinical trial.

Rituximab is a mouse/human chimeric monoclonal antibody targeting the CD 20 antigen. Among the lymphomas that occur in children, diffuse large B cell NHL (DLBCL) and Burkitt lymphoma both express high levels of CD 20. Data from adult clinical trials have demonstrated that rituximab is active against DLBCL. Rituximab has been safely combined with standard doxorubicin, cyclophosphamide, vincristine, and prednisone (CHOP) chemotherapy; in a randomized trial of adults with DLBCL comparing CHOP with CHOP plus rituximab, the rituximab arm demonstrated a superior outcome. In an adult study, rituximab has also been safely combined with an intensive chemotherapy regimen used to treat patients with Burkitt lymphoma. A Children's Oncology Group pilot study (COG-ANHL 01P1) is evaluating rituximab in combination with the intensive chemotherapy regimen based on the French LMB-89 protocol.

Standard Treatment Options

FAB/LMB 96: Cyclophosphamide, vincristine, prednisone, methotrexate (IT), high-dose methotrexate, doxorubicin, cytarabine, etoposide. Reduced intensity arm for Group B, and full intensity for Group C. NHL-BFM 95.

Treatment options under clinical evaluation:
COG-ANHL 01P1: Addition of rituximab to FAB/LMB-96–based therapy.

Disseminated Childhood Lymphoblastic Lymphoma

Patients with disseminated lymphoblastic lymphoma have long-term survival rates higher than 80%. As opposed to other pediatric non-Hodgkin lymphoma (NHL), it has been shown that lymphoblastic lymphoma responds much better to leukemia therapy with 2 years of therapy than with shorter, intensive, pulsed chemotherapy regimens. The best results to date come from the Berlin-Frankfurt-Munster (BFM) group. In NHL-BFM-90, the 5-year disease-free survival (DFS) was 90%. In NHL-BFM-95, the prophylactic cranial radiation was omitted, and the intensity of induction therapy was decreased slightly. There were no significant increases in central nervous system (CNS) relapses, but event-free survival (EFS) was worse in BFM-95 than in BFM-90 (90% vs 82%). All current therapies for advanced-stage lymphoblastic lymphoma have been derived from regimens designed for the treatment of acute lymphoblastic leukemia. Mediastinal radiation is not necessary for patients with mediastinal masses, except in the emergency treatment of symptomatic superior vena caval obstruction or airway obstruction, where low-dose radiation is usually employed.

Standard Treatment Options
- NHL-BFM-90
- NHL-BFM-95 protocol

Treatment options under clinical evaluation
COG A-5971: The Children's Oncology Group.

Disseminated Childhood Anaplastic Large Cell Lymphoma

Children and adolescents with disseminated childhood anaplastic large cell lymphoma (ALCL) have a disease-free survival (DFS) of approximately 60 to 75%. It is unclear which strategy is best for the treatment of disseminated ALCL. The French Society of Pediatric Oncology has treated patients with a cytoreduction phase followed by six cycles of intensive, pulsed chemotherapy (HM 89/91). The German Berlin-Frankfurt-Munster (BFM) group has also used six cycles of intensive pulsed therapy, similar to their B-NHL therapy (NHL-BFM-90). The Pediatric Oncology Group (POG) trial POG 9317 demonstrated no benefit to methotrexate and high-dose cytarabine added to 52 weeks of cyclic chemotherapy. The Italian Association of Pediatric Hematology/Oncology used a leukemia-like regimen for 24 months in LNH-92. Although uncommon, when leukemic peripheral blood involvement is present, it appears to be associated with an unfavorable prognosis. One study suggested that the amount of marrow involvement as measured by polymerase chain reaction is predictive for relapse.

Standard Treatment Options

HM 89/91: Vincristine, cyclophosphamide, prednisone, methotrexate, doxorubicin, etoposide (vinblastine and bleomycin HM 91)
NHL-BFM-90 (ALCL): Dexamethasone, cyclophosphamide, methotrexate, cytarabine, prednisolone (IT), ifosfamide, etoposide, doxorubicin.

APO: Doxorubicin, prednisone, vincristine.
LNH-92: Cyclophosphamide, vincristine, dexamethasone, daunorubicin, thioguanine, cytarabine, asparaginase, methotrexate, and intrathecal methotrexate/cytarabine/prednisolone.
Treatment options under clinical evaluation
ANHL 0131: The Children's Oncology Group
International ALCL 99: Dexamethasone, cyclophosphamide, methotrexate, cytarabine, prednisolone (IT), ifosfamide, high-dose methotrexate, etoposide, doxorubicin, vincristine.

Recurrent Childhood Non-Hodgkin Lymphoma (Fig. 9.8)

For recurrent or refractory B-lineage non-Hodgkin lymphoma (NHL) or lymphoblastic lymphoma, survival is generally 10 to 20%. For recurrent or refractory anaplastic large cell lymphoma, as many as 60% of patients can achieve long-term survival. A Children's Cancer Group study (CCG-5912) was able to achieve complete remission in 40% of NHL patients. Radiation therapy may have a role in treating patients who have not had a complete response to therapy. If remission can be achieved, high-dose therapy and stem cell transplantation are usually pursued. The benefit of autologous versus allogeneic stem cell transplantation is unclear. All patients with primary refractory or relapsed NHL should be considered for clinical trials.

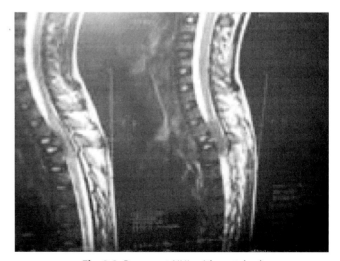

Fig. 9.8: Recurrent NHL with vertebral involvement and destruction

Standard Treatment Options

Allogeneic or autologous bone marrow transplantation.
DECAL: Dexamethasone, etoposide, cisplatin, cytarabine, and L-asparaginase.
ICE: Ifosfamide, carboplatin, and etoposide.
Treatment options under clinical evaluation
ANHL 0121: Rituximab, ifosfamide, carboplatin, and etoposide (mature B cell only).

Lymphoproliferative Disease Associated with Immunodeficiency in Children

Regardless of the etiology of the immune defect, immunodeficient children with lymphoma have a worse prognosis than does the general population with non-Hodgkin lymphoma (NHL). Most NHL in this population is disseminated and requires systemic cytotoxic therapy. These patients usually tolerate cytotoxic therapy poorly.

In the era of highly active antiretroviral therapy, children with HIV and NHL should be treated with standard chemotherapy regimens for NHL, but careful attention to prophylaxis against and early detection of infection is warranted. Patients with primary immunodeficiency can achieve complete and durable remissions with standard chemotherapy regimens for NHL, though again toxicity is increased. Immunologic correction through allogeneic stem cell transplantation is often required to prevent recurrences. In post-transplant lymphoproliferative disease (PTLD), first-line therapy is the reduction of immunosuppression, as much as can be tolerated. Rituximab, an anti-CD 20 antibody, has been used with some success, but data for its use in children are sparse.

Standard Treatment Options

Standard chemotherapy regimens for specific histology.
Low-dose cyclophosphamide and prednisone.
Treatment options under clinical evaluation
COG-ANHL 0221: Addition of rituximab to low-dose cyclophosphamide and prednisone.

Adoptive immunotherapy with either donor lymphocytes of *ex vivo*–generated Epstein-Barr virus–specific cytotoxic T cells have been effective in treating PTLD following blood or bone marrow transplant; however,

this has not been shown to be as effective or practical in patients with PTLD following solid organ transplant.

SUGGESTED READING

1. Abla O, Weitzman S. Primary central nervous system lymphoma in children. Neurosurg Focus. 2006;21:E 8.
2. Anderson JR, Jenkin RD, Wilson JF, et al. Long-term follow-up of patients treated with COMP or LSA 2 L 2 therapy for childhood non-Hodgkin's lymphoma: a report of CCG-551 from the Childrens Cancer Group. J Clin Oncol. 1993;11:1024-32.
3. Attarbaschi A, Dworzak M, Steiner M, et al. Outcome of children with primary resistant or relapsed non-Hodgkin lymphoma and mature B-cell leukemia after intensive first-line treatment: A population-based analysis of the Austrian Cooperative Study Group. Pediatr Blood Cancer. 2005;44:70-6.
4. Bea S, Zettl A, Wright G, et al. Diffuse large B-cell lymphoma subgroups have distinct genetic profiles that influence tumor biology and improve gene-expression-based survival prediction. Blood. 2005;106:3183-90.
5. Burkhardt B, Zimmermann M, Oschlies I, et al. The impact of age and gender on biology, clinical features and treatment outcome of non-Hodgkin lymphoma in childhood and adolescence. Br J Haematol. 2005;131:39-49.
6. Cairo MS, Gerrard M, Sposto R, et al. Results of a randomized international study of high-risk central nervous system B non-Hodgkin lymphoma and B acute lymphoblastic leukemia in children and adolescents. Blood. 2007;109:2736-43.
7. Cairo MS, Raetz E, Lim MS, et al. Childhood and adolescent non-Hodgkin lymphoma: new insights in biology and critical challenges for the future. Pediatr Blood Cancer. 2005;45:753-69.
8. Claviez A, Meyer U, Dominick C, et al. MALT lymphoma in children: a report from the NHL-BFM Study Group. Pediatr Blood Cancer. 2006;47:210-4.
9. Dalle JH, Mechinaud F, Michon J, et al. Testicular disease in childhood B-cell non-Hodgkin's lymphoma: the French Society of Pediatric Oncology experience. J Clin Oncol. 2001;19:2397-403.
10. Damm-Welk C, Busch K, Burkhardt B, et al. Prognostic significance of circulating tumor cells in bone marrow or peripheral blood as detected by qualitative and

quantitative PCR in pediatric NPM-ALK-positive anaplastic large-cell lymphoma. Blood. 2007;110:670-7.

11. Dave SS, Fu K, Wright GW, et al. Molecular diagnosis of Burkitt's lymphoma. N Engl J Med. 2006;354:2431-42.

12. Duyster J, Bai RY, Morris SW. Translocations involving anaplastic lymphoma kinase (ALK). Oncogene. 2001;20:5623-37.

13. Harris NL, Jaffe ES, Diebold J, et al. World Health Organization classification of neoplastic diseases of the hematopoietic and lymphoid tissues: Report of the Clinical Advisory Committee meeting-Airlie House, Virginia, November 1997. J Clin Oncol. 1999;17:3835-49.

14. Kirk O, Pedersen C, Cozzi-Lepri A, et al. Non-Hodgkin lymphoma in HIV-infected patients in the era of highly active antiretroviral therapy. Blood. 2001;98:3406-12.

15. Kobrinsky NL, Sposto R, Shah NR, et al. Outcomes of treatment of children and adolescents with recurrent non-Hodgkin's lymphoma and Hodgkin's disease with dexamethasone, etoposide, cisplatin, cytarabine, and l-asparaginase, maintenance chemotherapy, and transplantation: Children's Cancer Group Study CCG-5912. J Clin Oncol. 2001;19:2390-6.

16. Lorsbach RB, Shay-Seymore D, Moore J, et al. Clinicopathologic analysis of follicular lymphoma occurring in children. Blood. 2002;99:1959-64.

17. Murphy SB, Fairclough DL, Hutchison RE, et al. Non-Hodgkin's lymphomas of childhood: an analysis of the histology, staging, and response to treatment of 338 cases at a single institution. J Clin Oncol. 1989;7:186-93.

18. Neth O, Seidemann K, Jansen P, et al. Precursor B-cell lymphoblastic lymphoma in childhood and adolescence: Clinical features, treatment, and results in trials NHL-BFM 86 and 90. Med Pediatr Oncol. 2000;35:20-7.

19. Oschlies I, Klapper W, Zimmermann M, et al. Diffuse large B-cell lymphoma in pediatric patients belongs predominantly to the germinal-center type B-cell lymphomas: a clinicopathologic analysis of cases included in the German BFM (Berlin-Frankfurt-Munster) Multicenter Trial. Blood. 2006;107:4047-52.

20. Patte C, Auperin A, Gerrard M, et al. Results of the randomized international FAB/LMB 96 trial for intermediate risk B-cell non-Hodgkin lymphoma in children and adolescents: It is possible to reduce treatment for the early responding patients. Blood. 109 2007;2773-80.

21. Patte C, Auperin A, Michon J, et al. The Société Française d'Oncologie Pédiatrique LMB 89 protocol: highly effective multiagent chemotherapy tailored to the tumor burden and initial response in 561 unselected children with B-cell lymphomas and L 3 leukemia. Blood. 2001;97:3370-9.

22. Percy CL, Smith MA, Linet M, et al. Lymphomas and reticuloendothelial neoplasms. In: Ries LA, Smith MA, Gurney JG, et al. Eds.: Cancer incidence and survival among children and adolescents: United States SEER Program 1975-1995. Bethesda, Md: National Cancer Institute, SEER Program, 1999. NIH Pub. No. 99-4649, pp 35-50.

23. Reiter A, Schrappe M, Ludwig WD, et al. Intensive ALL-type therapy without local radiotherapy provides a 90% event-free survival for children with T-cell lymphoblastic lymphoma: a BFM group report. Blood. 2000;95:416-21.

24. Reiter A, Schrappe M, Tiemann M, et al. Improved treatment results in childhood B-cell neoplasms with tailored intensification of therapy: a report of the Berlin-Frankfurt-Münster Group Trial NHL-BFM 90. Blood. 1999;94:3294-306.

25. Reiter A. Diagnosis and treatment of childhood Non-Hodgkin's lymphoma. American Society of Hematology Education Program Book, 2007.

26. Rooney CM, Smith CA, Ng CY, et al. Infusion of cytotoxic T cells for the prevention and treatment of Epstein-Barr virus-induced lymphoma in allogeneic transplant recipients. Blood. 1998;92:1549-55.

27. Rosolen A, Pillon M, Garaventa A, et al. Anaplastic large cell lymphoma treated with a leukemia-like therapy: report of the Italian Association of Pediatric Hematology and Oncology (AIEOP) LNH-92 protocol. Cancer. 2005;104:2133-40.

28. Salzburg J, Burkhardt B, Zimmermann M, et al. Prevalence, clinical pattern, and outcome of CNS involvement in childhood and adolescent non-Hodgkin's lymphoma differ by non-Hodgkin's lymphoma subtype: a Berlin-Frankfurt-Munster Group Report. J Clin Oncol. 2007;25:3915-22.

29. Sandlund JT, Bowman L, Heslop HE, et al. Intensive chemotherapy w33. Griffin TC, Children's Oncology Group: Phase II Study of Ifosfamide, Carboplatin, and Etoposide Combined with Rituximab in Pediatric Patients with Recurrent or Refractory B-Cell

Non-Hodgkin's Lymphoma or Acute Lymphoblastic Leukemia, COG-ANHL 0121, Clinical trial, Completed.

30. Sandlund JT, Downing JR, Crist WM. Non-Hodgkin's lymphoma in childhood. N Engl J Med. 1996;334:1238-48.

31. Savage KJ, Monti S, Kutok JL, et al. The molecular signature of mediastinal large B-cell lymphoma differs from that of other diffuse large B-cell lymphomas and shares features with classical Hodgkin lymphoma. Blood. 2003;102:3871-9.

32. Seidemann K, Tiemann M, Schrappe M, et al. Short-pulse B-non-Hodgkin lymphoma-type chemotherapy is efficacious treatment for pediatric anaplastic large cell lymphoma: a report of the Berlin-Frankfurt-Münster Group Trial NHL-BFM 90. Blood. 2001;97:3699-706.

33. Thomas DA, Faderl S, O'Brien S, et al. Chemo-immunotherapy with hyper-CVAD plus rituximab for the treatment of adult Burkitt and Burkitt-type lymphoma or acute lymphoblastic leukemia. Cancer. 2006;106:1569-80.

34. Woessmann W, Seidemann K, Mann G, et al. The impact of the methotrexate administration schedule and dose in the treatment of children and adolescents with B-cell neoplasms: a report of the BFM Group Study. NHL-BFM 95. Blood. 2005;105:948-58.

10 Myeloid Leukemia in Children

Mousumi Nandi, Sandip Samanta

INTRODUCTION

Leukemia is a disease in which there is abnormal proliferation of hematopoietic cells which cause progressively increasing infiltration of the bone marrow. Acute leukemia consists of 97% of childhood leukemia with acute myeloid leukemia to be 20%. Chronic leukemia is myeloproliferative disorder characterized by predominance of relatively mature cells. In contrast to the acute leukemias, these diseases are indolent, with a natural history usually spanning over several years. Chronic leukemia is uncommon in children. They include adult type chronic myeloid leukemia (CML) and juvenile myelomonocytic leukemia (JMML), previously termed as juvenile chronic myeloid leukemia (JCML). Chronic myeloid leukemia accounts for 2% of childhood leukemias and 60% of cases occur after 6 years.

Acute myeloid leukemia is the heterogeneous group of leukemia that arises in precursors of myeloid, erythroid, megakaryocytic and monocytic cell lineage. This leukemia results from clonal transformation of hematopoietic precursor through the acquisition of chromosomal rearrangements and multiple gene mutations. New molecular technologies have allowed a better understanding of the molecular events with improved classification and new targeted therapy.

ACUTE MYELOID LEUKEMIA (AML) IN CHILDREN

Epidemiology and Risk Factors

The incidence of pediatric AML is estimated to be 5–7 cases per million people. There is no difference in incidence between male or female and black or white population. AML is an over production of immature myeloid cells with increasing incidence after exposure to chemotherapy and radiation. The risk remains high among children exposed to cyclophosphamide, melphalan, chlorambucil and nitrogen mustard, ionizing radiation, benzene and organophosporus pesticides.

A large number of inherited conditions which predispose to the development of AML are Down Syndrome, Fanconi's anemia, severe congenital neutropenia, Shwachman-Diamond Syndrome, Diamond-Blackfan Syndrome, Neurofibromatosis Type-I, Ataxia Telangiectasia, Klinefelters Syndrome and Bloom Syndrome. Finally, AML has been associated with aplastic anemia and myelodysplastic syndrome.

Classification of AML

There are several classifications and the most commonly used is the French-American-British (FAB) system which is based on type of cell from which leukemia has evolved and also maturity of the cell (Table 10.1).

Table 10.1: FAB classification of AML	
FAB Subtype	Name
M 0	Undifferentiated acute myeloblastic leukemia
M 1	Acute myeloblastic leukemia with minimal maturation
M 2	Acute myeloblastic leukemia with maturation
M 3	Acute promyelocytic leukemia
M 4	Acute myelomonocytic leukemia
M 5	Monocytic leukemia
M 6	Acute erythroid leukemia
M 7	Acute megakaryoblastic leukemia

World Health Organization recently proposed a newer system of classification for AML:

- AML with certain genetic abnormalities
- AML with a translocation between chromosomes 8 and 21
- AML with a translocation or inversion in chromosome 16
- AML with changes in chromosome 11
- APL (M 3), which usually has translocation between chromosomes 15 and 17
- AML with multilineage dysplasia
- AML related to previous chemotherapy or radiation
- AML not, otherwise, specified (includes cases of AML that don't fall into one of the above groups)
- Undifferentiated or biphenotypic acute leukemias.

Pathogenesis

AML is due to a clonal disorder caused by malignant transformation of a bone marrow derived self-renewing stem cell or progenitor which demonstrates a decreased rate of self-destruction and also aberrant differentiation. These events lead to increased malignant myeloid cell accumulation in the bone marrow and other organs. This self-renewing leukemia initiating cell is located within CD 34^+ and CD 34^- cell compartments. Some children with AML have a mutation in FLT 3 gene and these patients have a poor outcome. Patients with normal cytogenetics or with favorable cytogenetic abnormalities e.g. t (15;17) and t (16;16) have better prognosis. Patients with deletions in the long arm of chromosome 7 and 5, deletion or inversions of chromosome 3 have relatively poor prognosis.

Clinical Presentation and Diagnosis

The presentation of childhood AML reflects signs and symptoms that result from leukemic infiltration of the bone marrow and extramedullary sites (Figs 10.1 to 10.3). Children may often present with fever with or without infection, fatigue, pallor, night sweats, shortness of breath, pain in bones and joints, petechiae and bleeding manifestations. DIC is frequently seen in childhood acute promyelocytic leukemia (APL). Infiltration of extramedullary sites results in lymphadenopathy, hepatosplenomegaly, chloromatous tumors (myeloblastomas) and diseases in the skin (leukemia cutis), orbit, epidural space and rarely testicular involvement are seen. CNS involvement is seen in 15% of the cases at diagnosis.

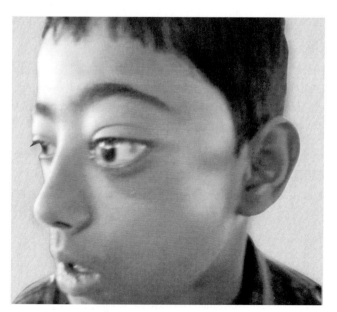

Fig. 10.1: AML with deposits

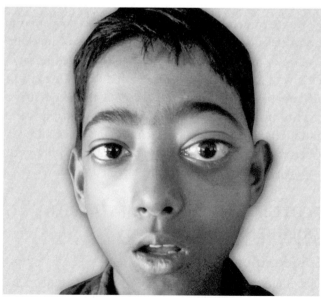

Fig. 10.2: AML with proptosis due to retro-orbital deposit

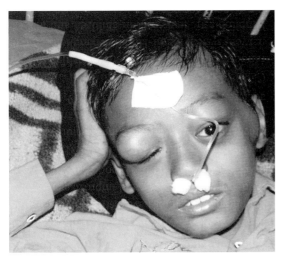

Fig. 10.3: AML with chloroma

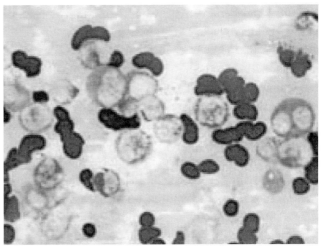

Fig. 10.4: Bone marrow picture of MPO positive myeloblast with Auer rod *(For color version, see Plate 2)*

Diagnosis of AML

Clinical suspicion of AML from history and physical examination should be followed by complete blood count. This reveals anemia, thrombocytopenia, abnormal WBC count with presence of myeloblasts. The other tests are bone marrow aspiration, trephine biopsy, blood biochemistry (Fig. 10.4). The diagnosis and subtype classification of AML is based on morphological and cytochemical study of the leukemic cells. The diagnosis is also based on cytogenetic, flow cytometric immunophenotyping, fluorescent *in situ* hybridization analysis and molecular testing (e.g. FLT 3 mutation analysis) (Fig. 10.5).

Management

The prognosis of AML has greatly improved with complete remission as high as 80–90% and overall survival rate is 60%. This success rate is due to intensive induction chemotherapy followed by postremission treatment. During induction therapy drugs used are cytarabine, anthracyclines like daunorubicin and etoposide. Postremission treatment with additional anthracyclines, high dose cytarabine or myeloablation followed by stem cell transplantation. Good results are seen with AML BFM 93 (1993–1998), CGG 2891 (1989–1995) and UK MRC AML 12 (1995–2002) regimens. In general, treatment for AML consists of an induction phase followed by consolidation phase. This

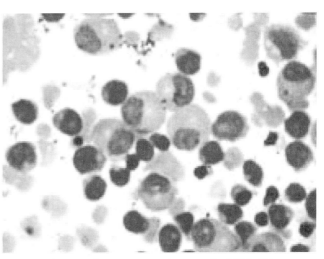

Fig. 10.5: Bone marrow photograph of AML M4 *(For color version, see Plate 3)*

is followed by intrathecal therapy with methotrexate for CNS prophylaxis. Children who are diagnosed to have AML with CNS involvement should receive intrathecal methotrexate along with radiotherapy.

The standard chemotherapy regimen for standard risk patient during induction phase is the use of daunorubicin for three days at a dose of 45 mg/m sq. IV slowly on day 1, day 2, day 3 along with cytosine arabinoside as continuous infusion in a dose of 100 mg/m sq/day IV in normal saline over 24 hours. Daunorubicin is cardiotoxic drug and so it has to be used with caution in children. The role of etoposide in AML was further evaluated in a large randomized trial conducted by MRC-UK but it was proved to have no additional benefit. APL which commonly presents with coagulopathy and DIC appear to resolve with ATRA (All Trans Retinoic Acid) and anthracyclins than with conventional chemotherapy. Patients must be monitored for development of hyperleukocytosis and respiratory distress, which are characteristic of retinoic acid syndrome. The other side-effect of chemotherapy for AML includes alopecia, anemia, neutropenia, nausea, vomiting and infection.

After completion of induction therapy, bone marrow examination is done to see whether the patient is in remission or not. Those patients who do not achieve remission a second cycle of induction chemotherapy can be tried. It is presumed that most patients after induction therapy need consolidation therapy. Consolidation therapy is done with high dose cytarabine at 3 gm/m sq IV in normal saline over 2–3 hours twice daily on day 1, day 3 and day 5. This consolidation regimen shows great success. After induction of remission and completion of consolidation phase, if there is failure, then stem cell transplantation can improve survival. Those patients who have greater risk of failure should not be offered standard therapy. The treatment of AML is advancing rapidly due to further insight into the genetic and molecular pathways of leukamogenesis.

The treatment of life threatening complications like bleeding, leukostasis and tumor lysis syndrome are platelet transfusion, leukopheresis, proper hydration and prompt initiation of chemotherapy. As there is high risk of febrile neutropenia and septicemia AML children should be hospitalized and receive broad spectrum IV antibiotics like third or fourth generation cephalosporin. For fungal infection in an AML child IV amphotericin or voriconazole should be used. Cytokines like GMCSF and GCSF are needed to correct leukopenia and neutropenia. So all children of AML should be treated in a medical unit, which has a multi-disciplinary team comprising pediatrician, hematologist, pathologist and oncologist. The other categories of staff needed are specialized nurses, dieticians, social workers, psychologists and counselors.

CHRONIC MYELOID LEUKEMIA (CML) IN CHILDREN

CML is a clonal panmyelopathy involving all the hemic lineages and at least some of the lymphoid. It is characterized by myeloid hyperplasia of the bone marrow, extramedullary hematopoiesis, expansion of the total body granulocyte pool, elevation of the leukocyte count (with appearance of the complete range of granulocyte precursor cells in the peripheral blood), and a specific cytogenetic marker, the Philadelphia (Ph1) chromosome.

Epidemiology and Risk Factor

CML is primarily a disease of middle age; the peak incidence is in the fourth and fifth decades. Although CML has been diagnosed in infants as young as 3 months, more than 80% of pediatric cases of CML are diagnosed after age 4 years and 60% age, 6 years. No significant racial or hereditary component exists. There is no difference in incidence between male and female.

The only environmental factor implicated in the etiology of CML is ionizing radiation. An increased incidence of CML has been reported in radiologists, in survivors of atomic bomb explosions, and in persons exposed to therapeutic radiation for treatment of ankylosing spondylitis and other disorders. However, only 5 to 7% of all patients with CML have documented exposure to excessive radiation, and radiation is rarely implicated in CML.

Pathology

The cytogenetic hallmark of CML is the ph-chromosome. Initially described as a truncated chromosome 22 (22q-), this anomaly is now recognized to result from the reciprocal translocation t (9; 22) (q34; q11). The C-able proto-oncogene is transposed from its normal position on chromosome 9 to a new position on chromosome 22, adjacent to the breakpoint cluster region (BCR) of the BCR gene. The hybrid BCR/ABL oncogene encodes a 210-k Da protein (p-210), which appears to have the major role in the pathogenesis of CML (changes normal hematopoietic cell into CML cell, through its properties of increased tyrosine kinase activity and ability to autophosphorylate).

The average half-life of CML granulocytes is 5–10 times longer than normal granulocytes. The BCR-ABL positive clone has a distinct survival advantage over normal progenitors and ultimately dominates hematopoiesis. As the diseases evolve, this leukemic clone acquires additional oncogenic mutations (multistep pathogenesis). The CML progenitor cell produces excessive quantities of CFU-GM resulting in hyper-production. P 210- BCR/ABL together also result in inappropriate expansion of the myeloid cell compartment, alteration of cyto-adhesive properties, impairment of maturation programs, disruption of cell cycle regulation and relative resistance to programed cell death.

Clinical Features of CML

The natural history of CML is divided into chronic, accelerated and blast phase.

Chronic Phase

Approximately 90% of patients with CML present in the chronic phase and almost half of these are detected incidentally when blood counts are performed for an unrelated reason. Symptomatic patients usually present with splenomegaly, anemia or increased cell. These include left upper quadrant pain or fullness, fatigue, lethargy, fever, weight-loss, night sweat and bone pains. Rarely, patients may have symptoms of hyperleukocytosis like respiratory distress, visual difficulties, priapism, etc. The usual physical finding includes pallor, splenomegaly, and sometimes hepatomegaly. On an average, the chronic phase lasts for approximately 3 years. The differential diagnosis of chronic phase CML includes leukemoid reaction, JMML, and other myeloproliferative disorders. The combination of low LAP score and the presence of the ph-chromosome usually distinguish CML from these conditions.

In leukemoid reaction, splenomegaly is usually not marked, the LAP score is high, the ph-chromosome is absent and an inflammatory focus is often demonstrable. In JMML, the LAP may be low, but the ph-chromosome is absent. Leukocytosis and splenomegaly are less marked than in CML, and involvement of skin, lymphoid tissue, and the monocytic lineage is more pronounced. CML can be distinguished from other myeloproliferative disorders by the disproportionate involvement of the granulocyte series and the presence of the ph-chromosome.

Metamorphosis

After approximately 3 years, the chronic phase of CML undergoes a metamorphosis into a more aggressive, phase this may occur gradually or abruptly. In approximately 5% of cases, the evolution is explosive, with a rapidly increasing blast cell population in the peripheral blood and concurrent neutropenia and thrombocytopenia (blast crisis). Approximately 50% of patients develop a progressive maturation defect resulting in a hematologic picture similar to that of de Novo acute leukemia. The remaining 45% have the gradual evolution of a myeloproliferative syndrome.

The onset of metamorphosis is characterized by progressive symptoms (e.g. fever, night sweats, and weight loss). Increasing leukocyte count with a high proportion of immature cells, like basophils, and increasing resistance to chemotherapy are other features. Along with these features, is evidence of karyotypic evolution. Mutation in the anti-oncogene p53 may play a significant role in transformation; p53 mutation is detectable in the late chronic phase of CML only and may indicate genomic in stability and progression to blast transformation.

Blast Phase

The blast phase is characterized by loss of the leukemic clones capacity to differentiate. As a consequence, the clinical picture resembles that of an acute leukemia, with anemia, thrombocytopenia, and increased numbers of blast cells in both the peripheral blood and the bone marrow. A marrow blast percentage of 30% or more is diagnostic of blast phase.

In approximately 60 to 70% of cases the blast cell morphology is myeloblastic; unlike to de Novo acute myelocytic leukemia, however, the blast cells are usually peroxides negative and rarely have Auer rods.

Definitions of accelerated and blastic phase of CML: Myelogenous leukemia

A. Blastic phase CML
- 30% or more blasts in the marrow or Peripheral blood
- Extramedullary disease with localized
- Immature blasts

B. Accelerated phase CML
Multivariate analysis—deserved criteria
- Peripheral blasts 15% or more
- Peripheral blasts plus promyelocytes 30% or more
- Peripheral basophils 20% or more
- Thrombocytopenia less than 100,000/mm^3 unrelated to therapy
- Cytogenetic clonal evaluation.
• Other criteria used in common practice are:
- Increasing drug dosage requirement
- Splenomegaly unresponsive to therapy
- Marrow reticulating or collagen fibrosis
- Marrow or peripheral blasts 10% or more
- Marrow or peripheral basophils + eosinophils 10% or more
- Triad of WBC greater than 50,000/mm^3
- Hematocrit less than 25%, and platelets less than 100,000/mm^3 not controlled with persistent unexplained fever or bone pain.

Laboratory Findings

A mild normochromic, normocytic anemia, marked leukocytosis with shift to the left, and thrombocytosis are common laboratory findings. The hematocrit at presentation in children is significantly less than that seen in adult. The leukocyte count at diagnosis ranges from approximately 8,000 to 800,000 per mm, the median count in children (approximately 250,00 per mm) is higher than that seen in adult. Extreme hyperleukocytosis (greater then 500,000 per mm) is also more common in children. The peripheral blood smear shows myeloid cells at all stages of differentiation; myeloblasts and promyelocytes generally comprise less then 15% of the differential count. And no hiatus leukemicus in maturation occurs. An absolute increase in the number of basophils and eosinophil is noted. Hybrid eosinophil-basophil granulocytes may also be seen, because similar chimeric granules may be found in normal immature granulocytes, this phenomenon may reflect incomplete maturation. The mean platelet count in children is approximately 50,00,000 per mm, which is not significantly higher than that in adults. Other finding includes elevation of uric acid, lactate dehydrogenase, vitamin B$_{12}$, and vitamin B$_{12}$ binding protein (transcobalamin).

The bone marrow is hypercellular mainly reflecting granulocytic (and often megakaryocytic) hyperplasia, orderly granulocytes maturation, eosinophilia, and basophilia are present. Myelofibrosis, which occurs in 30 to 40% of patients during the course of the disease, is uncommon in the early chronic phase. The bone marrow and spleen occasionally contain lipid-aden histiocytes that resemble Gaucher cells or sea-blue histiocytes.

The characteristic histochemical features of the granulocytes population is reduction in leukocytic alkaline phosphatase (LAP) activity. Although this abnormality does not appear to affect PMN function adversely, it has a diagnostic utility in distinguishing the leukocytosis of CML from that of inflammation. Low LAP activity is also seen in paroxysmal nocturnal hemoglobinuria, JMML, CMML, and Fanconi's anemia. Under normal condition, LAP activity appears very late in the development of granulocytes, and indeed, may be a terminal marker of granulocytes maturation. In CML, there appears to be no intrinsic defect in the synthesis and translation of LAP mRNA or transport of LAP protein to the plasma membrane, furthermore, LAP activity can be upregulated under a variety of conditions, e.g. inflammation, leuko-reduction disease progression, and administration of granulocyte colony stimulating factor (G-CSF)]. Thus, the low LAP levels in CML cells may result from granulocytes immaturity or hypo-production of G-CSF due to a relative decrease in monocyte mass.

LAP activity increases with infection or with a reduction of the granulocytes count after chemotherapy or progression to a more acute phase of the diseases. Although subtle functional abnormality of PMN adherence, bactericidal activity, and membrane sialylation can be demonstrated in chronic phase CML, the PMNs are sufficiently effective to prevent infectious complication. PMN function deteriorates progressively as the disease evolves.

PCR and FISH analysis are other molecular tests which confirm the disease.

Prognosis

With recent advances median survival is 5 years (previously 3–4 years). 40% patients survive up to 7–8 years. In blast phase/accelerated phase patients die in a few months.

- Other determinants: (Adult data)
  - Splenomegaly (>15 cm)
  - Hepatomegaly (> 6 cm)
  - Platelet ↑ (> 500,000) or thrombocytopenia
  - Blast cell (> 1%) or immature granulocyte (> 20%)
  - Role of these factors in pediatric patients with CML is less clear.

Treatment

True remission would require destroying all ph-positive cell and replace them with cytogenetically normal precursor, which is rarely accomplished with conventional therapeutic approach. Initial goal (for chronic phase) has been to provide symptomatic relief by decreasing leukocytes and organomegaly.

Cytoreduction

Standard approach (single agent chemotherapy) with hydroxyurea or busulfan and recently these agents are becoming replaced with interferon-α (INFα) and STI -571 (imatinib mesylate). In most cases, bone marrow continues to manifest granular hyperplasia and ph–positive, though blood count normalizes. Leukocytes are less deformable than RBC (myeloblasts are larger and more rigid) so if leukocyte greater than 200,000 (or blast > 50,000/mm) leukopheresis (or exchange transfusion) in combination with cytotoxic drug (hydroxyurea inflation) is required.

Several group used aggressive multiagent chemotherapy ± splenectomy in an effort to ablate ph–positive clone with shortlasting remission to ph-negative status or to stable mosaicism (ph-positive and negative) but without significant impact on duration of chronic phase.

Splenic irradiation/splenectomy; nowadays only considered for transient palliation of symptomatic massive splenomegaly and refractory to systemic chemotherapy as may result in profound myelo-suppresion. Splenectomy helpful in selected patients only with painful splenomegaly ± hypersplenism. It may also help in reducing the leukemic burden and in some cases blast transformation.

Blasts phase is generally a treatment resistant state that terminates fatally within weeks to months. Regimens developed for the treatment of acute myelogenous leukemia have proved disappointing in blasts phase CML. A regimen of alternate day mithramycin and daily hydroxyurea has been reported to convert myeloid blast phase back to chronic phase in occasional cases. The subset of patients with lymphoblastic transformation is more sensitive to chemotherapy; approximately two-thirds of such patients revert to chronic phase after treatment with vincristine and prednisone regimens.

STEM CELL TRANSPLANT (SCT)

The source for hematopoietic stem cell for transplantation can be autologous (from the patients), syngeneic (from an identical twin) or allogeneic (from HLA-identical sibling or matched related donor). However due to the presence of ph-positive cells in the graft, the result of this approach are poor.

Allogeneic stem cell transplantation: Allogeneic BMT remains the only proven curative therapy for patients with CML. Data series of adult patients undergoing SCT have identified a number of prognostic factors for allogeneic SCT. These include disease stage, degree of HLA, disparity, recipient/donor sex mismatch and duration of disease before transplantation. Indian data for MSD SCT from Tata Memorial Hospital, Mumbai has reported 50% DFS in adults with chronic phased CML.

Fortunately, relapse after allogeneic transplantation can be salvaged with donor lymphocyte infusion (DLI). Infusion of donor lymphocytes helps to mount a graft versus leukemia effect, which can effectively destroy the leukemic clone. Reduced intensity conditioning transplantation (RIC) is a relatively newer technique of SCT wherein the conditioning regimen is non-myeloablative and the success of the transplant depends on the gradual ablation of host hematopoiesis by donor T cells present in the original graft, or arising in the post-transplant period or by additional donor lymphocytes infusions (DLI).

Individual Drugs

Busulfan: An alkylating agent is a cell cycle phase none specific agent that has potent myelosuppressive action. The usual dosage is 0.06 to 0.10 mg/kg/daily orally. It produces clinical and hematological remission within 4–6 weeks. The dose should be titrated daily. It should be reduced to 50% when the WBC count reaches 30,000/cmm to 40,000/cmm and should be stopped when the WBC count drops below 20,000/cmm. Side effects of busulfan include Addisonian-like syndrome.

Hydroxyurea: The recommended beginning dose is 10–20 mg/kg/daily orally and should be adjusted according to hematological response. It is a short-acting drug, which is as effective as busulphan but with a greater margin of safety.

Interferon Alpha: IFN has direct anti-proliferate effect against both normal and myeloid precursors. It also brings about immune-modulation through increase in LFA-3 expression, decreased ability of CML cells to attach to bone marrow stoma and modification of expression of HLA-DR antigens. Dose of IFN is 3–5 million u/dose subcutaneously every day. The addition of low dose cytosine arabinoside to a regimen of interferon, improves the complete cytogenetic response rate of patients treated in early chronic phase. The hematological remission rate for patients in late chronic phase and overall survival rate. Very little published information is available addressing IFT, IFN plus low dose AraC treatment of a small number of children, which show an outcome and side effects profile similar to adults.

Imatinib Mesylate: Imatinib mesylate is amongst the first of molecular level targeted drugs. It is a tyrosine kinase inhibitor and works through competitive inhibition by occupying the ATP binding site in the SHI domain of the BCR/ABL oncoprotein. This prevents the transfer of the phosphate groups to the tyrosine residues on the substrate molecules involved in downstream single transduction pathways. This inhibitor of phosphorylation causes arrest of growth or apoptosis in cells that express BCR-ABL.

After phase I and phase II, trials proved the safety and efficacy of imatinib mesylate. It helps achieving complete hematologic responses and major cytogenetic responses in interferon intolerant and interferon unresponsive patents (it was approved by the FDA in May 2001 for use in upfront treatment of adults with chronic phase CML).

Table 10.2: Clinical characteristics of adult-type chronic myelogenous leukemia (ACML) and juvenile myelomonocytic leukemia (JMML) in childhood

	JMML	ACML
Characteristics at diagnosis		
Age	Usually > 4 years	Usually > 4 years
Lymphadenopathy	Common	Unusual
Skin lesions	Common	Unusual
Bleeding	Common	Unusual
Bacterial infection	Common	Unusual
White blood cells count >1000, 000 cells/μl	Unusual	Common
Hemoglobin (Hg) < 12 g/dl	Common	Variable
Platelets (low)	Unusual	Unusual
	Decreased	Increased
Monocytosis	Common	Unusual
Circulating pronormoblasts	Common	Unusual
HbF (% increased)	Common	Unusual
Philadelphia chromosome	Absent	> 90%
BCR-ABL, fusion gene	Absent	Present
Leukocyte alkaline phosphatase decreased	Variable	Common
Clinical course		
Median survival	1–2 years	4–5 years
Blastic phase	Unusual	Common

Five major trials have proved the efficacy of imatinib in different phase of CML. Imatinib is active in all phases of CML, but it is most effective in newly diagnosed chronic phase patients. Patients in accelerated phase and blast crisis are more likely to develop resistance to imatinib.

The IRIS study (the International Randomized Study of Interferon and STI 571) was a pivotal phase III study compared the efficacy of the combination of interferon alpha and low dose cytarabine with imatinib mesylate. In this trial, 1106 newly diagnosed chronic phase adult CML patients were randomized to receive interferon with low dose cytarabine or imatinib. It demonstrated the superiority of imatinib compared with IFN alpha/cytarabine (rates of complete hematological response, major and complete cytogenetic response freedom from progression to accelerated phase or blast crises and tolerance of therapy).

Juvenile CML

Juvenile CML (JMML): Beside the ph-positive CML, JMML constitute the most common form of MPS in childhood. JMML is probably a bridging disorder between MPS (Myeloproliferative) and MDS (Myelodysplastic) disease (Fig. 10.6).

JMML has been variously called juvenile granulocytic leukemia, infantile monosomy 7 syndrome, chronic myelomonocytic leukemia and more commonly used term Juvenile CML (JCML). Because of the similarity of the name JCML to ph-CML many clinicians inappropriately consider JMML to be the childhood form of adult ph-CML. Despite a similarity in the name, JMML and the adult form of CML have few clinical or biological similarities.

Clinical Presentation

European working group or myelodysplastic syndromes in childhood recommended diagnostic criteria for juvenile myelomonocytic leukemia.

Laboratory Criteria

- No Philadelphia chromosome or BCR/ABL rearrangement
- Peripheral blood monocyte count greater than 1
- Bone marrow blast density less than 20%

Clinical Findings

- Hepatomegaly
- Lymphadenopathy
- Pallor
- Fever
- Rash

Additional (Minimum of Two Required)
- Increased fetal hemoglobin
- Myeloid precursors in peripheral blood
- White blood cell count greater than 10,000/CMM
- Clonal abnormalities
- Granulocyte-macrophage colony-stimulating factor
- Hypersensitivity of myeloid progenitors *in vitro*.

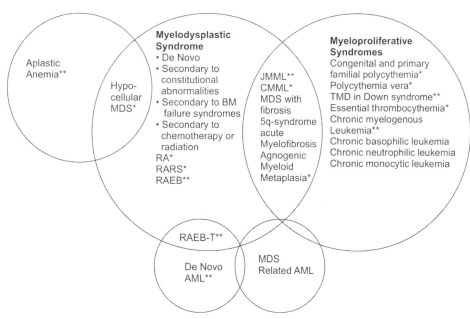

Fig. 10.6: Conceptual model for myeloproliferative (MPS) and myelodysplastic (MDS) disorders. *Reported incidence. ** Common form of MDS or MPS. AML, acute myeloid leukemia; BM, bone marrow; CML, chronic myelomonocytic leukemia; JMML, juvenile myelomonocytic leukemia; RA, refractory anemia; RAEB refractory anemia with excess blast, RAEB-T, refractory anemia with excess blast in transformation; RARS, refractory anemia with ringed sideroblasts; TMD, transient myeloproliferative disorder

Although early clonality studies suggested that JMML arose at the level of immature myeloid precursor cell, but recent data suggested that JML may arise in pluripotent stem cell with involvement of myeloid, erythroid and megakaryocyte lineages as well as B and T lymphocyte. JMML cells maintain their clonality when grow in long-term assays in contrast to Ph-chromosome positive CML cells, which become polyclonal in similar culture assays. Several recurrent chromosomal abnormality or causative mutation has been associated with JMML, (like Rae mutation activities heterozygosity of NFI). JMML is a progressive and often rapidly fatal disease particularly in older children. In children, younger than 2 years of age have more indolent phase. The accelerated blast phase characteristic of adult CMML is unusual in children with JMML.

Treatment: Several treatment regimens have been used to improve survival, including low dose chemotherapy, intensive AML type therapy and 13-cisretinoic acid. Oral 6-mercaptopurine, either alone or combination with subcutaneous cytarabine, has produced symptomatic relief in some patients, but supportive care has been as effective as vigorous chemotherapy in most cases. Durable remissions have been reported in a minority of patients, but the response to these agents is usually transient, and the long-term survival is poor. The only known curative therapy for JMML is Stem Transplantation (SCT). Survival rates of 35 to 55 percent have been reported with SCT, but treatment-related mortality and relapse rates remain high, particularly for patients with unrelated donor transplants.

SUGGESTED READING

1. Acute Myelogenous Leukemia. In: Nelson Textbook of pediatrics. Vol 2. 18th Edition. Robert M Kliegman, Richard E Behrman, Hal B Jenson, Bonita F Stanton Eds. Saunders Elsevier, Philadelphia, 2008;2120-21.
2. Benett JM, Young ML, Anderson JW. Long-term survival in acute myeloid leukemia. The eastern co-operative oncology group experience. Cancer 1997;80:2205-9.
3. Beverly J Lange. Acute myeloid leukemia in children and Adolescents. In: Leukemia. 7th Edn, Editor: Edward S Henderson, T Andrew Lister, Mel F Greaves. Saunders, Philadelphia, 2002;519-27.
4. Broker A. Adult type chronic myeliod leukemia in children. Chap 29 in pediatric hematology and oncology IAP specialty series. Editor MR Lokeshwar 2006;324-31.
5. Jeffrey E Rubnitz, Brenda Gibson, Franklin O Smith. Acute myeloid leukemia. Pediatr Clin N Am. Pediatric Oncology, 2008;55:21-39.
6. Kaspers GJ, Creutzig U. Pediatric acute myeloid leukemia international progress and future directionaries. Leukemia 2005;19:2025-9.
7. Lanzkowsky P. Leukemias. In: Manual of Ped Hem and Oncol Acad. 3rd Edn. 2000;359-409.
8. Mahapatra M, Choudhury VP, Saxena R, Pati HP. Management of AML in recent advances in hematology VP Choudhury (Ed). Jaypee Brothers, New Delhi, 2004;112-28.
9. Michael J Barnett, Connie J Eaves. Chronic myeloid leukemia. In: Leukemia. 7th Edn, Editor: Edward S Henderson, T Andrew Lister, and Mel F Greaves. Saunders, Philadelphia, 2002;583-94.
10. Mondal R, Sarkar S, Ghosh J, Sasen A. Macrocephaly and acute myeloid leukemia. J Pedtr Neurol. 2012;10:147-9.
11. Nathan and Oski's. Hematology of infancy and childhood. 6th Ed. Saunders-Elsevier, Philadelphia: 1183-90.
12. Philip A Pizzo Ed. Principle and practice of pediatric oncology. 4th Ed. Lippincott William and Wilkins, Philadelphia, USA 2002;591-628.
13. Rai KR, Holland JF, Glidewell OJ. Treatment of acute myelocytic leukemia: a study by cancer and leukemia group B Blood. 1981;58:1203.
14. Rubnitz JE, Look AT. Molecular genetics of childhood leukemia. J Ped Hem Oncol 1998;20:1-11.
15. Sartani PCE, Taylor MH, Stevens MCG, Darbyshire PJ. Treatment of childhood acute leukemia using BFM-83 protocol. Med Pediatr Oncol 1993;21:8-13.

11

Pediatric Myelodysplastic Syndrome

Rajib De

INTRODUCTION

The myelodysplastic syndromes (MDSs) are clonal bone marrow (BM) disorders characterized by ineffective hematopoiesis, a variable degree of cytopenia, and an increased risk of developing acute leukemia. MDS was probably first described in 1900 by Leube as 'leukanamie'(a macrocytic anemia progressing to acute leukemia). Many decades later, groups of patients who developed acute leukemia after having a macrocytic anemia were reported with common clinical features. These patients were given a diagnosis of 'pre-leukemia' until the 1970s, when it was realized that many such patients never developed leukemia but instead died of complications from the cytopenias. Then the term 'myelodysplastic syndromes' became widely accepted in place of 'pre-leukemia'. These are mainly viewed as disease of adults, particularly, the elderly. The term pediatric myelodysplastic syndrome appeared in the literatures in the early 1970s. Pediatric MDS is an uncommon disorder with an estimated annual incidence of 0.5–4 per million compared with adult MDS (20–40 per million). MDS comprises less than 5% of hematopoietic malignancies in children and adolescents.

DIFFERENCE FROM ADULT MDS

Pediatric MDS appears to differ from adult MDS in several aspects. In young children, dysplastic features are common and may be associated with infections, pre-existing bone marrow failure syndromes, nutritional deficiencies, immune cytopenias and medications, which may mimic MDS. Several entities like MDS refractory anemia with ringed sideroblasts (RARS), MDS with isolated deletion of long-arm of chromosome 5 (5q-syndrome) are rarely found in children. Specific entities like juvenile myelomonocytic leukemia (JMML) are unique to this age group. The prognostic significance of blast percentage in children is as yet unclear. Most importantly, the treatment goal is curative, not palliative. These made pediatric MDS to be considered as separate entity from adult MDS.

DIAGNOSIS OF MDS

National Comprehensive Cancer Network (NCCN) recommended that the minimal initial evaluation for patients clinically suspected to have MDS include—comprehensive history, physical examination, complete blood count, reticulocyte count, bone marrow aspiration and biopsy with iron stain, cytogenetic studies, erythropoietin level and iron studies (Fig. 11.1).

CLINICAL FEATURES

MDS patients manifest as isolated symptomatic anemia, neutropenia with infections, thrombocytopenia with bleeding manifestations or as multiple cytopenias. As there is no specific clinical feature for MDS, diagnosis mainly depends on laboratory findings.

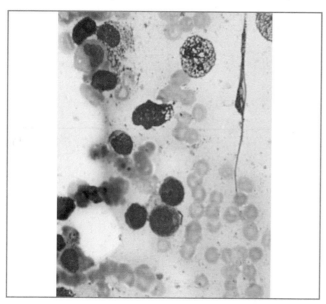

Fig. 11.1: Bone marrow microphotograph of a child with myelodysplastic syndrome (For color version, see Plate 3)

MORPHOLOGIC CONSIDERATION

The blood and marrow aspirate smears should be examined for dysplasia, the percentage of blasts and monocytes, and for ringed sideroblasts. Cells counted as blasts include myeloblasts, monoblasts and megakaryoblasts. Promonocytes are also considered as 'blast equivalents'.

Morphologic features in bone marrow aspirate smear show megaloblastic or megaloblastoid erythroid precursors. There may be multiple nuclei or asynchronous maturation of the nucleus and cytoplasm. Occasionally ringed sideroblasts, which are erythroid precursors with iron laden mitochondria can be identified, but these are extremely rare in pediatric MDS. Ringed sideroblasts are defined as the presence of at least five Prussian blue staining iron granules encircling more than one-third of nucleus of an erythroid precursor. Other possible causes of dyserythropoiesis should be excluded like—vitamin B_{12} and folic acid deficiency, viral infections (EBV/CMV/HIV), exposure to drugs such as antibiotics, chemotherapeutic drugs, ethanol, benzene and lead.

Abnormalities in myeloid series include both quantitive (most commonly neutropenia) and qualitative abnormality. A left shift with or without increased blast population is seen. Other features include asynchronous maturation of nucleus and cytoplasm, hypogranularity, hypolobated and Pseudo Pelger Huet cells.

Thrombocytopenia found in approximately 50% of patients and is the only cytopenia in 5% of cases. As in myeloid series both quantitative and qualitative abnormalities in platelet component are seen. These are giant or agranular platelet, micromegakaryocytes, hypolobated or multinuclear megakaryocytes.

Although bone marrow biopsy is not always necessary to establish a diagnosis of MDS, particularly in elderly, it is a very important diagnostic tool in pediatric population, specially to exclude inherited bone marrow failure syndrome. Dysplasia, particularly of megakaryocytes, evidence of disruption of normal marrow architecture, such as abnormal localization of immature precursors (ALIP), and an estimate of blast percentage and exclusion of hypoplastic bone marrow are important diagnostic findings in bone marrow biopsy.

Immunophenotype

Detection of CD 34 + cells by flowcytometry or immunohistochemistry may provide diagnostic and prognostic information. There is no single immunophenotypic parameter which is specific for MDS, but abnormal light scatter properties of dysplastic cells, abnormal antigen density, loss of antigen, and dysynchronous expression of antigens that are normally co-expressed during myeloid maturation have all been reported in MDS.

Cytogenetic Studies

A cytogenetic clone is detected in 50–70% of children with MDSs. Monosomy 7 is the most common abnormality. On the other hand, clonal cytogenetic abnormalities are present in approximately 90% of secondary MDSs. Next common abnormality is trisomy 8. Compared with adult MDS, loss of chromosome 5 or a del(5q) is rare in pediatric MDS, and when observed, generally occurs in the context of complex aberrations. The unique – 5 q syndrome is virtually absent in pediatric MDS. Other favorable cytogenetics, which are commonly found in adults (– Y, – 20q) are also generally absent in pediatric MDS. In MDS numerical chromosomal abnormalities are common rather than balanced translocations, which are common in de novo leukemias. Although chromosomal changes are not thought to be initiating events, they are probably involved in disease progression. Karyotype evolution is generally accompanied by progression to more advanced form of MDS.

CLASSIFICATION

To date, there have been 4 main classification schemes for pediatric MDSs:
- The FAB classification
- The World Health Organization (WHO) classification
- The category, cytology, cytogenetics (CCC) system
- The modified WHO classification for pediatric MDSs

FAB Classification

FAB classification for adult MDS has provided the first comprehensive criteria for diagnosis and classification of MDS patients. This classification depends on morphology of hematopoietic cells and blast cell percentage (Table 11.1).

Although the FAB classification has been used for pediatric patients with or without modifications, it became evident that approximately one-third of pediatric patients with MDS remain unclassified by this system.

WHO Classification

The adult WHO classification improved the terminology and allowed more pediatric patients to be classified (Table 11.2).

Although this classification retained some of the FAB categories, it adopted the term refractory cytopenia with multilineage dysplasia (RCMD) to incorporate a substantial proportion of previously unclassified cases. Here CMML & JMML were placed in a new category-MDS/MPD. The classification eliminated RAEB-T and lowered the threshold of the blast percentage for the diagnosis of acute leukemia to 20%. But the adult WHO classification fell short in addressing pediatric MDS that was associated with constitutional/inherited abnormalities. The threshold for recognizing dysplasia was 10%, which was considered too sensitive in pediatric age group. One group has proposed a threshold of 20% dysplasia for any cell line for diagnosis.

CCC Classification

It classifies patients according to etiologic, morphologic and cytogenetic criteria (Table 11.3).

The classification acknowledged the impact of constitutional/inherited disorders on pediatric MDS (Table 11.4). They didn't include JMML as they considered it as MPD and not MDS. This classification created a controversial new category of refractory single/multilineage cytopenia without obvious dysplasia (RC),which made diagnosis of MDS from inherited BM failure syndrome rather difficult in absence of dysplasia. This classification didn't provide any criteria or threshold for establishing the diagnosis, and Down's syndrome was included in syndrome related category despite its clearly different biologic behavior.

Table 11.1: FAB classification (1982)

Subtype	Peripheral blood	Bone marrow
Refractory anemia (RA)	< 1% blasts	Dyserythropoiesis < 5% blasts
Refractory anemia with ringed sideroblasts (RARS)	< 1% blasts	As for RA and > 15% ringed sideroblasts
Refractory anemia with excess blasts (RAEB)	< 5% blasts	Dyshematopoiesis 5–20% blasts
Refractory anemia with excess blasts in transformation (RAEB-T)	> 5% blasts	Dyshematopoiesis 21–30% blasts ± Auer rods
Chronic myelomonocytic leukemia (CMML)	> 1 × 10^9/L monocytes < 5% blasts	0–20% blasts

Table 11.2: WHO classification (2001)

Myelodysplastic syndrome/myeloproliferative disease

Chronic myelomonocytic leukemia (CMML)
Atypical chronic myeloid leukemia (aCML)
Juvenile myelomonocytic leukemia (JMML)
MDS/MPD, unclassified

Table 11.3: CCC system (2002)

Category
Idiopathic/de Novo Syndrome related Treatment/toxin related

Cytology
Refractory single/multilineage cytopenia without obvious dysplasia (RC) Refractory single/multilineage cytopenia with obvious dysplasia (RCD) Refractory single/multilineage cytopenia with ring sideroblasts (RCRS) Excess blasts (EB) 5–30%: RCEB, RCDEB, RCRSEB

Cytogenetics
CG + : Abnormal cytogenetics (abnormality should be specified) CG – : Normal cytogenetics CG 0 : Cytogenetics unknown

Modified WHO Classification of Pediatric MDS (Table 11.5)

This classification provided minimal diagnostic criteria for MDS diagnosis (Table 11.6).

This classification removed Auer rods as a discriminator of subtypes. As there are no data to indicate whether 20% blast count cut off is useful in pediatrics they retained RAEB-T category, which has been removed from adult WHO MDS classification. Although this classification disagreed with the 10% dysplasia threshold, it didn't recommend an alternative. RARS are extremely rare in children and as there are no data to document whether patients with RARS share distinctive clinical features, RARS is included in the category of refractory cytopenia. It also provided strict criteria for the diagnosis of MDS evolving from IBMFS. These criteria included increased BM blasts, persistent clonal chromosomal abnormalities and the development of hypercellular marrow accompanied by persistent peripheral cytopenia. This classification did not clarify categories of secondary MDSs.

JMML and Other MDS/MPD Disorder

JMML is a bridging disorder between MDS and MPDs (Table 11.7).

JMML includes patients with monosomy 7, previously considered to represent a distinct hematological disorder described as 'monosomy 7 syndrome'. But now it is found that there are no major clinical differences between JMML in children with and without monosomy 7.

The term CMML is included in the classification but is reserved for cases secondary to previous chemotherapy.

BCR-ABL negative CML is extremely rare in children and most cases are probably JMML.

Down syndrome (DS) disease: Individuals with DS have > 50 fold increased risk of leukemia during the first 5 years of life with about half the leukemias being myeloid.

Transient Abnormal Myelopoiesis (TAM)

Newborn with DS may show a clinical and morphological picture indistinguishable from AML. Blasts often have characteristics of megakaryoblasts. Spontaneous remission appears in the majority within 3 months. AML develops 1–3 years later in about one quarter of children. It is uncertain whether TAM should be considered a malignant disease.

Myeloid Leukemia in Down Syndrome

Occurs in children with DS outside the neonatal period. Mostly blast cells show features of megakaryoblasts. In contrast to TAM, MDS/AML in older children is fatal if untreated but responds well to AML treatment with a very favorable prognosis. There are no biological differences between MDS and AML in DS and have got no difference in prognostic or therapeutic consequences. Myeloid leukemia in DS children ≥ 3 years behaves more like de novo AML and doesn't fulfill the criteria for myeloid leukemia of DS.

Table 11.4: Myelodysplastic syndrome

Subtype	Peripheral blood	Bone marrow
Refractory anemia (RA)	Same as FAB	Same as FAB
Refractory anemia with ringed sideroblasts (RARS)	Same as FAB	Same as FAB
Refractory cytopenia with multilineage dysplasia (RCMD)	Cytopenia	Bi/trilineage dysplasia
RCMD with ringed sideroblasts (RCMD-RS)	Similar to RCMD	Similar to RCMD with ≥ 15% ringed sideroblasts
Refractory anemia with excess blasts 1 (RAEB-1)	Cytopenia, < 5% blasts	Uni/multilineage dysplasia, 5–9% blasts
RAEB-2	Cytopenia, 5–19% blasts	Uni/multilineage dysplasia, 10–19% blasts, ± Auer rods
MDS-unclassified	Cytopenia	Unilineage dysplasia other than Erythroid, blast count as in RA
MDS associated with isolated del (5q)	Anemia, increased platelet count, no Auer rods < 5% blasts	< 5% blasts hypolobated Megakaryocytes

Table 11.5: The modified WHO classification for pediatric MDSs (2003)

MDS/MPD

JMML
CMML(secondary only)
Ph- CML
Down syndrome (DS) disease
Transient abnormal myelopoiesis (TAM)
Myeloid leukemia of DS

MDS

Refractory cytopenia (RC) (PB blasts < 2% and BM blasts < 5%)
Refractory anemia with excess blasts (RAEB) (PB blasts 2–19% or BM blasts 5–19%)
RAEB in transformation (RAEB-T) (PB or BM blasts 20–29%)

Table 11.6: Minimal diagnostic criteria for MDS

At least two of the following

1. Sustained unexplained cytopenia
2. At least bilineage morphologic myelodysplasia
3. Acquired clonal cytogenetic abnormality in hematopoietic cells
4. Increased blasts (≥ 5%)

Table 11.7: Diagnostic guidelines for JMML

Suggestive clinical features	Hepatosplenomegaly Lymphadenopathy Pallor Skin rash
Laboratory criteria Minimal criteria (all 3 must be fulfilled)	No ph chromosome, no bcr-abl rearrangement PB monocyte count > 1 × 10^9/L Bone marrow blast count < 20%
Criteria for definite diagnosis (at least 2 must be fulfilled)	HbF increased for age Myeloid precursors in blood smear White cell count > 10 × 10^9/L Clonal abnormality GM-CSF hypersensitivity of myeloid progenitors

Myelodysplastic Syndrome (MDS)

Refractory Cytopenia

Persistent cytopenia with hypo or hypercellular BM and a blast count < 5% may indicate RC when infectious disease, metabolic disorder, and other causes of cytopenia and dysplasia have been ruled out. Anemia (Hb < 10 g/dl) is found around 60% patients of RC. Hematopoiesis is often dysplastic in IBMFS. Diagnosis of MDS in these patients should be done only if the BM blast count is increased, a persistent clonal chromosomal abnormality is present or hypercellularity in the BM develops in the presence of persistent PB cytopenia. RARS is extremely rare in children and should be included in RC category.

Refractory Anemia with Excess of Blasts (RAEB)

Bone marrow blast count between 5–20%. Subdivision of adult RAEB to RAEB 1 and RAEB 2 warrants further investigation in pediatrics to see whether they represent different entities in pediatric population.

Refractory Anemia with Excess of Blasts in Transformation (RAEB-T)

The recent WHO classification suggested abolition of the category of RAEB-T including most of these patients as AML. With multilineage dysplasia the cut off point for diagnosis of AML was lowered from the traditional 30 to 20% blast cells. The distinction is clearly an arbitrary one. There are no data to indicate whether a 20% blast cell cut-off is useful in pediatrics. Until more data are available RAEB-T category is maintained in pediatric group. In patients with BM blasts 20 to 30% and no clinical or cytogenetic changes characteristic of MDS or de novo AML, it is recommended to repeat BM examination 2 weeks later. If the blast count has increased to above 30%, the patient most likely has de novo AML. If the blast count is stable, an arbitrary period of 4 weeks is suggested before establishing a diagnosis of RAEB-T.

SECONDARY MDS

MDS may occur secondary to a constitutional or acquired abnormality. It is essential to note whether MDS is primary or secondary, as preceding events may affect treatment decisions and alter outcome.

Pathophysiology

Most of the studies on pathophysiology of MDS are on adults. The nature of putative stem cell and MDS initiating events are largely unknown. The incidence of MDS increase with age, suggesting that several cooperating events may be acquired during disease evolution. Exposure to genotoxic damage, germline polymorphisms affecting the activity of detoxifying enzymes, and/or cellular response to oxidative stress and the ability of the call to repair DNA damage all likely influence MDS pathogenesis. The cellular elements of blood originate from pluripotent hematopoietic stem cells. These stem cells have extensive regenerative and differentiating capacity and produce different cellular elements. In MDS, possibly dysregulation occurs in the differentiation process. The bone marrow failure that is seen in MDS, is due to ineffective hematopoiesis and not due to lack of hematopoiesis.

Chromosomal abnormalities (Table 11.8) are frequently found in MDS, but there causal relationship to disease remains unclear. The common chromosomal abnormalities identified are those involving chromosomes 7, 8 and 5. Monosomy 7 or del 7q can be found in de novo, secondary and constitutional forms (Fanconi anemia, Shwachmann-Diamond syndrome, severe congenital neutropenia) of MDS. These observations suggest that loss of one or several genes from the long arm of chromosome 7 is involved in the pathogenesis of childhood MDS. The segment of chromosome commonly deleted is 7q 22.

Cytogenetics and deletion mapping show that a loss of tumor suppressor gene within the deleted segment of chromosome 7 occurs. Compared to adult MDS, loss of chromosome 5 or a del 5 q is rare in childhood MDS.

Mutations in RAS oncogene have been found in 20–30% of childhood cases. RAS mutations disturb differentiation and lead to a proliferative advantage of hematopoietic precursor cells, ineffective erythropoiesis, and anemia. This is one mechanism thought to be responsible for the increased incidence of MDS in children with neurofibromatosis. Here NF-1 gene product loss occurs, which results in loss of negative feedback via guanosine 5 triphosphate (GTP) of oncogenic N-RAS, resulting in unregulated proliferation of an abnormal clone.

Table 11.8: Abnormalities associated with JMML and MDS in children

A. Associated with JMML

- Constitutional conditions
  - Neurofibromatosis type 1 (NF 1)
  - Noonan syndrome
  - Trisomy 8 mosaicism

B. Associated with MDS

- Constitutional conditions
  - Congenital bone marrow failure syndrome
  - Fanconi anemia
  - Kostmann syndrome
  - Shwachman- diamond syndrome
  - Blackfan-diamond anemia
  - Trisomy 8 mosaicism
  - Familial MDS (at least one first degree relative with MDS/AML)

- Acquired conditions
  - Prior chemotherapy/radiation
  - Aplastic anemia

A mutation of the transcription factor, RUNX1 (AML 1), has been described in MDS; loss of function of this gene may be critical in transformation to leukemia. Exposure to alkylating agents and/or radiation may lead to therapy related MDS. Deletions in chromosome 7 and/or 5 are often encountered in these cases. Chromosome 7 abnormalities observed in therapy related MDS are associated with methylation of CDKN 2 B promoter and mutations of RUNX 1. Additionally, chromosome 5 abnormalities are associated with mutations of P 53. The risk of MDS peaks at 5–7 years after alkylator treatment and is related to cumulative dose.

Scoring System

The international prognostic scoring system (IPSS) for MDS (Table 11.9) is based upon data on bone marrow blast percentage, cytopenia, and cytogenetics, separating patients into four prognostic groups. This scoring system has been developed mainly based on data of adult patients. However, this system has also been applied to pediatric patients to assess prognosis in this group of patients.

International Prognostic Scoring System (IPSS)

Poor: Complex (> 2), chromosome 7 abnormalities

Good: Normal, – y, 5q –, 20q–; intermediate: other abnormalities.

Cytopenia: Hb < 10 g/dl, neutrophil count < 1.5 × 10^9/L, platelet count <100 × 10^9/L.

Patients enrolled in studies of the European Working Group on childhood MDS (EWOG-MDS) showed among the criteria considered by the IPSS score, only BM blasts < 5% and platelets >100 × 10^9/L were significantly associated with a superior survival in MDS. There was no significant association with any other IPSS factors including cytogenetics. So the IPSS is of limited value in pediatric MDS. A new scoring system for pediatric MDS using HbF, platelet count, and cytogenetics (FPC score) as proposed by Passmore et al was not confirmed by other studies.

Treatment

The goal of pediatric MDS is curative and not palliative. The hematopoietic stem cell transplantation (HSCT) is a curative treatment and has emerged as the therapy of choice for almost all forms of MDS in children. Within the last few years, treatment of adult MDS patients has been changed considerably. A number of novel therapeutics is now in use. Examples include lenalidomide, which has been shown to be effective in MDS patients with isolated –5q and other chromosomal abnormalities associated with –5q; and several demethylating agents, such as decitabine and azacitidine, which are effective in high grade adult MDS patients. The azanucleosides have demonstrated particular efficacy in MDS with sole monosomy 7. Studies to investigate the value of these epigenetic drugs in children with MDS prior to HSCT or in a relapsed setting are highly attractive but have not been initiated yet.

Watch and Wait Strategy for Patients with Refractory Cytopenia without Monosomy 7 or Complex Karyotype

These patients can appropriately be followed up with a careful wait and watch strategy if the patients are neither transfusion dependent nor endangered by low-neutrophil count. Yearly BM examination is recommended to allow early recognition of disease progression. Most of these children may eventually need HSCT.

Immunosuppressive Therapy for Children with Refractory Cytopenia

Immunosuppressive therapy (IST) has been successful in some adults with low blast count, especially in patients

Table 11.9: International prognostic scoring system (IPSS) for MDS

Score value					
Prognostic variable	0	0.5	1.0	1.5	2.0
Marrow blasts (%)	< 5	5–10		11–20	21–30
Karyotype	Good	Intermediate	Poor		
Cytopenia	0/1	2/3			
Risk group					
Low	0				
Intermediate 1	0.5–1.0				
Intermediate 2	1.5–2.0				
High	2.5–3.5				

with BM hypoplasia and HLA DR 15. Few trials involving children, treated with IST (anti-thymocyte globulin and cyclosporine) suggest that IST can be a treatment option for selected patients with hypoplastic RC and normal karyotype. However, further observation is necessary to evaluate the long-term outcome of patients treated with IST specifically in comparison with the outcome of patients treated with an allograft as first choice of therapy.

Intensive Chemotherapy for Patients with Advanced MDS

The importance of cytoreductive therapy prior to the HSCT remains controversial. Data from EWOG-MDS indicate that intensive chemotherapy prior to HSCT will not improve survival and it is associated with low CR rate (< 60%), more relapse and low overall survival (< 30%). This study also showed that survival after HSCT was not influenced by marrow blast percentage at the time of HSCT. Well-controlled clinical trials will have to be designed to resolve the issues concerning pre-HSCT remission induction therapy.

Allogeneic HSCT for Patients with RC

For patients with RC HSCT from a HLA-identical sibling donor or HLA-compatible unrelated donor should be performed early in the course of disease. Probability of EFS is around 75%.

Allogeneic HSCT for Patients with Advanced Primary MDS

Treatment of choice in advanced MDS is HSCT. Procedure related mortality and disease recurrence remain the main cause of treatment failure. Intensive chemotherapy prior to HSCT is not routinely employed. 5 years probability of leukemia recurrence is approximately 25%. In the EWOG-MDS studies the EFS at 5 years is approximately 60%. Relapse following HSCT is associated with a poor outcome.

Therapy of Children with Secondary MDS

Children with MDS secondary to chemo or radiation have a poor survival rate. HSCT offers a probability of cure, with an EFS of 20–30%.

HSCT in MDS arising from IBMFS and acquired aplastic anemia indicate a poor outcome. Early HSCT

before neoplastic transformation or during less advanced MDS may be associated with improved survival.

CONCLUSION

Although significant progress has been made in the classification and treatment of childhood MDS, knowledge on initiating events and pathogenesis of pediatric MDS is still incomplete hampering a molecular classification of this rare disorder. Future studies should concentrate on understanding the molecular mechanisms underlying MDS in this age group. Clinical progress will only be possible in the context of enrolling patients in large prospective cooperative studies like those of EWOG-MDS or Children Oncology Group (COG).

SUGGESTED READING

1. Bennett JM, et al. Proposal for the classification of the myelodysplastic syndromes. Br J Haematol. 1982;51:189-99.
2. Charlotte M Niemeyer, et al. Myelodysplastic syndrome in children and adolescents. Seminars in Hematology. 2008;45:60-70.
3. Greenberg P, et al. International scoring system for evaluating prognosis in myelodysplastic syndromes. Blood. 1997;89:2079-88.
4. Greenberg PL. NCCN panel national comprehensive cancer network clinical practice guidelines in oncology. Myelodysplastic syndrome (sep 2004). Chicago IL; 2005;1.
5. Hassle H, et al. A pediatric approach to WHO classification of myelodysplastic and myeloproliferative disease. Leukemia. 2003;17:277-82.
6. Humbert JR, Hathway WE, Robin A, Peakman DC, Githens JH. Preleukemia in children with missing bone marrow C chromosome and a myeloproliferative disorder. Br J Haematol. 1971;21:705-16.
7. Jaffe ES, et al. Pathology and genetics of tumours of haematopoietic and lymphoid tissues. Lyon, France: IARC press; World Health Organization classification of tumours; 2001;3.
8. Jekic B, et al. Low frequency of NRAS and KRAS 2 gene mutations in childhood myelodysplastic syndrome. Cancer Genet Cytogenet. 2004;154:180-2.
9. Kardos G, et al. Refractory anemia in childhood: a retrospective analysis of 67 patients with particular reference to monosomy 7. Blood. 2003;102:1997-2003.

10. Le Beau MM, et al. Cytogenetics and molecular delineation of a region of chromosome 7 commonly deleted in malignant myeloid disease. Blood. 1996;88:1930-5.

11. Mandel K, et al. A practical comprehensive classification for pediatric myelodysplastic syndrome the CCC system. J Pediatr Hematol Oncol. 2002;24:596-604.

12. Muller CI, et al. DNA hypermethylation of myeloid cells, a novel therapeutic target in MDS and AML. Current Pharmaceutical Biotechnology. 2006;7:315-21.

13. Niemeyer CM, et al. Paediatric myelodysplastic syndromes and juvenile myelomonocytic leukemia: molecular classification and treatment options. BR J Haematol. 2008;140:610-24.

14. Passmore SJ, et al. Paediatric myelodysplastic syndromes and juvenile myelomonocytic leukemia in the UK: a population based study of incidence and survival. Br J Haematol. 2003;121:758-67.

15. Passmore SJ, et al. Pediatric myelodysplasia: a study of 68 children and a new prognostic scoring system. Blood. 1995;85:1742-50.

16. Ruter B, et al. Preferential cytogenetic response to continuous intravenous low dose decitabine administration in myelodysplastic syndromes with monosomy 7. Blood. 2007;110:1080 2.

17. Settler-stevenson M, et al. Diagnostic utility of flow cytometric immunophenotyping in myelodysplastic syndromes. Blood 2001;98:979-87.

18. Steensma DP, Tefferi A. The myelodysplastic syndrome(s): a perspective and review highlighting current controversies. Leuk Res. 2003;27:95-120.

12

Pediatric Histiocytic Disorders

Madhusmita Sengupta, Rakesh Mondal

The histiocytoses are a diverse group of hematological disorders identified by the pathologic infiltration of normal tissues by cells of the mononuclear phagocyte system. There is heterogeneity in this family of disorders, a result of the biologic variability of the cells they inhabit. Advances in basic hematology and immunology over the last two decades have significantly enhanced our understanding of the histiocytic disorders. It is now accepted that the pathogenic cells central to the development, arise from a common hematopoietic progenitor. Molecular identification of the hematopoietic cells has enabled to classify the histiocytoses based on the cellular basis of the disease.

These pathologic cells phenotypically resemble immature mononuclear phagocytes at specific stages of differentiation.

The Histiocyte Society, 1985, has served as a forum for enhanced collaboration between international histiocytosis experts. The Histiocyte Society has used the cellular based classification of the histiocytoses as a guideline for therapeutic studies.

In this chapter, we use the cellular classification of histiocytic disorders, as adopted by the Histiocyte Society, to present each subgroup of this family of disorders, describes their natural history and presents current therapeutic approaches and outcomes.

The importance of dendritic cells in presenting antigens to T and B lymphocytes is increasingly recognized. Immature dendritic cells respond to GM-CSF and become committed to generating dendritic cells, which are "professional" antigen-presenting cells (APCs). These cells can capture antigen and migrate to lymphoid organs, where they present the antigens to naive T cells and also stimulate B lymphocytes.

CLASSIFICATION OF HISTIOCYTOSIS SYNDROMES IN CHILDREN

Table 12.1 shows the classification of histiocytic and dendritic cell disorders proposed by World Health Organization (WHO).

CLASSIFICATION OF HISTIOCYTOSIS SYNDROMES FROM THE HISTIOCYTE SOCIETY

Table 12.2 shows the working classification of histiocytosis syndromes from the Histiocyte Society.

Definitive diagnosis of histiocytosis includes light microscopic characteristics plus Birbeck granules in the lesional cell on electron microscopy and/or positive staining for CD1a antigen on the lesional cell. The chapter focuses mainly on LCH. A brief discussion on Rosai-Dorfman disease has been incorporated at the end.

Langerhans Cell Histiocytoses

LCH is usually sporadic and non-hereditary condition. LCH formerly was divided into 3 disease categories: Eosinophilic granuloma, Hand-Schüller-Christian disease, and Letterer-Siwe disease, depending on the

Table 12.1: Classification of histiocytosis syndromes in children

Class	Syndromes
I	• LCH
II	• Histiocytosis of mononuclear phagocytes other than Langerhans cells • Familial and reactive hemophagocytic lymphohistiocytosis (HLH) • Sinus histiocytosis with massive lymphadenopathy (SHML/Rosai-Dorfman disease) • Juvenile xanthogranuloma (JXG) • Reticulohistiocytoma
III	• Malignant histiocytic disorders • Acute monocytic leukemia (FAB M 5) • Malignant histiocytosis • True histiocytic lymphoma

Table 12.2: Histiocyte Society classification of histiocytosis syndromes

Class	Syndromes
Dendritic-cell related	LCH
Macrophage related	HLH, Rosai-Dorfman disease
Malignant disorders	Monocyte related, monocytic leukemia (Malignant histiocytosis)

severity and extent of involvement. This classification and its related risk groups are no longer used.

Langerhans cell histiocytoses are traditionally divided into four groups.

a. **Unifocal (Eosinophilic granuloma):** A slowly progressing disease, characterized by an expanding proliferation of Langerhans cells in various bones, skin, lungs or stomach.

b. **Multifocal unisystem:** Characterized by fever and diffuse eruptions, usually on the scalp and in the ear canals, as well as bone lesions seen in children. There may be involvement of stalk of the pituitary gland, leading to diabetes insipidus. Hand-Schuller-Christian triad includes the triad of diabetes insipidus, proptosis, and lytic bone lesions.

c. **Multifocal multisystem (Letterer-Siwe disease):** A rapidly progressing disease where Langerhans cells proliferate in many tissues. It is mostly seen in children under two years, and the prognosis is poor even with aggressive chemotherapy, with 5-year survival is only 50%.

d. Pulmonary Langerhans cell histiocytosis (PLCH): A long-term complications like LCH histiocytosis usually affects children between 1 and 15 years old and peak incidence is between age 5 and 10.

A clinical-grouping system for LCH based on age, extent of the disease, and organ dysfunction, can provide a means to compare patient data and prognosis. Various categories, such as restricted and extensive multiorgan involvement, have also been proposed similarly.

When the disease is focal, establishing the diagnosis of LCH depends on a high level of suspicion. When advanced multisystem involvement is observed, diagnosis is often easy. Adequate workup to determine the extent of the disease and possible complications is essential. Biopsy and pathologic evaluation are needed to establish the diagnosis.

Bone involvement is observed in 78% of patients with LCH and often includes the skull (49%), innominate bone (23%), femur (17%), orbit (11%), and/or ribs (8%) (Fig. 12.1A). Upon clinical evaluation, the lesions can be single or multiple. Asymptomatic or painful involvement of vertebrae can occur and can result in collapse. Long-bone involvement can induce fractures. The lesions sometimes cause a clinically significant periosteal reaction. Extension to the adjacent tissues can produce symptoms that may be unrelated to the bone involvement. Purulent

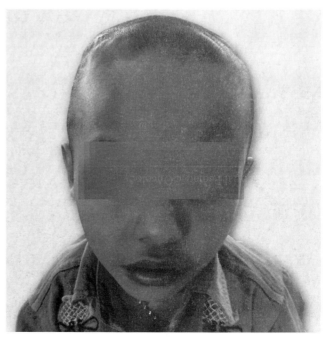

Fig. 12.1A: Histiocytosis presented with osteolytic nodules

otitis media may occur and may be difficult to distinguish from infectious etiologies. Orbital involvement may cause proptosis. Involvement of the eyes in the form of uveitis and iris nodules are reported.

Diabetes insipidus and delayed puberty are observed in as many as 50% of patients. Hypothalamic disease may also result in growth-hormone deficiency and short stature.

Maxillary, mandibular, and gingival disease may cause loss of teeth, hemorrhagic gum, and mucosal ulceration and bleeding. Cutaneous LCH is observed in as many as 50% of patients with LCH. Rash is a common presentation, and skin lesions may be the only evidence of the disease or may be part of systemic involvement. Skin infiltrates have a predilection for the midline of the trunk and the peripheral and flexural areas of skin. Skin infiltrates can be maculoerythematous, petechial xanthomatous, nodular papular, or nodular in appearance (Fig. 12.1B).

Pulmonary involvement is observed in 20–40% of patients and may result in respiratory symptoms, such as cough, tachypnea, dyspnea, and pneumothorax. Imaging studies may reveal cysts and micronodular infiltrates. Pulmonary function tests may reveal restrictive lung disease with decreased pulmonary volume. GI bleeding may be the presenting sign of patients with GI involvement. Appropriate imaging studies, endoscopy, and biopsy may be helpful to confirm the diagnosis. Liver involvement is characterized by elevated transaminase levels, and less commonly, increased bilirubin levels (Figs 12.2A and B).

Marrow involvement or enlargement of the spleen may cause hematologic changes. Lymph node enlargement is observed in approximately 30% of patients. Lymph node enlargement surrounding the respiratory tract may result in pulmonary-related symptoms, such as cough, dyspnea, or cyanosis. Infiltration of various areas of the brain gives rise to corresponding signs and symptoms, including cerebellar dysfunction and loss of coordination. Disruption of hypothalamic and pituitary function is most common. This includes symptoms secondary to diabetes insipidus and, to a lesser extent, growth-hormone deficiency and hypopituitarism. Other symptoms, such as seizures and

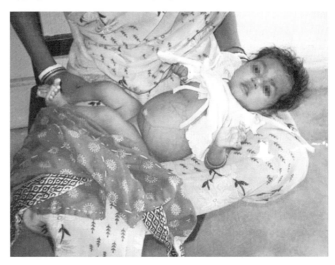

Fig. 12.2A: Clinical photograph of a child showing characteristic skin rash and huge hepato-splenomegaly of LCH

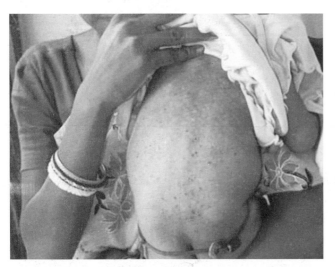

Fig. 12.1B: Clinical photograph of a child showing characteristic skin rash of LCH

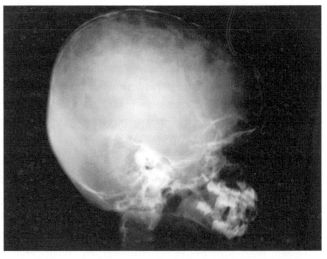

Fig. 12.2B: X-ray skull of histiocytosis presented with osteolytic nodules

those related to increased intracranial pressure, depend on the site and volume of the space-occupying lesion. Anemia, leukopenia, thrombocytopenia, and their related symptoms are uncommon.

Laboratory investigations and diagnostic tests should partly be tailored to the extent of disease suspected on the basis of the patient's history and physical findings (Table 12.3).

Laboratory and Imaging Studies

Histologic Findings

Regardless of the clinical severity, the histopathology of LCH is generally uniform. To some extent, the location and age of the lesion may influence the histopathology of the disease. Early in the course of the disease, lesions tend to be cellular and contain aggregates of

Table 12.3: Laboratory and imaging studies in patients with Langerhans cell histiocytosis (LCH)

a. Hemoglobin and hematocrit
b. Leukocyte count and differential cell count
c. Liver function tests
d. Coagulation studies
e. Urine osmolality
f. Chest, posteroanterior and lateral
g. Skeletal survey (Fig. 12.2A)
h. Bone marrow aspiration biopsy
i. Pulmonary function tests
j. Lung biopsy and bronchoalveolar lavage
k. Small bowel series, endoscopy and biopsy
l. Hepatic ERCP, angiography, or biopsy
m. MRI of brain and hypothalamic-pituitary axis
n. Endocrine investigation

pathologic Langerhans cells (PLCs), intermediate cells, interdigitating cells, macrophages, T cells, and giant histiocytes. Multinucleated giant cells are common, and some may exhibit phagocytosis. Lesions may also include eosinophils, necrotic cells, and LCH cells. With time, the cellularity and number of LCH cells are reduced, and macrophages and fibrosis become eminent. The infiltrates tend to destroy epithelial cells. Cell markers and phenotypes of histiocytic disorders along with specialized stains are described in the tables 12.4 and 12.5.

Treatment

The aim of therapy in histiocytosis is to relieve clinical symptoms and prevent complications of the disease. For single-system disease, no therapy or only local therapy may be necessary, although further treatment may be needed in certain circumstances.

Topical Therapy

Localized skin lesions, especially in infants, can spontaneously regress. If treatment is required, topical corticosteroids may be tried. Low-dose radiation therapy to the local lesions is often effective but is rarely needed. For unresponsive skin lesions, low-dose mild systemic therapy can be used.

Chemotherapy for multisystemic disease with local or constitutional symptoms is used. Single agents or adjuvant use of several chemotherapeutic agents and/or biologic-response modifiers may be effective. Published therapies include corticosteroids, vinca alkaloids,

Table 12.4: Cell markers and phenotypes of histiocytic disorders

Cell marker	LCH	SHML	Follicular dendritic tumor	Histiocytic sarcoma	Acute monocytic leukemia	Anaplastic large-cell lymphoma
CD 1a	+	−	−	−	−	−
CD 4	+	+	−	+	+	+
CD 21	−	+/−	+	−	−	−
CD 25	−	+	−	+	+	++
CD 30	−	−	−	−	−	++
CD 35	−	+	+	−	−	−
CD 45	−	+	−	+/−	+	+/−
CD 68	−	+	−	+	+	+/−
S-100	+	+	−	+/1	−	−

Table 12.5: Shows specialized stains for diagnosing these disorders

Type of test	Stain	Mononuclear phagocytic system	Langerhans cells	Dendritic cells	Dendritic reticulum cells
Frozen-section histochemisty	Nonspecific esterase	–	–	–	–
	Acid phosphatase	+	–	·	–
	ATPase	–	+	+	–
	Lambda-mannosidase	–	+	–	–
	Nucleotidase	–	–	–	+
Immunohistochemistry	CD 14	+	+	+	+
	CD 11 C	+	+	+	+
	CD 68	+	–	–	–
	CD 1a	–	+	+	–
Paraffin-section immunohistochemistry	HLA-DR	+	+	+	+
	CD 68	+	–	–	–
	Alpha-antitrypsin	+	–	–	–
	S-100	–	+	+	–

Note—ATPase = adenosine triphosphatase; HLA = human leukocyte antigen.
In LCH, the cytoplasm and, rarely, the nucleus contain the characteristic structures termed Birbeck granules. These trilaminar organelles are 190–360 nm long and approximately 33 nm wide, with a central striated line. These are derived from cytoplasmic membrane and are involved in receptor mediated and non-receptor-mediated endocytosis. An electron microscopic finding of racquet-shaped granules in the cells can be helpful in confirming the pathologic diagnosis. Birbeck granules are the products of internalization of complexes originating from cell-membrane antigens and corresponding antibodies.

antimetabolites-nucleoside analogs, immune modulators such as cyclosporine, antithymocyte globulin, biologic-response modifiers such as IL-2 and INFs, cellular treatment, and exchange transfusion. Most reports of treatment modalities lack controls, with most authors citing the rarity of the disease as justification for the lack.

Single-agent Therapy

Purine analogs with activity for treatment of Langerhans cell histiocytosis (LCH) include 2-chlorodeoxyadenosine and 2-deoxycoformycin (CDF). In a review of 15 patients with multiorgan involvement receiving 2 CdA and 2 receiving 2 CDF, 6 had complete responses, 3 had partial responses, 5 had no response, and 1 died early. As a single agent, cyclosporine has been used in pretreated patients with advanced LCH. Cyclosporine, a cyclic undecapeptide immunosuppressant of fungal origin, inhibits immune responses. The proposed mechanism of action is blockage of the transmission and synthesis of lymphokines, such as IL-2 and INF.

Cyclosporine is postulated to disrupt abnormal cytokine-dependent activation of lymphocytes and histiocytes in the liver, spleen, lymph nodes, and bone marrow. The activation of lymphocytes is presumed to be secondary to uncontrolled proliferation of Langerhans cells. Furthermore, cyclosporine can inhibit cytokine-mediated cellular activation that potentially contributes to phagocytosis and disease progression. Partial and complete responses have been recorded in a small number of patients. Patients with partial response had achieved a complete response with prednisone and vinblastine chemotherapy. Cyclosporine A has also been used in familial erythrophagocytic lymphohistiocytosis (FEL). INF-alpha had some effect in anecdotal cases of LCH. Treatment of multifocal relapsing and resistant bone lesions in LCH is challenging. Langerhans cells are capable of releasing cytokines, which are potent activators of osteoclasts and can result in the lytic lesions seen in the disease. Pamidronate, a bisphosphonate agent, has been reported to induce response or result in disease stability in a very small group of patients.

Multiagent Therapy

Most chemotherapy agents for the treatment of LCH are used in combination. The length of therapy is arbitrarily chosen. In some studies, patients were stratified by risk factor. Use of a combination of cytarabine arabinoside (Ara-C), vincristine, and prednisolone to treat disseminated LCH with organ dysfunction has been reported. An organized international approach to LCH has been successful. Using the Histiocyte Society's LCH I protocol 1994, investigators prospectively and randomly assigned patients with multisystemic LCH who met criteria based on standard diagnostic evaluation. Patients received vinblastine (6 mg/m^2 intravenously weekly for 24 weeks) or etoposide (150 mg/m^2 intravenously on 3 consecutive days every 3 weeks for 24 weeks). All patients received methylprednisolone (30 mg/kg intravenously for 3 consecutive days. Of the 447 patients who were registered from various countries, 192 had multisystemic disease, and 136 were randomly assigned (72 to the vinblastine arm and 64 to the etoposide arm). Patients were evaluated at predetermined intervals. Responses at 6 weeks appeared to differentiate responders from nonresponders, who had poor outcomes. Neither the patients' ages nor the number, type, or dysfunction of the organs differentiated the groups. At 6 weeks, 51 (50%) of 103 patients achieved a complete response or substantial disease regression, whereas 32 (31%) had stable disease or partial or mixed responses. Disease progression was reported in 19 patients. At 26 months, the mortality rate was 18%. Among the patients who died, 4 had an initial response, 5 had intermediate responses, and 9 had initial nonresponses.

The randomized LCH II study of the Histiocyte Society was performed to compare the effects of oral prednisone with vinblastine (with or without etoposide) in patients with multisystemic disease. Patients were divided into low- or high-risk groups. All patients received prednisone (40 mg/m^2/d for 28 d with weekly reduction afterward) and vinblastine (6 mg/m^2 intravenously weekly for 6 weeks). The low-risk group received continuation therapy with vinblastine (6 mg/m^2 during weeks 9, 12, 15, 18, 21, and 24), as well as 5-day pulses of prednisone during the same weeks. Patients in the low-risk group were excluded from randomization.

Patients in the high-risk group were randomly assigned to treatment A or B. Treatment consisted of an initial 6 weeks of therapy with prednisolone and weekly vinblastine and continuation therapy, pulses of vinblastine and/or oral prednisone as in the low-risk group, and daily doses of 6-mercaptopurine (50 mg/m^2 during weeks 6–24). Treatment B was the same as treatment A, with the addition of etoposide (150 mg/m^2 administered on day 1 of weeks 9, 12, 15, 18, 21, and 24). Results of this protocol have not yet been published.

Radiation Therapy

Radiation therapy is effective in LCH. Doses ranging from 750–1500 cGy are usually administered, resulting in good local control of single lesions or metastasis, which can occur in critical areas or cause permanent damage. Fractionated doses of radiotherapy have also been used.

Treatment for Recurrent or Refractory Disease

The severity of the recurrent disease often dictates the type of therapy that is most likely to be helpful. For example, recurrence of an isolated bone lesion can often be treated with nonsteroidal anti-inflammatory drugs (NSAIDs) or intralesional steroid injections. When bone lesions are multiple and cause clinically significant morbidity, systemic therapy can be helpful. In such circumstances, patients often respond to the same drugs that they previously received, such as vinblastine and/or corticosteroids. Extensive recurrence of skin disease, including refractory perianal or vulvar involvement, often requires systemic chemotherapy. When patients do not have an early response to vinblastine, corticosteroids, methotrexate, 6-mercaptopurine, or even etoposide, alternate therapies should be administered. Although several immunomodulatory agents, such as cyclosporine, have been used in patients with refractory disease, the results have been inconsistent. Cytotoxic chemotherapy often needs to be administered as well.

Other approaches to the treatment of patients with refractory LCH that are being tested or developed and include agents such as thalidomide, which is used to inhibit TNF-alpha and INF-gamma production. In some studies, only patients with low-risk disease were likely to respond to thalidomide, whereas high-risk patients with organ involvement were not. Further recognition of NF-kappa B pathway may improve the success of targeted therapy for LCH.

Targeting humanized antibodies against lineage-specific antigens, such as CD1a antigens on LCH cells, is another treatment being developed. The application of inhibitors of activated cytokine receptors and their downstream signal-transduction pathways is also an important area of future therapeutic trials. Although hematopoietic stem-cell transplantation has been successful in some patients with refractory LCH, identifying patients who might benefit from such high-risk therapy is difficult, and this treatment is associated with significant acute and chronic complications. Specific therapies, including monoclonal antibodies against the CD1a or CD 52 epitopes found on Langerhans cells, are emerging.

Local therapy with various agents has been reported. Intralesional infiltration of corticosteroids for treatment of localized LCH has been advocated.

Myeloablative therapy followed by bone marrow or stem cell transplantation in disease refractory to the conventional therapy has been reported. However, reporting of positive results are likely to bias such reports. Intravenous immunoglobulin has been used to treat neurodegenerative LCH. However, to the authors' knowledge, no formal study has been done to conclusively affirm the benefit of such a treatment.

HEMOPHAGOCYTIC LYMPHOHISTIOCYTOSES (HLH)

Hemophagocytic Lymphohistiocytoses (HLH) are heterogeneous group of clinical syndromes characterized by uncontrolled and ineffective hyperinflammatory response due to activation and non-malignant proliferation of T-lymphocytes and macrophages, leading to a cytokine storm.

Types of HLH: It includes two different conditions that may be difficult to distinguish from each other:

1. **Primary HLH:** Familial hemophagocytic lymphohistiocytosis (FHL, FHLH, or FEL)—this is an autosomal recessive disorder

2. **Secondary HLH:** Infection-associated hemophagocytic syndrome (IAHS or VAHS) and malignancy-associated hemophagocytic syndrome (MAHS). The main focus of discussion here is the primary, e.g. FHL.

Clinical Features: The most common presenting features are pyrexia of unknown origin, respiratory symptoms, hepatosplenomegaly and cytopenias.

Diagnosis: Absent or decreased lymphocyte cytotoxicity is the cellular hallmark of FHL.

Bone marrow aspirate may demonstrate the characteristic hemophagocytes, but may not be found initially in two-thirds of patients (Figs 12.3 and 12.4). Diagnosis can be made by a set of definite criteria, formulated and revised by Histiocytic society as follows: Diagnostic criteria for hemophagocytic lympho-histiocytosis (HLH)

HLH can be diagnosed if either of the following two are met:

1. A gene mutation consistent with familial HLH is present (these include mutations of PRF, UNC13D and STX11), or

2. At least five out of the eight following diagnostic criteria for HLH are fulfilled:
   – Fever
   – Splenomegaly
   – Cytopenias (affecting ≥2 of 3 lineages in the peripheral blood): Hemoglobin <90 g/L (in infants <4 weeks: hemoglobin <100 g/L); Platelets <100 x10^9/L; Neutrophils <1.0 x10^9/L
   – Hypertriglyceridemia and/or hypofibrino-genemia: Fasting triglycerides ≥3.0 mmol/L (≥265 mg/dl), OR fibrinogen ≤1.5 g/L
   – Hemophagocytosis in bone marrow or spleen or lymph nodes
   – Low or absent NK-cell activity (according to local laboratory reference)
   – Ferritin ≥500 ug/L
   – Soluble CD25 (i.e., soluble IL-2 receptor) ≥2,400 U/ml

Treatment and prognosis: Unlike the secondary HLH, where underlying causes are to be treated, FHLH, when diagnosed, needs to be treated with etoposide, corticosteroid and intrathecal methotrexate. Antithymocyte globulin and cyclosporine may be used

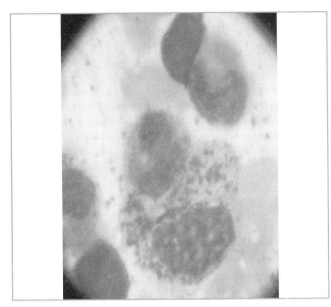

Fig. 12.3: Microphotograph of bone marrow slide showing phagocytosis of neutrophils in hemophagocytic lymphohistiocytosis (HLH) *(For color version, see Plate 3)*

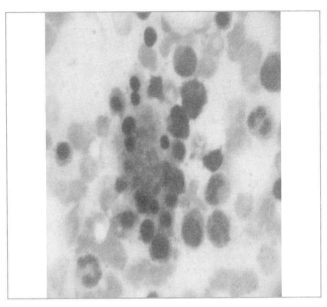

Fig. 12.4: Microphotograph of bone marrow slide showing phagocytosis of erythrocytes in hemophagocytic lymphohistiocytosis (HLH) *(For color version, see Plate 3)*

for maintenance therapy. Definitive therapy of this potentially fatal condition is hematopoietic stem cell transplantation (HSCT). The introduction of HSCT has dramatically improved the prognosis of the disease curing approximately 60% of patients.

ROSAI-DORFMAN DISEASE

Rosai-Dorfman disease is a rare, benign histiocytic disorder of children and young adults, described initially as a separate entity in 1969 by Rosai and Dorfman under the term sinus histiocytosis with massive lymphadenopathy (SHML). The etiology is not fully understood and it may co-exist with other autoimmune diseases, hematological malignancies and infections (Herpesvirus 6 and Epstein Barr virus E). The accumulation and activation of of histiocytes may be caused by cytokine mediated migration of monocytes.

Clinical features: Bilateral and painless cervical lymphadenopathy with fever, night sweats and weight loss are common features (Fig.12.5). Other lymphnode areas may also be involved. Extranodal sites of involvement are skin, urogenital tract, breast, gastrointestinal tract, liver, pancreas, lung, bone, parotid, eye and retro-orbital tissue (Fig.12.6). The clinical course is unpredictable with occasional exacerbations.

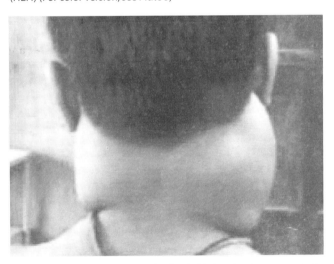

Fig. 12.5: Clinical photograph of a child showing huge cervical adenopathy bilaterally following Rosai-Dorfman's disease

The disease is often self-limiting. Cutaneous RDD, a distinct entity, is confined to the skin with papular or nodular lesions without lymphadenopathy. Spontaneous regression is seen in most cases.

Diagnosis

A normochromic/normocytic or autoimmune hemolytic anemia with elevated serum ferritin are observed. Radiography shows osteolytic lesions. Diagnosis is

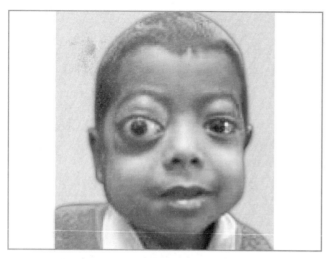

Fig. 12.6: Clinical photograph of a child showing bilateral proptosis following Rosai Dorfman's disease

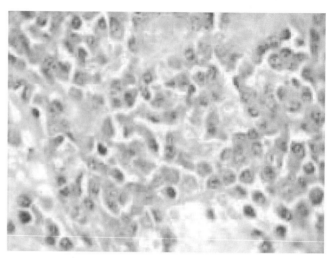

Fig. 12.7: Microphotograph of lymph node biopsy of Rosai-Dorfman's disease *(For color version, see Plate 4)*

confirmed by histology characteristically showing emperipolesis, or the engulfment of lymphocytes and erythrocytes by histiocytes that express S-100 (Fig.12.7). Pericapsular fibrosis and dilated sinuses along with infiltration of large histiocytes, lymphocytes and plasma cells are also found. Immunohistochemical stains of RDD cells are also positive for CD68, CD163, α1-antichymotrypsin, α1-antitrypsin, IL-1β and TNF-α and HAM-56 while CD1a is typically negative.

Treatment

RDD has a benign course and treatment is necessary only in case of life-threatening complications or extra-nodal RDD having vital organ involvement.

Surgery is occasionally required. Role of radiotherapy is limited.

Systemic corticosteroids can reduce nodal size and relieve symptoms.

Chemotherapy options include with methotrexate (MTX), 6-mercaptopurine (6 MP), etoposide, vinblastine.

Others include interferon-α, thalidomide and tyrosine kinase inhibitor imatinib.

SUGGESTED READING

1. Harris NL, et al. World Health Organization classification of neoplastic diseases of the hematopoietic and lymphoid tissues: report of the Clinical Advisory Committee Meeting. Airlie House, Virginia, November, 1997. J Clin Oncol. 1999;17:3835.
2. Nandi M, Mondal RK, Datta S, Karmakar BC, Mukherjee K, Dhibar TK. Rosai-Dorfman disease. Indian J Pedtr. 2008;75(3):290-4.
3. Pediatric blood and cancer. 2007;48:124-31.
4. Sieff CA, Nathan DG, Clark SC. The anatomy and physiology of hematopoiesis. In: Nathan DG, Orkin SH (eds): Hematology of Infancy and Childhood, 5th ed. Philadelphia, WB Saunders, 1997.
5. Vassallo R, et al. Clinical outcomes of pulmonary Langerhans'-cell histiocytosis in adults. N Engl J Med. 2002;346:484.

13 Pediatric Solid Tumors

Bishwanath Mukhopadhyay

Pediatric solid tumors constitute a major cause of morbidity and mortality, next to congenital malformations and trauma. There tumors make up about one third of all pediatric cancers. The common solid tumors include brain tumors neuroblastoma, rhabdomyosarcoma, Wilms' tumor, bone tumors and germ cell tumors. If we exclude brain and spinal cord tumors (treated by Neurosurgeons) and bone tumors (managed by Orthopedic Surgeons), the most common solid tumors we come across are renal tumors (mainly Wilms' tumors), neuroblastoma, Hodgkin's and non-Hodgkin's lymphoma, rhabdomyosarcoma, liver tumors, teratomas and germ cell tumors.

Incidence of childhood solid tumors is highest between 1 and 3 years. More than 80% of children with cancer live in developing countries. It is obvious that there is remarkable improvement in the survival of childhood solid tumors. It is from 30% in 1960 to more than 80% in 2000.

WILMS' TUMOR OR NEPHROBLASTOMA

It was described by Max Wilms (1867–1918). It is the most common type of renal tumor in children. The incidence of Wilms' tumor is remarkably constant among the different countries of the world. The incidence in India is reported as one in 10 children below 15 years (reported from Mumbai). Usual presentation is a painless abdominal mass. Hematuria, hypertension and pain occur in some cases. The tumor is often discovered on routine clinical examination. Neurological findings are common in metastatic disease. Rarely these tumors may present with stroke (Figs 13.1 and 13.2). Different renal tumors have been classified as follows:

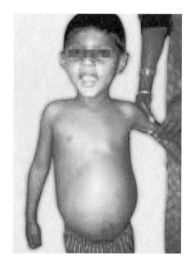

Fig. 13.1: The child with huge abdominal swelling following mesoblastic nephroma

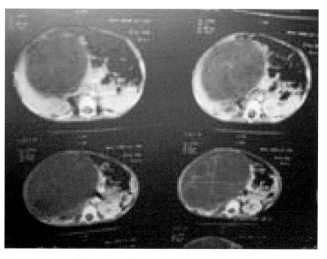

Fig. 13.2: CT scan of abdomen showing huge renal mass following mesoblastic nephroma

Low-risk tumors:

1. Cystic partially differentiated nephroblastoma.
2. Nephroblastoma completely necrotic after pre-operative chemotherapy.
3. Mesoblastic nephroma.

Intermediate risk tumors:

1. Nephroblastoma—epithelial type
2. Nephroblastoma—stromal type
3. Nephroblastoma—mixed type
4. Nephroblastoma—regressive type
5. Nephroblastoma—with focal anaplasia.

High-risk tumors:

1. Nephroblastoma with diffuse anaplasia.
2. Nephroblastoma with blastemal type.
3. Clear cell sarcoma of kidney.
4. Rhabdoid tumor of kidney.

Wilms' tumor may be associated with different syndromes like WAGR syndrome (Wilms' tumor, aniridia, genitourinary anomalies and mental retardation), Beckwith Wiedemann syndrome (exomphalos, visceromegaly, Macroglossia and hyperinsulinemic hypoglycemia), Denys–Drash syndrome (pseudohermaphroditism, progressive glomerulopathy and Wilms' tumor). Chromosomal abnormalities i.e. gene deletion at 11p13 and 11p15 are associated with development of Wilms' tumor. In such syndromes, genetic counseling is an important part of overall management. With the improvement in diagnostic facilities, pre-and post-operative care, more than 95% of children can expect cure.

Treatment

The role of surgery in Wilms' tumor is to excise the tumor, accurate histopathological diagnosis with post-surgical staging/lymph node sampling. The principal line of management is nephrectomy followed by chemotherapy and/or radiotherapy as indicated (Fig. 13.3). As per protocol of SIOP (International Society of Pediatric Oncology), pre-operative chemotherapy has remarkably improved the overall results of Wilms' tumors. Wilms' tumor is an ideal model for the study of basic mechanism of carcinogenesis. The present policy in treating Wilms' tumor can be summarized as follows:

1. Complete surgical excision depending upon operative staging and histopathology (favorable/unfavorable), chemotherapy and radiotherapy.

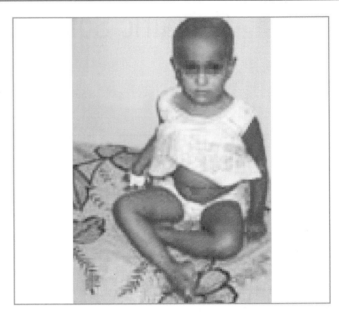

Fig. 13.3: The clinical photograph of the child with operated nephroblastoma

2. Pre-operative chemotherapy if the presentation is late with very big tumors, tumors with metastases, involving inferior vena cava and bilateral Wilms' tumors.
3. Decreased treatment intensity for patients with favorable histology.
4. Decreased cost of therapy in pulse intensive regimen.

From the different study groups and reports from different centers in India, 90% of children with Wilms' tumors can be cured. It has become important to look into life-threatening medical conditions in survivors of Wilms' tumors and the quality of life of the survivors.

NEUROBLASTOMA

Neural origin was first described by Virchow in 1864. Hypothesis of maturation of neuroblastoma to ganglioneuroma was given by Cushing in 1927. In spite of tremendous advancement in the understanding of the disease and its molecular biology, investigations and overall outcome of neuroblastoma is still not encouraging. Though the survival of neuroblastoma in stage I and stage II is around 90%, the outcome is poor in stage III and IV patients (20–40%). Neuroblastoma is a tumor that arises from developing sympathetic nerve tissue. It is a cancer that occurs most frequently in infants and young children and is rarely seen in children older than ten years of age. It is the leading form of cancer in infants and is the most common type of solid extra-cranial tumor in children. Prognosis depends on age, spread of disease, and the absence/presence of molecular and genetic markers in tumor cells.

Symptoms

Most patients with neuroblastoma present with signs and symptoms that are related to primary and metastatic tumor growth. Tumors located in the abdomen can cause abdominal pain, constipation, bladder dysfunction and abdominal swelling. Tumors located in the thorax can cause breathing difficulties, facial swelling, and droopy eyes due to the superior vena cava syndrome and Horner's syndrome, respectively. Tumors located along the spinal cord or along various nerve fibers can present with any type of neurologic dysfunction including weakness, loss of sensation, pain, bladder and bowel incontinence, or paralysis. Other symptoms that can be seen in association with neuroblastoma include bulging, complaints of back pain or limb pain from bone metastases, watery diarrhea from elevated levels of the substance vasoactive intestinal polypeptide (VIP), jerky body movements or uncontrolled eye movements called opsoclonus "opsoclonus-myoclonus syndrome", hypertension.

Diagnosis

Imaging Tests

Ultrasound: This is often the first imaging study to be done if a tumor is appreciated in the abdomen because it is painless and noninvasive.

CT/CAT-scan/MRI: MRI gives more detailed images than CT and ultrasound (Fig. 13.4).

Metaiodobenzylguanidine (MIBG): MIBG is a compound similar to the hormone norepinephrine, which is found specifically in sympathetic nervous tissue. MIBG can be labeled with radioactive iodine allowing it to then be visualized with scintigraphy. Thus, MIBG scans can show "hot spots" throughout the body where tumor is located. Bone scans are often done in conjunction with MIBG scans to look for bone lesions.

Additional tests: Chest X-ray to look for cancer in the lungs, bone scan or bone radiographs to look for cancer in the bones, brain MRI to look for cancer in the brain.

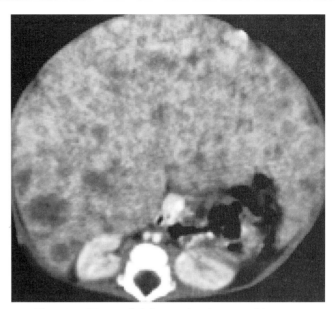

Fig. 13.4: CT scan of abdomen showing neuroblastoma with hepatic metastasis

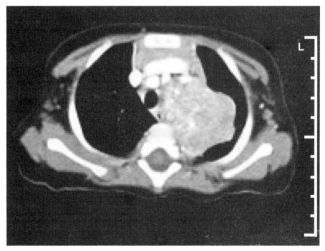

Fig.13.5: CT scan abdomen showing neuroblastoma with post-mediastinal mass

Lab Tests

Complete blood count (CBC): Blood chemistry and a blood sample is taken for estimation of two hormones, dopamine and norepinephrine, which when elevated can be a sign of neuroblastoma

24 hours urinalysis: Urine is collected for 24 hours to look for abnormal levels of homovanillic acid (HMA) and vanillyl mandelic acid (VMA), which when elevated can be a sign of neuroblastoma.

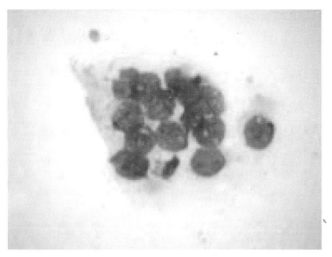

Fig. 13.6A: Neuroblastoma metastatic cell cluster in bone marrow
(For color version, see Plate 4)

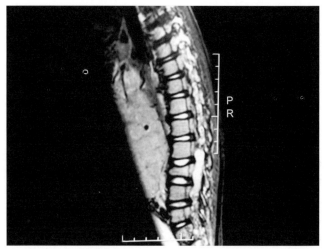

Fig. 13.6B: MRI of neuroblastoma extending to the spine

Biopsies

A tissue diagnosis is needed for definite diagnosis of neuroblastoma and to aid in staging and prognosis. Biopsies from the tumor site and bone marrow are done for specific histopathological, molecular and genetic tumor findings (Fig. 13.6A). On microscopy tumor cells are small, round and blue with rosette pattern (Homer-Wight).

Screening studies: The studies check the urine of infants for abnormal levels of catecholamines, in the hope of earlier detection to improve prognosis.

NSE: Neuron-specific enolase, is a serum marker. This is an enzyme specific to the sympathetic nervous cells from which the neuroblastoma derives.

CD44 antigen: The presence of this antigen indicates a particular developmental stage of the neuroblastoma cells.

Staging of neuroblastoma is described in the chapter of neoplasms in neonates.

Treatment

Treatment of neuroblastoma depends on stage. In low and intermediate-risk tumors, surgical removal of the primary tumor is the initial treatment and combinations of various chemotherapy drugs are added when needed. In high-risk tumors where the long-term probabilities of survival are less than 15%, treatment involves intensive combinations of chemotherapy agents, surgery, bone marrow transplantation, and radiation therapy. When these conventional modalities fail and disease recurs, novel therapies are attempted including anti-angiogenic agents, MIBG radionuclide therapy,

etc. Common chemotherapy agents are: daunorubicin, cyclophosphamide, carboplatin, and etoposide. Bone marrow transplantation with autologous BMT may be used following aggressive chemotherapy.

To detect neuroblastoma in early stage particularly during infancy, screening program was initiated in several countries, notably in Japan. But it has not improved the overall outcome of neuroblastoma.

There is also remarkable improvement in the long-term outcome of several other pediatric solid tumors, particularly in Hodgkin's and non-Hodgkin's lymphoma, rhabdomyosarcoma and different types of teratomas. Our primary aim now is to give a quality life to the survivors. To have good result, a team (Pediatric surgeon, Pediatric oncologist, Pediatric pathologist, Psychologist and Social worker) approach is essential. Pediatric pathologists play an important part in predicting the prognosis of the tumor. Immunohistochemistry is sometimes essential to identify the specific nature of the tumor. In general, risk-based strategy is planned on the basis of the stage of the tumor, age of the patient, histological features, tumor cell ploidy and molecular biology features.

Prognosis

Neuroblastoma is a clinically diverse disease. There are several factors that affect prognosis and response to therapy.

Age: Infants and younger children have a much more favorable prognosis. Children under the age of one year are more likely to have localized tumor while older children frequently have metastases at the time of diagnosis (Fig. 13.6B). In addition, younger children tend to have less aggressive tumors.

Stage: An important factor in prognosis is the extent of tumor spread at the time of diagnosis. Metastasis disease to distant organs or to the bone marrow brings a much worse prognosis with exception is stage 4 S disease. In this form of neuroblastoma found only in children less than one year of age, infants have primary tumors that can be removed by surgery and have metastases to the liver, skin, or bone marrow. Despite these metastases, the children do exceptionally well and have survival rates around 85% because the tumor often spontaneously regresses (Fig. 13.7).

Tumor histology and tumor biology: Favorable tumors are ones that are more differentiated. "Ploidy" and "MYC-N amplification" are two additional molecular genetic findings that affect prognosis.

Better prognosis has been reported in:
1. Low-stage tumor.
2. Age less than 12 months.
3. Mediastinal and pelvic tumors.
4. Hyperploidy.
5. CD 44 and PRKA expression.
6. Absence of MYCN oncogene.

SCOPE OF FURTHER IMPROVEMENT

Maintenance of cancer registry is poor in this part of the country. We must collect necessary data. It may take time but will definitely help us in long run. We must improve

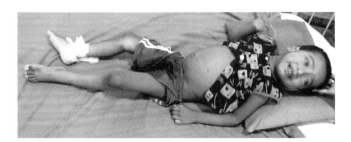

Fig. 13.7: Neuroblastoma showing good response

the supportive care. We must take part in research projects, particularly biological studies. Drugs are expensive for our poor patients. Cancer chemotherapeutic drugs must be declared as essential life-saving for children.

Availability of immunotherapy, different growth factors, stem cell therapy is likely to improve the long-term outcome of pediatric solid tumors.

SUGGESTED READING

1. Brodeur GM, Maris JM. "Neuroblastoma." In: Principles and practice of pediatric oncology. In Pizzo, PA, Poplack, DG (Eds), Lippincott Williams Wilkins, Philadelphia. 2006;933-70.
2. Goldsby RE, Matthay KK. Neuroblastoma: Evolving therapies for a disease of many faces. Goldsby and Matthay Paediatr Drugs. 2004;6:107-22.
3. Jan de Kraker. Wilms' tumor. SIOP education book published during 39th Congress of the International Society of Pediatric Oncology. 2007;38-41.
4. Katherine MK. Neuroblastoma today and tomorrow. SIOP Book. In: B Agarwal, G Perilongo, G Calminus, Tim Eden. 2007;42-6.
5. Krasin MJ, Davidoff AM. Principles of pediatric oncology, genetics of cancer and radiation therapy: Pediatric Surgery. In: Jay L Grosfeld, James A O'Neill Jr, Eric W Fonkalsrud, Arnold G Coran (Eds). Sixth edition Publishers- Mosby. 2006;1:412.
6. Matthay KK, Villablanca JG, Seeger RC, et al. Treatment of high-risk neuroblastoma with intensive chemotherapy, radiotherapy, autologous bone marrow transplantation, and 13-cis-retinoic acid. N Engl J Med. 1999;341:1165-73.
7. Parkins DM, Kramarova E, et al. International incidence of childhood cancers. Lyon, France, IARC Scientific. 1988;2:144.
8. Tagge EP, Thomas PB, Othersen HB Jr. Wilms' tumor. Pediatric Surgery. In: Jay L Grosfeld (Ed). Sixth edition, Mosby. 2006;445-66.
9. Yaris N, Mandieacioglu A, Buyukpama Kcu M. Childhood cancer in developing countries. Pediatric hematology and oncology. 2004;21:237-53.

14 Adrenal Tumors

Rakesh Mondal, Krishnendu Mukherjee

The adrenal glands are located on top of the kidneys and consist of two parts that function separately: The outer layer (cortex) and the inner area (medulla). The cortex produces three major hormones: cortisol (a glucocorticoid), aldosterone (a mineralocorticoid), and dehydroepiandrosterone (DHEA; an androgen). The medulla produces epinephrine (adrenaline), norepinephrine, and dopamine. Tumors originating from the adrenal glands are rare. Adrenal tumors, which increase hormone production, termed as functioning tumors, others are nonfunctioning. Symptoms of adrenal cancer and treatment for the condition depend on whether the tumor is functioning or nonfunctioning, and the particular type of hormone production.

INCIDENCE AND PREVALENCE

Worldwide, about 1 out of 1 million people develop adrenal cancer each year. Prevalence of the condition is slightly higher in children younger than 5 years old.

Causes and Risk Factors

The cause of adrenal cancer is unknown and most cases do not have identifiable risk factors. In some cases, heredity plays a role in the development of the disease. Li-Fraumeni syndrome and type 1 multiple endocrine neoplasia (MEN1) are genetic mutations in tumor suppressor genes that increase the risk for several types of cancer, including adrenal cancer. Genetic testing may be recommended in families with a high incidence of suspected tumor suppressor gene mutation. Other familial syndromes associated with adrenal cancer include: Gardner syndrome, Carney triad, Cowden syndrome, Familial polyposis, Turcot syndrome.

Types: Most (99%) adrenal tumors are non-cancerous adrenal cortical adenomas. These small tumors do not produce any symptoms and are diagnosed incidentally. The most common type of adrenal cancer develops in the adrenal cortex and is called adrenocortical carcinoma. Functioning adrenocortical carcinomas may produce symptoms related to increased hormone production. Nonfunctioning tumors may cause pain from pressure on abdominal organs and a mass in the abdomen. Cancers that develop in the adrenal medulla include neuroblastoma and pheochromocytoma. Only cortical tumors are described in this chapter. Other adrenal tumors are described elsewhere.

SIGNS AND SYMPTOMS

Both nonfunctioning adrenocortical carcinomas and large functioning tumors may cause the following: fever, palpable abdominal mass, persistent abdominal pain, sensation of abdominal "fullness", weight loss. Additional symptoms of functioning adrenocortical carcinoma depend on overproduction of specific hormones. Overproduction of androgens usually do not produce symptoms in men because the testicles produce testosterone, which is a more potent androgen. Rarely, gynecomastia occurs in men. Excess androgens may cause early puberty in children and masculinization in women.

A functioning adrenocortical tumor that produces excess cortisol may result in Cushing's syndrome. Approximately 30–40% of patients with Cushing's syndrome and an adrenal mass are diagnosed with adrenal cancer.

Symptoms of Cushing's syndrome include the following:
- Amenorrhea
- Bruising easily
- Excessive growth of facial and body hair in women (hirsutism)
- Flushing
- High blood pressure
- Increased blood sugar, and diabetes
- Increased body fat (adiposity) in the face, neck, and abdomen
- Loss of bone mass (osteoporosis); spinal curvature
- Severe acne
- Slowed growth rate in children
- Stretch marks (abdominal striae)
- Weakness and muscle wasting.

Conn's syndrome is caused by increased aldosterone production from a functioning tumor in the adrenal cortex. Symptoms of Conn's syndrome include the following:
- Chronic excessive thirst
- Excessive urination
- High blood pressure
- Hypokalemia.

Other symptoms include severe headaches, sweating, heart palpitations and nausea.

DIAGNOSIS

Diagnosis of adrenal cancer involves taking a medical history and performing a physical examination, blood and urine tests, imaging tests, and a biopsy. Medical history includes family history of adrenal cancer, menstrual and sexual history, and the patient's history of symptoms. Physical examination includes palpating the abdomen for evidence of an adrenal mass.

Blood and Urine Tests

Blood and urine tests are used to detect elevated levels of hormones, e.g. cortisol, aldosterone and potassium. The patient's symptoms determine which tests are performed.

Imaging Tests

Computed tomography (CT scan) and magnetic resonance imaging (MRI scan) are the imaging studies of choice used to produce images of the adrenal gland and identify abnormal enlargement or tumors. CT-scan produces detailed images of the adrenal glands, other abdominal organs, and lymph nodes. MRI uses magnetic fields to produce a cross-sectional image that detects abnormal enlargement of the adrenal gland. This test may be used to help determine if adrenal tumors are benign or cancerous.

Biopsy

Biopsy is the surgical removal of cells or tissue for microscopic evaluation. This procedure may be used to evaluate an adrenal mass for cancer cells. During biopsy, ultrasound or CT-scan is used to guide a needle into the tumor to remove cells or to do tissue biopsy. The cells are then examined under a microscope and if cancerous cells are found, the cancer is staged.

TREATMENT

Treatment for adrenal cancer depends on the stage of the disease at diagnosis. Options include surgery, chemotherapy, and radiation. Treatment for patients with functioning tumors usually involves using medications to manage symptoms.

Surgery

Surgical removal of the adrenal gland is the only cure for adrenal cancer. It is important to determine if the cancer has spread before surgery, because metastases to lymph nodes or other organs. Adrenal tumors that have not spread are sometimes removed using laparoscopic adrenalectomy.

Chemotherapy

Chemotherapy often uses a combination of drugs to destroy cancer cells. It is used as a palliative treatment for metastatic adrenal cancer and may also be used in addition to surgery (adjuvant therapy). Drugs may be administered orally or intravenously. Mitotane suppresses adrenal gland function and is the drug of choice to treat inoperable adrenal cancer. Approximately 20% of adrenal cancer patients respond to treatment with mitotane. Side-effects include gastrointestinal disturbances, e.g. loss of appetite, nausea, vomiting, diarrhea and neurological disturbances, e.g. depression, lethargy, sleepiness. When mitotane therapy fails, cisplatin may be tried, alone or combined with other agents. Drug combinations used include the following: cyclophosphamide, doxorubicin, cisplatin, fluorouracil, doxorubicin, cisplatin, cisplatin with VP-16.

Radiation Therapy

Radiation is not used as a primary treatment for adrenal cancer. It is sometimes used as a pain relieving (palliative) treatment for metastatic adrenal cancer.

Medical Management of Functioning Tumors

Treatment for patients with functioning tumors includes managing symptoms caused by increased hormone production. Increased cortisol production is often treated with aminoglutethimide or ketoconazole to inhibit cortisol synthesis. They may be used alone, or in combination with chemotherapy. Excess aldosterone production is usually treated using spironolactone. Aromatase inhibitors such as anastrozole and anti-androgens such as bicalutamide may be used to treat excessive androgen production.

PROGNOSIS

The prognosis for adrenal tumor depends on the stage of the disease. Metastatic tumors have a poor prognosis. The 5-year survival rate when surgical removal of the cancer is achieved in approximately 40%.

SUGGESTED READING

1. Kercher KW, et al. Laparoscopic adrenalectomy for pheochromocytoma. Surg Endosc. 2002;16:100.
2. Lenders JWM, et al. Biochemical diagnosis of pheochromocytoma. JAMA. 2002;287:1427.
3. Newell Price J, et al. Diagnosis and management of Cushing's syndrome. Lancet. 1999;353:2087.
4. Young WF. Minireview: Primary aldosteronism—changing concepts in diagnosis and treatment. Endocrinology. 2003;144:2208.

15 Pheochromocytomas

Rakesh Mondal, Pranab Sahana

Pheochromocytomas are tumors of adrenal medulla derived from chromaffin cells. The production of catecholamines can cause hypertensive crisis and sudden death. Patients experience symptoms that are often mistaken for other common conditions, leading to delayed diagnoses. Adrenal pheochromocytoma (PHEO) and extra-adrenal pheochromocytoma (paraganglioma, PGL) are rare tumors and malignant PHEOs and PGLs are extremely rare.

INCIDENCE

The yearly incidence of pheochromocytoma has been reported to be 1 per million population in world literature. About 40 to 45% of these cases were diagnosed at autopsy. Ten to twenty percent of all tumors in children reported to have pheochromocytoma.

At least 8% of incidentally discovered tumors have metastasized by the time of their detection. Genetic syndromes, predisposing to bilateral pheochromocytoma or multiple PGLs, commonly present in childhood. Approximately, 20 to 30% of all patients with pheochromocytoma have been found to harbor germline mutations.

Rule of 10: Approximately, 10% of pheochromocytomas are extra-adrenal. Ten percent of them encountered in children. Ten to twenty percent had familial association. 10% of them had either bilateral or multiple. Recurrence is seen in 10% commonly in extra-adrenal. 10% had malignant potential. 10% of them discovered incidentally during radioimaging for other reasons.

CLINICAL FEATURES

They usually present between 6 to 14 years of age. Male to female ratio is 2:1. The classical triad of symptoms are described as headache, palpitations and perspiration. Paroxysmal hypertension, blurring of vision, nausea, vomiting, anxiety, chest pain, flushing, paresthesia, etc. are other common symptoms. Unlike the case in most other tumors, histopathology cannot accurately determine whether a given pheochromocytoma is benign or malignant. Even the presence of vascular invasion does not predict metastases. Efforts have been made to predict the metastatic potential of adrenal pheochromocytoma on the basis of histology. The Pheochromocytoma of the Adrenal Gland Scaled Score (PASS) considers multiple factors in assessing a given adrenal pheochromocytoma's likelihood of having metastasized. Pheochromocytomas were found to be more aggressive and likely to metastasize when they had a combination of the following characteristics: vascular or capsular invasion, increased mitotic rate, atypical mitoses, necrosis, high cellularity, hyperchromasia, tumor cell spindling, large nests of diffuse growth, cellular monotony, and profound nuclear pleomorphism.

Other methodologies have been used to determine a given tumor's potential for metastasis. Serum levels of catecholamines, metanephrines, and chromogranin.

One cannot reliably distinguish benign from malignant tumors prior to resection. However, when tumor markers are found to be persistently or recurrently high, months or years after the pheochromocytoma resection, metastases or new primary tumors must be suspected.

Neuron-specific enolase (NSE) is a neuroendocrine glycolytic enzyme. Serum levels of NSE have been reported to be normal in patients with benign pheochromocytoma and elevated in about half of the patients with malignant pheochromocytoma. However, NSE levels are related to tumor burden, rather than malignancy therefore, the clinical utility of NSE levels remains unproven. At this point, only the presence of detectable metastases defines a pheochromocytoma as being malignant. However, even this feature may be misleading, because metastases may not be detected at the time of the primary tumor resection. Also, patients with familial germline mutations can develop PGLs at a later date in different locations, which may be mistaken for metastases or which may themselves metastasize.

DIFFERENTIAL DIAGNOSIS

The differential diagnosis includes benign paragangliomas, multicentric paragangliomas, second pheochromocytomas, other malignancies, etc. Patients with MEN-2 may have concurrent medullary thyroid carcinoma. Patients with NF-1 usually have concurrent neurofibromas and may develop gliomas and malignant peripheral nerve sheath tumors. Any suspicious mass lesion that is not demonstrated on 132I-MIBG or18F-dopamine PET scanning should be considered for a CT-guided fine-needle aspiration biopsy for definitive diagnosis. von-Hippel Lindau disease has association with pheochromocytoma.

DIAGNOSIS

Urine and Blood Tumor Markers

Most patients with recurrent or metastatic pheochromocytoma have elevations in plasma or urinary normetanephrine, but some metastases from adrenal pheochromocytomas secrete mostly epinephrine and metanephrine. Plasma fractionated free metanephrine is probably the most sensitive test. Other important tests are measurement of vanillylmandelic acid (VMA). Plasma free metanephrine is one of the best biochemical markers of tumor. The sensitivity of tests increases with collection at the onset of paroxysm. Some conditions like excercise,

renal failure, psychosis, drugs like acetaminophen, captopril, metodopramide, labetalol, etc. foods like bananas, tea, coffee, coco, etc. increase catecholamine measurements. Drugs like clonidine, MAOI, salicylates, etc. decrease catecholamine measurements.

Some patients with "nonsecretory" metastases have normal plasma and urine fractionated metanephrines. Serum chromogranin A (CgA) is usually elevated in patients with both secretory and "nonsecretory" variety. Serum CgA is usually elevated in patients with clinically significant metastases. It is an excellent tumor marker for most patients, reflecting tumor burden. Fractionated urine and plasma metanephrines and serum CgA usually normalize by two weeks after a successful resection. However, patients with normal postoperative tests may still harbor small or nonsecretory metastases.

Scanning

MIBG and 111In-DTPA-Octreotide Scanning. Benzylguanidine was first developed as a guanethidine derivative for potential use as an adrenergic-blocking antihypertensive agent. 131I-metaiodobenzylguanidine (131I-MIBG) was developed for detecting adrenal pheochromocytomas. Most pheochromocytoma metastases can be detected on whole-body scintigraphy with MIBG, tagged with a radioisotope of iodine. 123I-MIBG scanning with single-photon emission computed tomography (SPECT) is more sensitive than 131I-MIBG. MIBG is excreted in the urine, bladder paragangliomas may not be visualized. 123I-MIBG SPECT imaging of the bladder during bladder irrigation is sometimes required to clarify. Another nuclear imaging technique used to locate metastases is 111In-DTPA-octreotide.

DRUG THERAPY

About 50% of patients have persistent hypertension after resection of the tumor. Phenoxybenzamine is effective and tolerable for short periods preoperatively, most patients experience side effects from phenoxybenzamine, such as fatigue and nasal congestion, making the drug less suitable for chronic therapy usual dose is 40–120 mg daily. Phenoxybenzamine accumulates in the fetus more than the mother, with a fetal-maternal concentration ratio of 1.6:1 and has been associated with neonatal hypotension. Calcium channel blockers are effective and tolerated better than alpha-blockade. They may be used alone or in combination with tolerated doses of alpha-blockers or other antihypertensives. Other antihypertensive medications may be effective as add-on therapy for hypertensive patients with malignant pheochromocytoma or paraganglioma. Elevated catecholamine levels stimulate renin secretion, which increases angiotensin II production and aggravates hypertension. Adding an angiotensin receptor blocker (ARB) or angiotensin-converting enzyme (ACE) inhibitor is often an effective measure. Beta-blocker therapy is given to patients with sustained tachycardia or intermittent tachyarrhythmias, after initiation of antihypertensive therapy with alpha-blocker. Labetalol is avoided, since it causes misleading elevations in urinary catecholamine determinations in some assays. Labetalol also interferes with norepinephrine uptake-1, and patients taking labetalol should discontinue the drug for at least one week before PET, MIBG scintigraphy. Patients with functioning malignant pheochromocytoma are advised to observe certain precautions. Patients are advised to avoid activities that might put physical pressure on large soft tissue tumors, precipitating catecholamine release, and hypertensive crisis. Patients must be counseled to avoid decongestants, cocaine, MAO inhibitors, and other drugs that can provoke a hypertensive crisis. Intravenous ionic contrast for CT scanning may precipitate hypertensive crisis in patients with secretory tumors in contrast to nonionic intravenous contrast.

The most commonly used chemotherapy regimen uses a combination of cyclophosphamide, vincristine, and dacarbazine/DTIC (CVD). Cyclophosphamide 750 mg/m^2 and vincristine 1.4 mg/m^2 are given on day 1, and dacarbazine 600 mg/m^2 is given on days 1 and 2. The cycle is repeated every 21 days. Chemotherapy regimen, given every 21 days, was reported to cause complete or partial remissions in majority of patients. Despite some success with chemotherapy for patients with malignant pheochromocytoma, continuous cycles must be given on a long-term basis, to avoid recurrence. Zoledronic acid is a third-generation bisphosphonate. Patients with bone metastases are empirically treated with zoledronic acid. Zoledronic acid inhibits osteoclastic bone resorption and has proven useful. Zoledronic acid therapy is generally well tolerated, with the exception of transient flu-like symptoms within a week following the infusion; hypocalcemia and thrombotic thrombocytopenic purpura, and jaw osteonecrosis.

SURGERY

For patients having with an isolated adrenal pheochromocytoma, a total adrenalectomy is more likely to prevent recurrence than a selective adrenal-sparing surgical procedure, which is attempted for patients with bilateral pheochromocytomas or familial disease. For patients who are found to have metastases at the time of diagnosis, it is usually best to resect the primary tumor as well as large metastases. The surgical reduction of tumor burden can reduce symptoms and is presumed to prolong survival. These tumors can be indolent and debulking improves local symptoms, catecholamine levels and hypertension. Some tumors, particularly retroperitoneal paragangliomas in the abdomen or pelvis, can become massive, encasing major blood vessels and other organs. Surgical resection of massive paragangliomas can be extremely difficult and the patients must be normotensive preoperatively before hand.

Large invasive pheochromocytomas and paragangliomas are extremely vascular, causing serious problems with hemostasis and making tumor resection difficult. Preoperative arterial embolization has proven feasible for some secretory tumors. However, large tumors, particularly massive retroperitoneal paragangliomas that have encased major blood vessels is difficult to operate.

RADIATION THERAPY

External beam radiation therapy completely abolishes tumoral avidity for MIBG and renders subsequent MIBG scanning insensitive and makes 131I-MIBG ineffective therapy. Therefore, if 131I-MIBG therapy is planned, radiation should not be given to metastases displaying

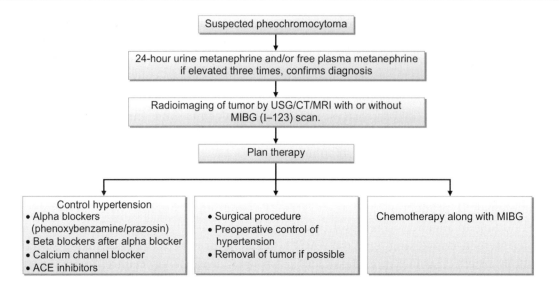

MIBG avidity prior to 131I-MIBG therapy. External beam radiation therapy may be given subsequently to osseous metastases, if 131I-MIBG therapy is ineffective. Radiation therapy has proven moderately efficacious for relieving pain and inhibiting the growth of bone metastases.

ADJUVANT THERAPIES

In inoperable or metastatic large tumors, high dose 1-131 MIBG is used with other therapy. Vascular endothelial growth factors (VEGFs) are pro-angiogenesis molecules. VEGFs bind to vascular VEGF receptors (VEGFRs), causing receptor dimerization and activation of receptor tyrosine kinase that induces vascular proliferation, a necessary process for tumorigenesis and metastasis. Potential anti-VEGF drug therapies include monoclonal antibodies against VEGF. A VEGF monoclonal antibody, bevacizumab, has been approved by the FDA as a first-line treatment for colorectal cancer.

New cancer therapies are targeting VEGF receptors (VEGFRs). Cyclooxygenase-2 is over-expressed in pheochromocytoma and Cox-2 inhibitors might be helpful in reversing resistance to chemotherapy. Clinical trials of such potential anti-VEGF/VEGFR and adjuvant therapies are required for patients with metastatic tumors.

PROGNOSIS

Patients with benign pheochromocytomas even have an increased mortality rate. Although the perioperative mortality rate for patients undergoing unilateral benign adrenal pheochromocytoma resection is low with optimal medical preparation, anesthesia, surgical, and postoperative care, these patients experience a long-term mortality rate that is higher than that of age-matched controls. Patients with metastatic pheochromocytoma, treated with conventional radiation and chemotherapy, have been reported to have a mean 5-year survival rate of about 44%. The prognosis is worse for those patients whose metastatic disease is discovered at a late stage. Malignant tumors vary tremendously in their aggressiveness, secretory capacity, and sites of metastases. Proper chemotherapy with adjuvant I–123MIBG treatment have increased 5 years survival rate to 75% in some center.

SUGGESTED READING

1. Argiris A, et al. PET scan assessment of chemotherapy response in metastatic paraganglioma. Am J Clin Oncol. 2003;26:563-6.
2. Averbuch SD, et al. Malignant pheochromocytoma: effective treatment with a combination of cyclophosphamide, vincristine, and dacarbazine. Ann Intern Med. 1988;109:267-73.

3. Baguet JP, et al. Circumstances of discovery of phaeochromocytoma: a retrospective study of 41 consecutive patients. Eur J Endocrinol. 2004;1 50:681-6.

4. Bravo EL. Pheochromocytoma: an approach to antihypertensive management. Ann NY Acad Sci. 2002; 970:1-10.

5. Ciftci AO, et al. Pheochromocytoma in children. J Pediatr Surg. 2001;36:447-52.

6. Diner EK, et al. Partial adrenalectomy: The National Cancer Institute Experience. Urology. 2005;66:19-23.

7. Fitzgerald PA, et al. Malignant pheochromocytomas and paragangliomas; A phase II Study of therapy with high-dose 131I-metaiodobenzylguanidine (131I-MIBG); Ann NY Acad. Sci. 2006;1073:465-90.

8. Ilias. Anatomical and functional imaging of metastatic pheochromocytoma. Ann NY. 2004;1018: 495-504.

9. Michalson MD. Bisphosphonates for treatment and prevention of bone metastases. J Clin. Oncol. 2005;23: 8219-24.

10. Minami T, et al. An effective use of magnesium sulfate for intraoperative management of laparoscopic adrenalectomy for pheochromocytoma in a pediatric patient. Anesth Analg. 2002;95:1243-4.

11. Misra AK, et al. Pheochromocytoma in children and adolescents. An institutional experience. Indian Pediatr. 2002;39:51-7.

12. Mukherjee JJ, et al. Pheochromocytoma: effect of nonionic contrast medium in CT on circulating catecholamine levels. Radiology. 1997;202:227-31.

13. Oishi S. Elevated serum neuron-specific enolase in patients with malignant pheochromocytoma. Cancer. 1988;61:1167-70.

14. Pacak K, et al. Functional imaging of endocrine tumors: role of positron emission tomography. Endocr Rev. 2004;25:569-80.

15. Patel SR, et al. A 15-year experience with chemotherapy of patients with paraganglioma. Cancer. 1995;76: 1476-80.

16. Rao F, et al. Malignant pheochromocytoma: chromaffin granule transmitters and response to treatment. Hypertension. 2000;36:1045-52.

17. Salmenkivi K, et al. Increased expression of cyclooxygenase-2 in malignant pheochromocytomas. J Clin Endocrinol Metab. 2001;86:5615-9.

18. Santeiro ML, et al. Phenoxybenzamine placental transfer during the third trimester. Ann Pharmacother. 1996;30:1249-51.

19. Thompson LDR. Pheochromocytoma of the adrenal gland scaled score (PASS) to separate benign from malignant neoplasms. Am J Surg Pathol. 2002;26: 551-6.

20. Zielke A, et al. VEGF-mediated angiogenesis of human pheochromocytomas is associated to malignancy and inhibited by anti-VEGF antibodies in experimental tumors. Surgery. 2002;132:1056-60.

16 Soft Tissue Sarcoma

Rakesh Mondal, Pradip Kumar Mitra

Sarcomas are large group of malignant tumors arising from primarily of mesenchymal cell origins in extra skeletal non-epithelial location with distinct clinical features. Sarcomas are broadly divided into two categories; sarcomas of soft tissues and sarcomas of bone. Soft tissue sarcomas can develop in every type of soft tissue in the body, including nerves, fat, muscle and blood vessels. Sarcomas can also occur in almost any organ, including the lungs, heart, gastrointestinal tract, liver, kidney and the extremities. The soft tissue sarcomas of children arise primarily from the connective tissues of the body, like fibrous tissue, adipose tissue, and muscle tissue.

Collectively sarcomas account for fifth most common solid pediatric malignancies. Rhabdomyosarcoma (RMS) is the most common soft tissue sarcoma among children 0–14 years, representing nearly 50% of soft tissue sarcomas for this age. There are two major types of rhabdomyosarcoma: embryonal and alveolar. These two subtypes tended to occur at different body sites. The incidence of embryonal rhabdomyosarcoma was higher among children 0–4 years, while the incidence of alveolar rhabdomyosarcoma was similar throughout childhood. Other types of soft tissue sarcomas are rare and the incidence is higher in adolescents compared to younger children. Among these are the fibrosarcomas, malignant fibrous histiocytoma, synovial sarcoma, leiomyosarcoma, liposarcoma, and others. For infants, the most common soft tissue sarcoma is embryonal rhabdomyosarcoma. Males have slightly higher incidence rates for soft tissue sarcomas than females.

The overall 5-year survival rate for children with rhabdomyosarcoma was good. Younger children had higher survival rates than older children and adolescents, and children with embryonal rhabdomyosarcoma had a more favorable prognosis than children with alveolar rhabdomyosarcoma. Congenital anomalies and genetic conditions are the only known risk factors.

More than half of soft tissue sarcomas occur in the arms and legs. Other common sites include the trunk, the abdomen and the head and neck region. Sarcomas can also occur in cartilage and bones are discussed in section of bone tumors.

RISK FACTORS FOR SOFT TISSUE SARCOMAS IN CHILDREN

a. Congenital anomalies: There is some concordance with the anatomic location of RMS and major birth defects. One autopsy study showed a significant percentage of children and adolescents with RMS to have at least one congenital anomaly.
b. Genetic conditions: Li-Fraumeni syndrome (associated with p53 mutations) and neurofibromatosis (associated with NF1 mutations).
c. Socioeconomic status: Low socioeconomic status is associated with increased risk.
d. Ionizing radiation: Diagnostic X-rays during pregnancy were associated with increased risk in one study.
e. Parental use of drugs: Parental use of marijuana and cocaine during the pregnancy was associated with increased risk. Prolonged exposure to vinyl chloride or chlorophenol, etc. may also predispose sarcomas.
f. Viral infection: Human herpesvirus and associated with Kaposi sarcoma.

SYMPTOMS OF SARCOMA

Sarcomas close to the surface of the skin may be easily detected, but those deeper in the body may not become apparent. Only about half of sarcomas are detected in the early stages before they spread. Symptoms may include:

a. A lump that appears to be growing in size
b. Abdominal pain
c. Blood in the stool or vomitus
d. Unexplained anemia
e. Uneven posture
f. Coincidental finding after some injury
g. Pressure symptoms

Differential diagnosis of soft tissue sarcomas includes lymphoma, melanoma, desmoids and benign lesions like leiomyomas, neuromas, lipomas, etc.

TYPES OF SARCOMA

More than fifty different histologic categories of soft tissue sarcoma have been recognized. Mesenchymal cells normally mature into skeletal muscle, smooth muscle, fat, fibrous tissue, bone and cartilage. The malignant counterparts of normal soft tissue cells include: fibrosarcomas (fibrous tissue), liposarcomas (adipose tissue), leiomyosarcomas (smooth muscle), rhabdomyosarcomas (striated muscle), angiosarcomas (vascular) and malignant hemangiopericytoma (blood vessels), synovial sarcomas (synovial tissue), and chondrosarcomas (cartilage). Tumors derived from peripheral nervous system tissues are also included within the soft tissue sarcoma category, including malignant peripheral nerve sheath tumors termed as malignant schwannoma and neurofibrosarcoma), and extraosseous Ewing's sarcoma. In children, soft tissue sarcomas generally are classified as either rhabdomyosarcomas (RMS) or non-rhabdomyosarcomas (non-RMS), with the non-RMS being further divided into multiple histologic subtypes.

International Classification of Childhood Cancer (ICCC): Soft Tissue Sarcomas

A. Rhabdomyosarcoma subcategory
  i. Embryonal rhabdomyosarcoma
  ii. Alveolar rhabdomyosarcoma
  iii. Rhabdomyosarcoma, NOS, pleomorphic, etc.

B. Fibrosarcoma subcategory
  i. Fibrosarcoma
  ii. Infantile fibrosarcoma
  iii. Malignant fibrous histiocytoma
  iv. Dermatofibrosarcoma
  v. Malignant peripheral nerve sheath tumor

C. Kaposi's sarcoma

D. Other specified soft tissue sarcoma
  i. Liposarcoma
  ii. Leiomyosarcoma
  iii. Malignant mesenchymoma
  iv. Synovial sarcoma
  v. Hemangiosarcoma and malignant hemangioendothelioma
  vi. Hemangiopericytoma, malignant
  vii. Alveolar soft part sarcoma
  viii. Chondrosarcoma
  ix. Ewing's (extraosseous) family.

E. Unspecified Subcategory

The various soft tissue sarcomas are associated with distinctive chromosomal alterations that can be used in some instances to support or confirm a specific diagnosis. Embryonal RMS tumor cells often show extra chromosome copies, i.e. hyperdiploidy and loss of heterozygosity involving a specific site on the short arm of chromosome 11. Alveolar RMS tumor cells have translocations involving the FKHR gene on the long arm of chromosome 13 with genes of the PAX family on either chromosome 2 (PAX 3) or chromosome 1 (PAX 7). Many of the non-RMS also show characteristic chromosome translocations. Infantile fibrosarcoma tumor cells contain the same chromosomal abnormalities as the tumor cells of congenital mesoblastic nephroma, with both possessing t(12;15)(p13;q25)-associated ETV6-NTRK3 gene fusions. Synovial sarcomas are virtually always associated with translocations that fuse the SYT gene on chromosome 18 with the SSX-1 or SSX-2 genes on the X chromosome. Extraosseous Ewing's sarcoma and peripheral neuroectodermal tumors have translocations involving the EWS gene on chromosome 22 and either the FLI1 gene on chromosome 11 or the ERG gene on chromosome 21. Malignant peripheral nerve sheath tumors known as neurofibrosarcomas, malignant schwannomas, and neurogenic sarcomas are associated with neurofibromatosis 1 (NF1), the gene for which is located on the long arm of chromosome 17.

Molecular characterization of soft tissue sarcomas and diagnostic chromosomal abnormality involved are:

a. Rhabdomyosarcoma, Embryonal: Hyperdiploidy, abnormality at chromosome 11p15. Unidentified gene at chromosome band 11p15.

b. Rhabdomyosarcoma, Alveolar: t(2;13) or t(1;13) FKHR on chromosome 13 and PAX 3 (chromosome 2) or PAX7 (chromosome 1).

c. Infantile fibrosarcoma: t(12;15) TEL (ETV6) gene on chromosome 12 and NTRK3 (TRKC) on chromosome 15.

d. Dermatofibrosarcoma protuberans: t(17;22) Platelet-derived growth factor b-chain (PDGFB) gene on chromosome 17 and collagen type I alpha 1 (COL1A1) on chromosome 22.

e. Malignant peripheral nerve sheath tumors, i.e. neurofibrosarcomas and malignant schwannomas: Abnormalities of chromosome 17. Neurofibromatosis 1 (NF1) gene.

f. Synovial sarcoma: t(X;18) SYT on chromosome 18 and SSX-1 or SSX-2 on the X chromosome.

g. Liposarcoma: t(12;16), FUS gene on chromosome 16 and CHOP gene on chromosome 12.

h. Chondrosarcoma, Myxoid: t(9;22) EWS gene on chromosome 22 and TEC gene on chromosome 9.

i. Extra-osseous Ewing's sarcoma and peripheral neuroectodermal tumor (PNET): t(11;22) EWS gene on chromosome 22 and FLI gene on chromosome 11.

j. Alveolar soft tissue sarcoma: t(X; 17) Unidentified gene at chromosome band 17q25.

There are more than 30 clinically different types of malignant soft tissue sarcoma. They can be simply categorized according to the types of cells affected: fat, smooth muscle, skeletal muscle, nerve tissue, joints, blood and/or lymph vessels and fibrous tissue. There is also a category for sarcomas of undetermined or mixed type. Some of the most common sarcoma types are listed below:

Liposarcoma appears as a malignant form of fatty tissue and is most often found in the legs, or the posterior abdominal area. Liposarcomas can be slow-growing or aggressive.

Leiomyosarcoma appears as a malignant form of smooth muscle, which is found in the lining of the gastrointestinal tract, uterus, blood vessels, skin and other organs. The abdomen, extremities, and posterior abdominal area are the most common site for leiomyosarcomas, but internal organs and blood vessels may also be affected.

Pleomorphic sarcoma and malignant fibrosarcoma occur in fibrous tissue in the extremities. It has a tendency to spread to distant areas of the body, particularly the lungs.

Rhabdomyosarcoma has the appearance of rhabdomyoblasts, immature cells that form the body's skeletal muscles. It occurs in two age groups: children under 5 years of age, and adolescents. It is the most common soft tissue cancer in children.

Fibrosarcoma originates in the fibrous tissue found at the end of long bones in the arms and legs, and in the trunk. Fibrosarcomas generally occur in adults, but infants and the elderly can also be affected.

Synovial sarcomas are composed of cells that are similar to cells that line joints. These tumors are usually found in the knees, ankles, hips and shoulders. Adolescents and young adults are most likely to have synovial sarcomas.

Gastrointestinal stromal tumors (GIST) occur in the interstitial cells of Cajal (ICC), which are special cells that line the walls of the gastrointestinal tract. These cells signal muscles to contract to move food and liquid along the digestive tract. More than half of GIST tumors are found in the stomach, but can also occur in the small intestine, esophagus, colon and rectum.

DIAGNOSIS AND TREATMENT

Soft tissue sarcomas can be difficult to classify, and the accurate diagnosis is possible with a biopsy. A sample of the suspected tumor is taken with a needle and inspected under a microscope. Images with a CT scan MRI or X-ray are generally taken after diagnosis to determine the size and location of the tumor. Biopsy may be incisional core or excisional type.

Surgery is the most common treatment for soft tissue sarcomas. Advances in surgical limb-sparing techniques have greatly reduced the need for amputations. Only about 5% of sarcoma patients will lose a limb to disease.

Evaluation for postoperative rehabilitation is needed for all patients with extremity sarcoma. If a patient cannot be surgically operated, preoperative RT and chemotherapy is to be considered as alternative option. The surgeon and pathologist should always try to include surgical margins in evaluating a resected specimen. Margins less than one cm is to be carefully evaluated for postoperative therapy. Resection may be required to get optimum margins. Amputation should only be done in presence of extensive soft tissue mass and or skin involvement, major arterial involvement, extensive bony involvement, failed preoperative therapy or recurrence after prior radiotherapy, etc.

Radiation therapy as a stand-alone treatment for sarcoma is not common, and may only be used in patients who are not healthy enough for surgery or to ease pain and other symptoms of disease. In some cases, radiation may be used before surgery to shrink the tumor. Total dose of RT should be determined by normal tissue tolerance. Usual dose of preoperative radiotherapy is 50 Gy. Intraoperative or postoperative boost with brachytherapy is recommended for positive margins. Preoperative radiotherapy has advantages like treatment volume is smaller reduce seeding during surgical manipulation, capsular thickening and subsequent easy resection and less recurrence. The disadvantages being problem in wound healing. A single intraoperative dose to the tumor bed of 10–16 Gy, based on margins can be delivered immediately after resection. External beam radiotherapy may be an alternative to brachytherapy or intraoperative radiation. The dose used are 10–14 Gy for close margins, 16–20 Gy for microscopically positive margins and 20–26 Gy for positive margins. Postoperative radiotherapy has been to improve local control in patients with high grade extremity soft tissue sarcomas with positive surgical margins. External beam radiotherapy is delivered to large fields after surgical healing is complete to doses of 50 Gy.

Chemotherapy may be used as a primary treatment for sarcoma or in combination with surgery or radiation. Treating soft tissue sarcomas usually requires a combination of two or more chemotherapy drugs. The commonly used drugs are:

A. Extremity/Retroperitoneal
  i. Combination regimens:
    a. AD (Adriamycin, Dacarbazine)
    b. AIM (Adriamycin, Ifosfamide, Mesna)
    c. MAID (Adriamycin, Ifosfamide, Mesna, Dacarbazine)
  ii. Single agents:
    a. Adriamycin
    b. Ifosfamide
    c. Epirubicin
    d. Dacarbazine
B. Angiosarcomas:
    a. Paclitaxel
    b. Docetaxel
    c. Vinorelbine
C. Gastrointestinal stromal tumor GIST
    a. Imatinib mesylate
    b. Sunitinib malate
D. Desmoids:
    a. Sulindac and NSAIDs
    b. Tamoxifen
    c. Adriamycin
    d. Imatinib mesylate.

RHABDOMYOSARCOMA

Rhabdomyosarcoma is thought to arise from immature mesenchymal cells that are committed to skeletal muscle lineage. Among the extracranial solid tumors of childhood, RMS is the third most common neoplasm after neuroblastoma and Wilms' tumor, comprising one- fifth of all solid tumors. Almost two-thirds of cases of RMS are diagnosed in children <6 years of age although there is another mid-adolescence peak (Fig. 16.1). It is slightly more common in males than in females (1.3–1.4:1). It is ubiquitous occurring almost everywhere but most commonly in the head and neck and the genitourinary (GU) areas. There are certain distinctive clusters of features regarding age at diagnosis, site of primary and histology. The head and neck tumors are most common in children younger than 8 years of age and if arising in the orbit, are almost always of embryonal histology (Fig. 16.2). On the other hand, the extremity tumors are more commonly seen in adolescents and are more frequently of alveolar histology.

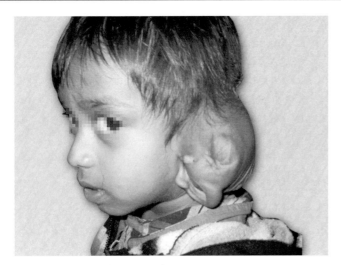

Fig.16.1: Soft tissue sarcoma

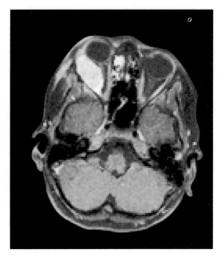

Fig.16.2: CT scan of brain showing orbital rhabdomyosarcoma

Pathology

Rhabdomyosarcomas are grossly firm, nodular and of variable size and consistency. They are well circumscribed but not encapsulated and often tend to infiltrate extensively into adjacent tissues. Sarcoma botryoides subtype has characteristic grape-like appearance arising from a mucosa lined area. Histologically RMS falls into the category of small round cell tumor. The standard classification is still the one proposed by Horn and Enterline in 1958, which divided the tumor into four subgroups: embryonal, alveolar, botryoid and pleomorphic and noted that botryoid was actually a subtype of embryonal. Since there was no overall agreement among the pathologists using the conventional classification, therefore, an international classification system for childhood RMS was proposed. This system is being used in all new IRS studies beginning IRS IV. The histologic distribution of the tumor in IRS III is shown in. Light microscopy diagnosis of RMS is based on the identification of cross-striations, characteristic of skeletal muscle, or characteristic rhabdomyoblasts. Cross-striations are seen in 50–60% of the cases. Histologically embryonal rhabdomyosarcoma (ERMS) is composed of rhabdomyoblasts and small round cells. Rhabdomyoblast, the more mature of the embryonal component, is characterized by bright eosinophilic cytoplasm. Sarcoma botryoides and spindle cell variant are two subtypes of embryonal RMS. Alveolar RMS

(ARMS) consist of rhabdomyoblasts mixed with a larger round cell with prominent eosinophilic cytoplasm. The tumor grows in cords and produces cleft like spaces, namely alveoli. The pleomorphic RMS, which is rare in children show anaplastic cells present in large aggregates or as diffuse sheets. It occurs in the extremities and the trunk. Electron microscopy and immunohistochemical analysis of tumors are now useful tools for demonstrating characteristics of RMS, especially when light microscopy is inconclusive. The diagnostic EM features of RMS are visible z-bands. Skeletal muscle or muscle-specific proteins, like antidesmin, muscle-specific actin and Myo D can be identified by immunohistochemical staining. Monoclonal antibodies, like those to desmin, muscle specific actin, sarcomeric actin and myoglogin have also been used to confirm the myogenic lineage with very good specificity and sensitivity. Monoclonal antibodies against Myo D can be used in frozen section analysis. The ERMS and ARMS have been associated with distinct clinical characteristics and genetic alterations. ARMS is associated with 2;13 or 1;13 chromosomal translocations, which generate PAX3-FKHR and PAX7-FKHR fusion proteins respectively.

International Classification System for Childhood Rhabdomyosarcomas

I. Superior Prognosis

a. Botryoid
b. Spindle cell

II. Intermediate Prognosis

a. Embryonal

III. Poor Prognosis

a. Alveolar

b. Undifferentiated sarcomas

Clinical Staging

It is critical to assess the extent of tumor in every patient as the therapy and prognosis depends on the degree to which the mass has spread beyond the primary site. Several surgicopathologic staging systems have been used historically, but the clinical group staging system, developed by IRS in 1972 has been most widely used.

Patterns of Spread

The tumor spreads locally to invade adjacent structures and may spread distantly via lymphatics and hematogenous routes. Approximately 15% children with RMS present with metastatic disease and their prognosis has not improved over the last few years. The most frequent sites of distant metastases are lymph nodes, lungs, bone marrow, bones, central nervous system, heart, liver and the breast. The lung is the most frequent site of metastases (40–50%) and majority (74%) of these have bilateral metastases. Less common sites, either isolated or in conjunction with multi-metastatic disease, are bone marrow (20–30%), bone (10%) and depending on the site of primary tumor, lymph node. Though visceral metastases are rare, but in cases of treatment failures, predominantly, visceral metastasis (e.g. brain or liver) may be seen.

Prognostic Factors

The most important prognostic variables identified appear to be the extent of disease, i.e. patients with TNM stage IV fares worse than others. Among localized RMS, those tumors, which are completely excised surgically have better survival rate than those with microscopic residue. Those with gross residual tumors fare less well. Histology is also an important prognostic factor. Five-year survival is related to the histology with 95% for sarcoma botryoides, 75% for pleomorphic sarcoma, 66% for embryonal, 54% for alveolar and 40% for undifferentiated

RMS. Other unfavorable prognostic variables are older age at diagnosis, presence of regional LN metastases for extremity and paratesticular tumors, presence of extensive bony erosions in cranial parameningeal tumors, DNA proliferative activity and diploid embryonal tumors.

Metastatic disease is the single most important predictor of clinical outcome in patients with RMS. Children with metastatic RMS have a poorer prognosis.

Principles of Treatment of RMS

There are three modalities of treating children with RMS. These are surgery, radiation therapy for control of residual bulk or microscopic tumor and systemic combination chemotherapy for primary cytoreduction and eradication of gross and micrometastases.

Surgical Management

Surgery includes complete resection of the primary tumor. If microscopic residual disease is found after initial resection, re-excision of the area is indicated before any other nonsurgical management. Debulking procedures have no value as initial biopsy and neo-adjuvant therapy results in shrinkage of the tumor allowing complete resection at second look operation.

Second-look procedures are required in two clinical situations: (1) to pathologically verify the completeness of an apparently complete clinical radiologic remission and (2) to resect any residual viable tumor cells that have survived induction chemotherapy and local RT.

Radiation Therapy

Radiation therapy (RT) is a major tool in the treatment of RMS. It can eradicate residual tumor cells, especially in the head and neck region and the pelvis. According to IRSG protocols all RMS should get RT to achieve long-term local control of tumors. The dose delivered may differ depending on many factors. The International Society of Pediatric Oncology (SIOP) differs in this as shown clearly by their study MMT-84. The major difference in therapeutic approach between MMT-84 and IRSG studies was the omission of radiotherapy in patients with nonmetastatic RMS who achieved complete remission with chemotherapy alone. However, RT was given to patients <5 years of age and having parameningeal tumors and to patients more than 12 years of age having tumors at any site.

Chemotherapy

All patients with RMS must receive combination chemotherapy as there is ample evidence that the adjuvant or neoadjuvant therapy significantly improves survival. The chemotherapy should begin as soon as possible after diagnostic studies are completed or primary excision done, as the major role of chemotherapy is the eradication of microscopic foci of disease, thereby improving both local control and survival. Preoperative chemotherapy may also be used in unresectable tumors to reduce their size. The current gold standard frontline chemotherapy consists of vincristine, actinomycin D and cyclophosphamide (VAC). Two conventional regimes, which are most commonly used are: intensive vincristine/actinomycin D and pulse vincristine/actinomycin D/cyclophosphamide (VAC).

Ifosfamide, as a single agent, is an active drug against RMS. Irinotecan, a topoisomerase I inhibitor, also appears to have promising activity against RMS, with minimal hematopoietic toxicity.

NON-RMS SOFT TISSUE SARCOMAS (NRSTS) IN CHILDREN

The rarity and histologic heterogeneity of NRSTS in children preclude study of their natural history and response to therapy. NRSTS like RMS can arise in any part of the body, but the most common sites are extremities, trunk, abdomen and pelvis. The most frequent histologic types are synovial sarcoma. Some common and uncommon NRSTS seen in children.

Common

- Synovial sarcoma
- Fibrosarcoma
- Peripheral neuroectodermal tumor
- Malignant fibrous histiocytoma
- Leiomyosarcoma
- Neurogenic tumors
  - Malignant schwanoma
  - Neurofibrosarcoma
  - Malignant peripheral nerve sheath tumor (PNET).

Rare

- Angiosarcoma
- Hemangiopericytoma
- Epithelioid cell sarcoma
- Malignant mesenchymoma
- Extraskeletal chondrosarcoma

In the extremities the tumor occurs mostly in the lower limbs. While most of the extremity NRSTS in children are synovial sarcomas, tumors of the trunk are predominantly malignant fibrous histiocytomas (MFH), or neurogenic in origin.

Prognostic Factors for NRSTS

The prognostic factors for children with NRSTS include the presence of or absence of metastatic disease, surgical respectability of the lesion, tumor histologic grade, tumor invasiveness and size of the lesion.

Clinical Evaluation and Staging of NRSTS

In all children suspected to have NRSTS the clinical evaluation should include routine hemograms, renal and liver function tests, bone scans and bone marrow examination. CT or MRI scan is considered the imaging modality of choice for the evaluation of local and regional disease, particularly in the extremities, the pelvis and head and neck regions.

The staging system currently used for NRSTS is the same as the modified TNM staging system used for RMS.

Treatment and Outcome of NRSTS

During the past few years, the surgical management of these tumors has undergone a considerable evolution with the realization that multimodal therapy provides the best chance for survival. Unlike that for RMS, which is a highly chemosensitive tumor, the mainstay of treatment of NRSTS is complete surgical resection with or without adjuvant radiotherapy to prevent local recurrence. The most active drugs against NRSTS include ifosfamide and doxorubicin. Currently pediatric oncology group is investigating the clinical activity of some combination chemotherapies for unresectable or metastatic NRSTS. Wide local excision or en bloc resection should be the primary form of treatment in children with NRSTS. RT has been used sparingly in children because of its long-term effects.

SUGGESTED READING

1. Agarwala S. Pediatric soft tissue sarcomas. J Indian Assoc Pediatr Surg. 2006;11:15-23.

2. Barr FG: Molecular genetics and pathogenesis of rhabdomyosarcoma. J Pediatr Hematol Oncol. 1997;19: 483-91.

3. Breneman J, Lyden E, Pappo A. Prognostic factors and clinical outcome in children and adolescents with metastatic rhabdomyosarcoma - a report from IRS-IV. J Clin Oncol. 2003;2178-84.

4. Brennan M, Casper E, Harrison L. Soft tissue sarcoma. In: Cancer, Principles and Practice of Oncology (DeVita V, Hellman S, Rosenberg S, eds). Philadelphia: Lippincott-Raven. 1997;1738-88.

5. Carli M, Passone E, Perilongo G, Bisogno G. Ifosfamide in pediatric solid tumors. Oncology. 2003;65:99-104.

6. Harms D. Soft tissue sarcomas in the Kiel Pediatric Tumor Registry. Curr Top Pathol. 1995;89:31-45.

7. Hibshoosh H, Lattes R. Immunohistochemical and molecular genetic approaches to soft tissue tumor diagnosis: a primer. Semin Oncol. 1997;24:515-25.

8. Kawai A, Woodruff J, Healey JH, et al. SYTSSX gene fusion as a determinant of morphology and prognosis in synovial sarcoma. N Engl J Med. 1998;338:153-60.

9. Kramarova E, Stiller CA. The international classification of childhood cancer. Int J Cancer. 1996;68:759-65.

10. Miser J, Triche T, Kinsella T, et al. Other soft tissue sarcomas of childhood. In: Principles and Practice of Pediatric Oncology (Pizzo P, Poplack D) (eds). Philadelphia: Lippincott-Raven Publishers. 1997; 865-88.

11. Pappo A, Lyden E, Breneman J, Wiener E, Teot L, Meza J, et al. Upfront window trial of topotecan in previously untreated children and adolescents with metastatic rhabdomyosarcoma: an intergroup rhabdomyosarcoma study. J Clin Oncol. 2001;19:213-9.

12. Rodeberg D, Arndt C, Breneman J, Lyden E, Donaldson S, Paidas C, et al. Characteristics and outcome of rhabdomyosarcoma patients with isolated lung metastasis from intergroup rhabdomyosarcoma study-IV. J Pediatr Surg. 2005;40:256-62.

13. Swanson P, Dehner L. Pathology of soft tissue sarcomas in children and adolescents. In: Rhabdomyosarcoma and Related Tumors in Children and Adolescents (HM M, FB R, CE P) (Eds). Boca Raton: CRC Press. 1991; 385-419.

14. Wexler L, Helman L. Rhabdomyosarcoma and the undifferentiated sarcomas. In: Principles and Practice of Pediatric Oncology (Pizzo P, Poplack D) (Eds). Philadelphia: Lippincott-Raven Publishers. 1997; 799-829.

15. Xia SJ, Pressey JG, Barr FG. Molecular pathogenesis of rhabdomyosarcoma. Cancer Biol Ther. 2002;1:97-104.

17 Brain Tumor

Rakesh Mondal, Amitava Chandra

A **brain tumor** is an abnormal growth in the brain. Primary brain tumors involve a growth that starts in the brain, rather than spreading to the brain from another part of the body. Tumors may be benign or malignant. Tumors may destroy brain cells or damage cells by producing inflammation, and by pressing on other parts of the brain. This pressure causes cerebral edema and increased intracranial pressure.

Central nervous system tumors make-up about 20 percent of all childhood cancers. Brain tumors are the most common solid tumor in children.

SIGNS AND SYMPTOMS

The symptoms of a brain tumor vary according to the size, type and location of the tumor. Symptoms may occur when a tumor presses on a nerve or damages certain parts of the brain. They may also occur when the brain swelling occurred.

The most common symptoms include:
a. Headaches (usually worse in the morning).
b. Nausea or vomiting
c. Changes in speech, vision, or hearing
d. Problems balancing or walking
e. Changes in mood, personality or ability to concentrate
f. Problems with memory
g. Seizures or convulsions
h. Numbness or tingling in the arms or legs

DIFFERENT TYPES OF TUMORS

The most common primary childhood brain tumors are astrocytoma, medulloblastoma, ependymoma and brain stem glioma. Gliomas account for 75 percent of brain tumors in young children. Tumors found in craniospinal cavities may arise from the brain and/or spinal cord, or from other tissues or structures near them. Secondary metastasis to the nervous system is rare except of neuroblastomas.

Gliomas: The most common type of brain tumor at all ages is glioma. Gliomas consist of glial cells, which form the supportive tissue of the brain. The two major types of glial tumors are astrocytomas and ependymomas.

Astrocytoma: Astrocytomas are the most common type of childhood glioma and favor the nervous system. They typically occur in the cerebellum, a part of the brain that coordinates voluntary muscle movements and maintains posture, balance and equilibrium. The majority are curable by surgery. Astrocytomas may arise in the optic nerve, especially in children with neurofibromatosis. Children may also suffer from gliomas in the brainstem.

Malignant gliomas: These tumors, including the anaplastic astrocytomas and glioblastomas, can arise anywhere in the brain and are much more aggressive than astrocytomas. They are never cured by surgery alone and require combination therapy with radiation and chemotherapy (Fig. 17.1).

Optical nerve glioma: These are slow growing tumors which form along the optic nerves. They usually occur in children under the age of 10. The common cell type is pilocytic astrocytoma (Figs 17.2 and 17.3).

Brainstem glioma: These tumors, located in the brain stem, can be either slow or fast growing. Depending on the type of supporting tissue from which they arise, they

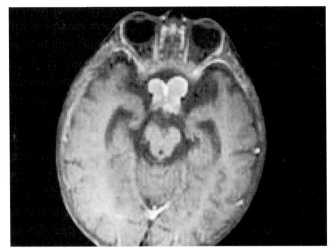

Fig. 17.1: Neuroimaging of optic nerve glioma

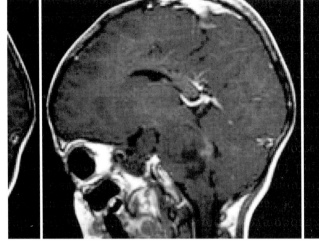

Fig. 17.2: Sagittal section of brain showing brain stem glioma

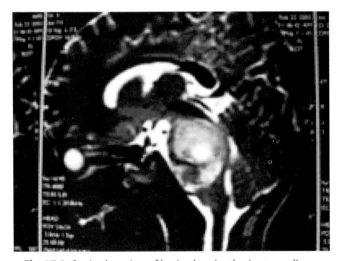

Fig. 17.3: Sagittal section of brain showing brain stem glioma

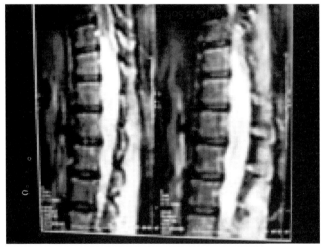

Fig. 17.4A: MRI of spinal cord showing photograph suggestive of ependymoma

can be either astrocytomas, anaplastic astrocytomas, glioblastoma multiforme, or a mixed tumor.

Oligodendroglioma: Slow growing tumors which arise from cells which make the myelin that insulates nerve fibers. They are located in the hemispheres of the brain, especially the frontal and temporal lobes, and in children are more common in the thalamus.

Ependymoma (Fig. 17.4A): This type of glial tumor usually arises from the cells lining the ventricles—the cerebrospinal fluid-filled cavities in the brain. Often slow growing, they may reoccur after treatment.

Mixed neuronal-glial tumors: Tumors containing a mix of glial cells and neurons occur more often in children than in adults. They may arise anywhere in the nervous system but most typically appear in the cerebrum, an area of the brain involved in motor function and personality. Surgery to remove the tumors is effective.

Ganglioglioma: This is the most common of the mixed neuronal-glial tumors and generally appears in childhood or the early teen years. The majority are benign and can usually be treated successfully by surgery.

Subependymal giant cell tumor: These tumors are common in children who have a genetic condition called tuberous sclerosis. These tumors are rarely malignant.

Pleomorphic xanthoastrocytoma: These tumors are most commonly seen in teens or young adults; most are benign.

Embryonal tumors: Up to 25 percent of nervous system tumors that occur in infants and children are tumors made up of poorly-differentiated neuroepithelial cells. When the nervous system develops, neuroepithelial cells differentiate into glial and nerve cells. The two main types of embryonal tumors are:

a. **Primitive neuroectodermal tumor (PNET):** This most common embryonal tumor can arise anywhere in the nervous system but typically appears in the cerebellum. When this happens, it is called medulloblastoma (Fig. 17.4B). New advances in therapy have made treatment more effective for these tumors. Medulloblastomas are usually located in the cerebellum and are fast growing and highly malignant. They frequently spread, invading other parts of the central nervous system via the spinal fluid. Medulloblastomas account for the largest percentage of pediatric brain cancers. It is more common in boys than girls; it usually occurs between the ages of 2 and 6 years.

b. **Atypical teratoid/rhabdoid tumor:** Ninety percent of patients with these tumors are below 2 years or younger. Approximately, 90 percent of these tumors have abnormality involving chromosome 22. The tumors may arise anywhere in the nervous system but typically appear in the cerebellum. They may also appear in the kidneys of infants. At the time of diagnosis, about one-third of these tumors have spread throughout the nervous system.

Choroid plexus papilloma/carcinoma: These tumors may also be found in ventricles. They may be both benign and malignant, and may spread throughout the nervous system. They are filled with blood vessels, making them difficult to remove because of their tendency to bleed.

Tumors arising from non-neuroepithelial tissue: The intracranial and intraspinal cavities contain tissues and structures that may give rise to tumors, a number of which are more common in children than adults. These tumors include:

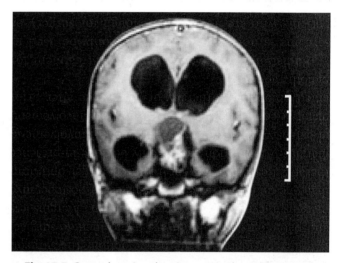

Fig. 17.5: Coronal section showing craniopharyngioma with obstructive hydrocephalus

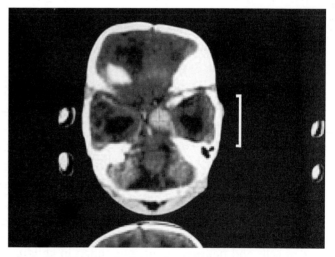

Fig. 17.6: Craniopharyngioma with hydrocephalus

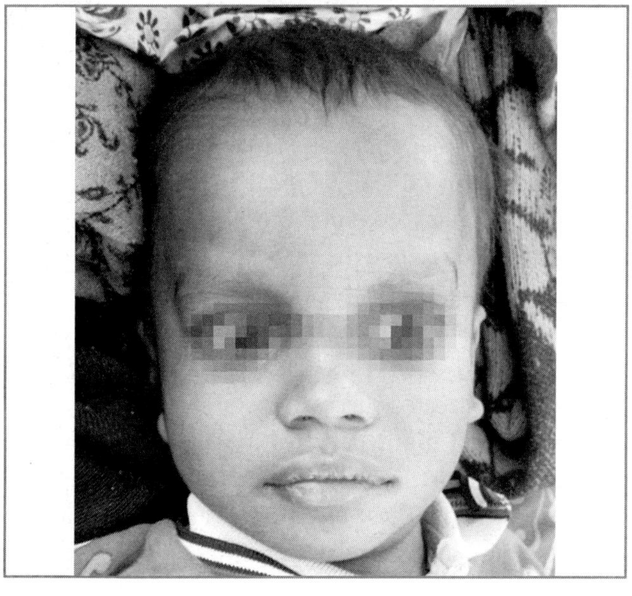

Fig.17.4B: Clinical photograph of child with medulloblastoma with hydrocephalus developing sun-setting sign

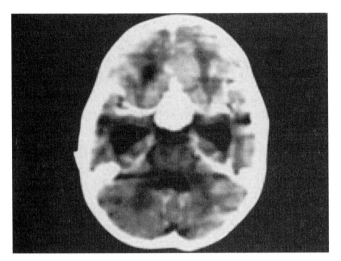

Fig. 17.7: Craniopharyngioma with hydrocephalus

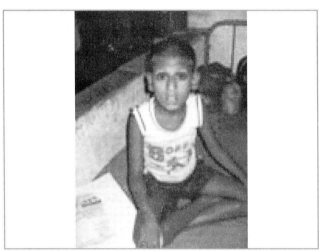

Fig. 17.8: Clinical photograph of a child with pineal gland tumor presented with raised ICT

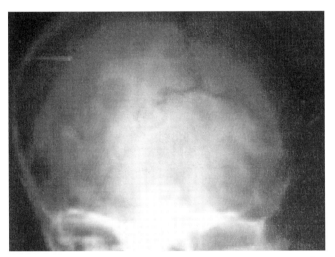

Fig. 17.9: X-ray picture of skull showing sellar calcification with moth beaten appearance following raised intra-cranial tension

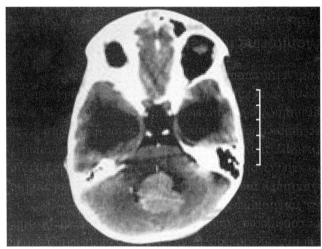

Fig. 17.10: CT scan of brain suggestive of post-fossa tumor

a. **Craniopharyngioma (Figs 17.5 to 17.7):** These benign tumors are thought to originate from residual tissue left behind following the development of the head. Because they occur at the front base of the brain near the pituitary gland and optic nerves, they may cause serious neurological and endocrine problems. Surgery may not be able to completely remove them.

b. **Pineal region tumors (Fig. 17.8):** Tumors can arise near the pineal gland at the base of the skull. The most common type, germinoma, is treated with radiation.

Meningeal tumors: The brain and spinal cord are covered with membranes called dura mater, arachnoid and pia mater. Tumors called meningiomas may develop in these membranes, but are more common in adults than children.

DIAGNOSIS OF BRAIN TUMORS

After taking a complete medical history and doing a physical examination, the following diagnostic tests may be done to determine if a brain tumor is present (Figs 17.9 and 17.10):

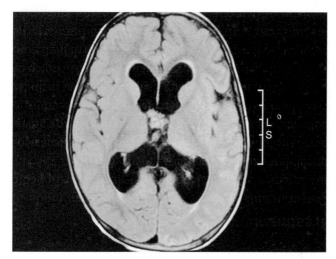

Fig. 17.11: MRI of choroid plexus papilloma with non-obstructive hydrocephalus

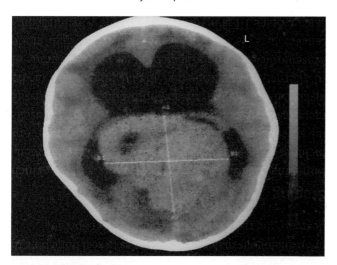

Fig. 17.12: CT scan head of medulloblastoma

a. **Neurological examination**
b. **X-ray**
c. **Computerized tomography scan (CAT scan or CT scan)**
d. **Magnetic resonance imaging (MRI) (Figs 17.11 and 17.12)**
e. **Lumbar puncture/spinal tap**
f. **Bone scan**
g. **Angiogram.**

MANAGEMENT OF BRAIN TUMORS

Surgery is usually the first step in treating brain tumors in children. The goal is to remove all or as much of the tumor as possible while maintaining neurological function. Surgery is also performed for a biopsy. This helps establish a diagnosis and treatment plan. This is frequently done when the tumor is surrounded by sensitive structures that may be damaged by surgical removal. Other therapies used to treat brain tumors include:

a. Chemotherapy
b. Radiation therapy (high-energy rays that kill or shrink cancer cells)
c. Steroids to treat and prevent swelling in the brain
d. High-dose chemotherapy and stem-cell rescue
e. Supportive care for the side effects of the tumor or treatment
f. Rehabilitation to regain lost motor skills and muscle strength
g. Continuous follow-up care to manage disease, detect recurrence of the tumor and manage late effects of treatment
h. Ventriculoperitoneal shunt to relieve obstructive hydrocephalus.

Children with brain tumors should be seen at a multidisciplinary medical center, staffed with the following: pediatric neurosurgeon, pediatric neuro-oncologist, pediatric, hemato-oncologist, pediatric neuroradiolgoist, and a pediatric neuropsychologist.

The treatment and prognosis depends on the type, grade, and location of the tumor. Tumors with distinct borders are considered "grade I", are sometimes referred to as benign or mildly malignant. These tumors either do not grow or grow very slowly. Infiltrating tumors are those that tend to grow into surrounding tissue. Of the infiltrating tumors, the terms low-grade, mid-grade, and high-grade are frequently used. A "high grade" tumor is considered highly malignant. However, the exact system used to grade tumors varies with each specific family of tumors. Depending on the type of tumor and the promptness of diagnosis, the 5-year survival rate is 40–80%.

Surgery: The purpose of surgery is to remove as much of the tumor as possible, to establish an exact diagnosis, to determine the extent of the tumor, and sometimes to provide access for other treatments, such as implants or radiation.

Radiation: Conventional radiation therapy uses external beams of radiation aimed at the tumor, a therapy which is given over a period of several weeks. Other types of radiation are also available. Because the developing brain of a child is so very sensitive to radiation therapy, it is deliberately limited or delayed until the child has grown older and the brain has sufficiently matured.

Chemotherapy: Chemotherapy is required for the more aggressive or higher grade tumors. Many drugs will kill brain cells, but it is difficult to predict which tumors will respond to which chemotherapy agents. Therefore, treatment often consists of a combination of drugs.

Shunting: Quite often childhood tumors block the CSF flow increasing the intracranial pressure when a shunt to divert CSF flow may have to be placed.

As with any cancer, prognosis and long-term survival vary greatly from child to child. Prompt medical attention and aggressive therapy are important for the best prognosis. Continuous follow-up care is essential for a child diagnosed with a brain tumor, because the side effects of radiation and chemotherapy as well as second malignancies can occur in survivors of brain tumors. Rehabilitation for lost motor skills and muscle strength may be required. Speech therapists and physical and occupational therapists specialize in the unique needs of children may help them.

Newer treatment: To date, minimal progress has been achieved in improving outcome for children with malignant supratentorial gliomas and brainstem tumors. The use of radiation therapy alone, at least for children and adolescents, is no longer accepted as the standard treatment for patients with nondisseminated medulloblastoma. The most recent published studies in children and adolescents receiving the now-standard dose of 2,340 cGy to the neuraxis with chemotherapy, are reporting 5-year event-free survival rates in excess of 75% with some sparing of cognitive function. The benefits of adjuvant chemotherapy added to irradiation in children and adolescents with disseminated medulloblastoma and with any stage of supratentorial PNET are indisputable. Publications over the past decade, utilizing full-dose irradiation and adjuvant chemotherapy, have produced 3-year survival rates ranging from 50 to 60%. Furthermore, the most recent analyses of the Children's Cancer Group (CCG) trial for ependymoma—a large experience with longer follow-up—confirm that children with incomplete resections

who received pre-irradiation chemotherapy enjoyed a 3-year event-free survival equivalent to that of children with complete resection treated with irradiation only. (UK-CCG) Marrow ablative chemotherapy and stem cell rescue, produced 5-year event-free survivals either superior to or equivalent to other infant ependymoma studies utilizing chemotherapy and irradiation.

Biologic

Clearly, much work lies ahead in improving the treatment of pediatric brain tumors. However, the work done on medulloblastoma needs to be expanded to identify molecular risk groups in all brain tumor patients using various technologies. The technologies used in identifying these molecular markers should include genomic markers (single nucleotide polymorphism [SNP] arrays of host and tumor), transcriptome markers (RNA arrays), and proteome markers (tissue microarrays, histologic evaluation). The combinations of these markers-especially the SNP information- may further facilitate our understanding of host-drug (pharmacodynamics/ pharmacokinetics) and tumor-drug (drug resistance) interactions. Use of biologic agents as therapies without accurate molecular classification of patients may lead to inaccurate assessment of their efficacy. The initial trials with antiangiogenic therapies, starting in the early 1990s, have been disappointing.

SUGGESTED READING

1. Cohen BH, Zeltzer PM, Boyett JM, et al. Prognostic factors and treatment results for supratentorial primitive neuroectodermal tumors in children using radiation and chemotherapy: A Children's Cancer Group randomized trial. J Clin Oncol. 1995;13:1687-96.

2. Jakacki RI, Zeltzer PM, Boyett JM, et al. Survival and prognostic factors following radiation and/or chemotherapy for primitive neuroectodermal tumors of the pineal region in infants and children: A report of the Children's Cancer Group. J Clin Oncol. 1995;13:1377-83.

3. Merchant TE, Wang MH, Haida T, et al. Medulloblastoma: Long-term results for patients treated with definitive radiation therapy during the computed tomography era. Int J Radiat Oncol Biol Phys. 1996;36:29-35.

4. Packer RJ, Goldwein J, Nicholson HS, et al. Treatment of children with medulloblastomas with reduced-dose craniospinal radiation therapy and adjuvant chemotherapy: A Children's Cancer Group Study. J Clin Oncol. 1999;17:2127-36.

5. Packer RJ, Gurney JG, Punyko JA, et al. Long-term neurologic and neurosensory sequelae in adult survivors of a childhood brain tumor: Childhood cancer survivor study. J Clin Oncol. 2003;21:3255-61.

6. Taylor RE, Bailey CC, Robinson K, et al. Results of a randomized study of preradiation chemotherapy vs radiotherapy alone for nonmetastatic medulloblastoma: The International Society of Paediatric Oncology/United Kingdom Children's Cancer Study Group PNET-3 Study. J Clin Oncol. 2003;21:1581-91.

Bone Tumor

Anirban Chatterjee, Alok Shobhan Datta

There are different types of bone tumor that occur in children out of which the most important are:

A. Osteosarcoma

B. Ewing Sarcoma.

OSTEOSARCOMA

In 1805, first time the term "osteosarcoma" was used by French surgeon Alexis Boyer who was also the private surgeon to Napoleon. The word sarcoma means in Greek language "fleshy excrescence." The most frequent malignant bone tumor is Osteosarcoma. It is responsible for 35% of primary bone cancer. It most commonly occurs in metaphysis of tubular long bones and 50% found around the knee. The hallmark of histological appearance is osteoblastic differentiation and the formation of malignant osteoid. Primitive mesenchymal cell is the cell of origin but may originate from pluripotential mesenchymal cells.

Osteosarcoma is a lethal variety of musculoskeletal cancer. That most common cause of mortality in osteosarcoma is pulmonary metastatic disease. Most osteosarcomas begin as single lesion within the most growing part of the long bones of children. Osteosarcoma most commonly present in the distal femur, the proximal tibia, and the proximal humerus, but almost any bone can be affected.

Not all arise in a solitary fashion, as multiple sites of osteosarcomas may occur. When it starts within 6 months it is called synchronous osteosarcoma or multiple sites may be found over a period more than 6 months is called metachronous osteosarcoma. Such multifocal osteosarcoma usually found in less than 10 years old children.

Under age group of 15, osteosarcoma is one of the sixth most important cancers. The incidence of osteosarcoma is slightly higher in males than in females. Osteosarcoma is very rare in children below five years. However, the incidence increases steadily with age, increasing more dramatically in adolescence, corresponding with the adolescent growth spurt.

Causes

The causes of osteosarcoma is still under in question. Possible explanations are:

Rapid bone growth: Rapid bone growth probably influence to form osteosarcoma, as it increases at the growth spurt of pubescent and osteosarcoma's characteristics affected area is the metaphysis close to the growth plate (physis) of long bones.

Environmental factors: There is controversy that radium, or fluoride, in drinking water can "trigger" for uprising incidence of osteosarcoma.

Genetic predisposition: Bone dysplasias, including Paget disease, fibrous dysplasia, enchondromatosis, and hereditary multiple exostoses and retinoblastoma are common occurrence of osteosarcoma. The mutation of the *RB* gene, which is a germline of retinoblastoma and radiation is correlated with a high-risk factor of osteosarcoma.

Li-Fraumeni syndrome where germline p53 mutation has occurred and Rothmund-Thomson syndromes are associated with osteosarcoma. A disbalance between cancer suppressor and cancer originator might have a noteworthy role in development of osteosarcoma. These can be measured by low selenium or Vitamin D-3 level and a high level of inflammation, interleukin-6, interleukin-8, tumor necrosis factor alpha respectively.

Pathology

It most commonly affects the long tubular bones close to metaphyseal growth plates. They most commonly affect the femur (42%) among which 75% are in the distal femur, tibia (19%) among them 80% are in the proximal tibia and humerus (10%) among which 90% in the proximal humerus. Other less common sites are the skull, jaw (8%) and pelvis (8%). The tumor is solid, hard, irregular due to the tumor spicules of calcified bone radiating in right angles which appear as "fir-tree" or "sun-burst"sign on X-rays. The distinguishing microscopic characteristic of osteosarcoma is the bone formation (osteoid) inside the tumor. Cancer cells are anaplastic, pleomorphic with numerous atypical mitoses and giant cell formation. These cells form osteoid. Osteoids are irregular amorphous trabeculae, which are eosinophilic/pink with or without central granular calcification, which are hematoxylinophilic/blue. Malignant cells are incorporated in the osteoid matrix. Stromal cells are atypical spindle-shaped with irregularly nuclei. There are various histologic types of osteosarcoma. The most common type in pediatric age is the conventional, which can be subdivided into different subtypes according to predominant cell-like osteoblastic, chondroblastic, fibroblastic. Other types of osteosrcoma are telangiectatic type with the large, blood-filled spaces are present, parosteal type which arise from bone cortex and periosteal osteosarcoma which develop from just beneath of periosteum.

Clinical Features

The most common clinical presentation of osteosarcoma is pain, which become extreme at night persist for weeks or months. Pain typically increases with activity. The history of trauma is not uncommon, but the trauma as cause of osteosarcoma is doubtful. Patients may be concerned that their child has a sprain, arthritis, or growing pains. Many patients first complain of pain that may be worse at night, and may have been occurring for some time. If the tumor is large, it can appear as a swelling. The affected bone is not as strong as normal bones and may fracture with minor trauma (a pathological fracture). Pathologic fractures also occur but uncommon and it commonly associated with telangiectatic type of osteosarcoma. Limp is due to pain. Swelling may appear if lesion is large. Systemic symptoms like fever and night sweats are rare. Pulmonary metastasis also found. A respiratory symptom implies huge pulmonary involvement. Metastatic involvement to other organ is extremely rare. Physical examination relate to the location of the primary tumor. Palpable swelling, which is hot, tender, increased skin vascularity and bruit may be presenting features. Close differential in this situation is osteomyelitis. Reduced range of motion of nearby joint common and local lymph node enlargement is uncommon. Over the years, many authors have suggested variable and arbitrary amounts of the normal tissue cuff to remove along with the primary tumor to increase the likelihood of negative margins.

Investigation

Blood Examination

Significant prognostic blood tests are lactic dehydrogenase (LDH) and alkaline phosphatase (ALP). At the point of diagnosis, an elevated ALP are indicated lung metastases. In patients without metastases, an elevated LDH have poor outcome than normal LDH if no metastasis have occur. Laboratory tests should be done to assess organ function before start of chemotherapy. These are complete blood cell (CBC) count, including differential, platelet count liver function tests: Aspartate aminotransferase (AST), alanine aminotransferase (ALT), bilirubin, and albumin electrolyte levels: Sodium, potassium, chloride, bicarbonate, calcium, magnesium, phosphorus renal function tests: blood urea nitrogen (BUN), creatinine urinalysis.

Imaging Studies

Plain films: Advise two plain films of the assumed primary lesions including total bone and nearby joint to determine the skip lesions and joint invasion. Posteroanterior (PA), and lateral chest X-ray should be done to exclude pulmonary involvement. Osteosarcoma can be present as purely osteolytic in 30% of cases and purely osteoblastic in 45% of cases . The typical Codman triangle is due rise of the periosteum. The "sunburst" sign is found in 60% of lesions due to expansion of cancer through the periosteum. The 'sunburst' sign is found in 60% of lesions due to expansion of cancer through the periosteum.

CT scanning: CT-scan is advised for suspected lesion due to delineate the site and size of the cancer which are important to plan the surgical resection. High resolution CT of the thorax is essential to detect pulmonary metastases. It should be done before pulmonary biopsy to avoid postanesthesia atelectasis, which may mimic metastasis.

MRI: MRI is the best modality to determine intramedullary extension, soft-tissue involvement and skip lesions. This imaging method is only the most important analysis for correct surgical staging.

Radionuclide bone scanning with technetium-99 (^{99m}Tc)-methylene diphosphonate (MDP/MDI). It is most important to detect metastatic and focal lesion at different site.

Other Tests

Echocardiography and audiography is usually done before administration of adriamycin and cisplatin.

Diagnostic Procedures

Biopsy: An orthopedic surgeon should perform biopsies. Open biopsy must be advocated and choice of biopsy as it reduces sampling error and to obtain sufficient tissue for histological examination. Trephine biopsy or core needle biopsy is well-accepted choice for vertebral bodies and pelvic bone, and fine needle aspiration is not an option. A frozen section of each sample must be examined and intraoperative opinion of pathologist should be sought for evaluation of the frozen-section specimen. It is always better to make the sample from the extraosseous portion than bone to reduce the risk of fracture. Gelfoam or an analogous material usually uses to seal bone hole to decrease the risk of hematoma and cancer spread.

Staging

Enneking, in 1980, described a staging system, which includes criteria of grade of cancer, extracompartmental spread, and status of metastasis, whether or not metastases are present. The system use to total musculoskeletal tumors that means both bone and soft tissue so alternatively its known as the staging system of the Musculoskeletal Tumor Society. Stage based on grade of cancer. Stage I is low-grade cancer. Stage II is high-grade cancer. Stage III is metastases. Substage A is intracompartmental tumor that means intramedullary osteosarcoma. Substage B is extracompartmental lesion, which is extramedullary extension of osteosarcoma.

Treatment

Osteosarcoma requires a multidisciplinary mode of management. Medical oncologist and an orthopedic oncologist expert in sarcomas management are the key personnel of management. At present, best mode is neoadjuvant chemotherapy in which chemotherapy advocated before surgery and thereafter-surgical resection.

Standard therapy is a surgical resection that includes either limb-salvage surgery, which is the best choice or amputation if necessary with a combination of high dose methotrexate with leucovorin rescue, and intra-arterial cisplatin, adriamycin, ifosfamide with mesna, etoposide, muramyl tri-peptide (MTP). Ifosfamide is usually used for adjuvant treatment when necrosis count is in lower range. Before introduction of chemotherapy, which was started in 1970, surgery particularly amputation was the mode of treatment and micrometastasis causes pulmonary recurrence. Neoadjuvant chemotherapy shows two facets of gain. One, it reduces the size of tumor to facilitate surgical resection. And another is, it provides a risk judgment by histologic response. There is more than ninety-five percent cell necrosis, which has better prognosis.

Definitive resection: The goal of resection is survival. Wide margin that means margin is surrounded by normal tissue usually preserved. Radical margin resection is resection of involved bone, joint to joint; muscle, origin to insertion. Radical margins are not essential for cure. Amputation may be the treatment of choice in some situations. In addition, limb-salvage reconstruction should be considered. Autologous bone graft, allograft, prosthesis, rotationplasty are the common example.

Auxiliary management: Additional cycles of methotrexate, cisplatin, doxorubicin, and ifosfamide chemotherapy may be necessary. A CBC measurement is recommended two times per week for those who are on granulocyte colony-stimulating factor (G-CSF) treatment. Fever and neutropenia require inpatient treatment with intravenous antibiotics and monitoring.

Monitoring for Recurrence

Visits: Every 3 months for the first year; every 6 months for the second and third year; and yearly thereafter.

Prognosis

After proper treatment, three-year event free survival is 50 to 75% and five-year survival is 60 to 85% in some studies. These rates are an average and vary enormously.

Prognosis is depending on stage and substage. In Stage I, it shows a very good outcome (> 90%) if wide resection has done. In Stage II b, the outcome with 2-year survival after the metastases is 50% and 5-year survival is 40% and 10 year, 20%. Initial presentation of stage III, overall outcome is 30% or more. It depends on resection can done in osteosarcoma or pulmonary metastasis, the number metastases, degree of necrosis of the primary tumor location of primary tumor. The best prognosis if site is distal part of limbs, distal femur has intermediate prognosis and axial skeleton is worst one. In a retrospect, the cancer size at initial stage is a significant prognostic factor in osteosarcoma.

EWING SARCOMA

Ewing sarcoma (ES) was first revealed in literature, in 1921, by James Ewing. James Ewing confirmed that ES was totally different from lymphoma and other tumors which were well-established at that time. ES primary bone tumor and highly malignant round-cell tumor. ES originates from red bone marrow. This tumor is most commonly seen in 4–15 years and rarely above than 30 years. Ewing sarcoma accounts for approximately 5% of biopsy-analyzed bone tumors and this is responsible for about 33% of primary bone tumors. This disease is the second most common malignant bone cancer in pediatric age group, and the most fatal bone cancer. Ewing sarcoma and primitive peripheral neuroectodermal tumor (PNET) are originated from a common genetic locus, so they are categorized as Ewing family of tumors. PNETs are usually not a bone tumor.

Pathology

ES is originated from red bone marrow. The histological features are similar to reticulum cell sarcoma. ES found as a monostotic lesion in the metaphysis or diaphysis of the long bones of the limbs and in the pelvic area, ribs, and scapulae. It is most frequently seen in the pelvis and proximal long tubular bones. The most common involved long bone is the diaphysis of the femur and less commonly the tibia and the humerus. Clinically, metastatic disease is found in thirty percent cases. It is positive for CD99 and negative for CD45. The characteristic of Ewing sarcoma is the periosteal reaction and new bone formation, which appears like an onion-skin. ES may be lytic or sclerotic. Ewing's sarcoma is caused by a translocation between chromosomes 11 and 22. This translocation combines the EWS gene of chromosome 22 to the FLI1 gene of chromosome 11. Moreover, EWS/FLI acts as the main regulator. Ewing's sarcomas show the features of both mesodermal and ectodermal cell of origin. Therefore, classification of ES is complex. Though it is recognized as primary bone tumor. Ewing sarcoma and peripheral neuroepithelioma grouped as the Ewing family of tumors (EFTs) and believed as neural tumors. Neuroepithelioma appears as more differentiated than Ewing sarcoma, where neuron-specific enolase and S-100 protein testing are positive.

Frequency

The annual incidence of Ewing sarcoma is less than two cases per 1 million children.

Race: Ewing sarcoma found commonly in whites and, to a less commonly, in blacks and Asians. ES in rare Chinese population.

Sex: ES occurrence is more in males than females. The M:F ratio is 1.5:1.

Age: Children and adolescents aged 4–15 years are the most common age group for ES with a peak between 10 and 20 years of age and rarely occur in adults older than 30 years.

Clinical Details (Figs 18.1 to 18.3)

The first and most significant symptom is pain. At early stage, pain is intermittent and extreme. The radiation of pain along the limbs is commonly found in the vertebral or pelvic ES. Neurologic presentation as nerve root signs and cord compression are found in 50% ES and it is commonly seen in the axial skeleton ES. Rarely, pathologic fracture is also a presenting feature. Uncommonly, ES can mimic as acute or chronic osteomyelitis and clinical features are remittent fever, increased total leukocyte count, weight-loss and an elevated erythrocyte sedimentation rate (ESR), increased serum lactic dehydrogenase (LDH) and it persists for weeks to months levels. Sooner large palpable tense and tender local swellings appear, and it grows quickly. The classification of ES is localized and metastatic disease. In localized lesion, there is no spread beyond the primary site or regional lymph node involvement by clinical and imaging techniques but continuous extension into adjacent soft tissue may occur. The local disease is usually subdivided by prognostic factors into two groups that is a high-risk group and a low-risk group. Ewing sarcoma showed that the following factors are correlate with a poor prognosis. Male sex, age older than 12 years, anemia, elevated LDH levels, radiation therapy only for local control, poor chemotherapeutic course.

Differential diagnosis: Osteomyelitis, round-cell tumors, osteosarcomas, osteolytic osteosarcoma and fibrosarcoma—(Difficult to differentiate between these 2 entities, because of lytic lesions, periosteal reaction) lymphoma.

Radiograph

ES can affect every bone. The ES is most commonly in metaphyseal or diaphyseal in long bone. A permeative lytic lesion with a prominent soft-tissue mass spreading from bone is the most commonly found in radiograph in the long bone. A sclerotic lesion, which has

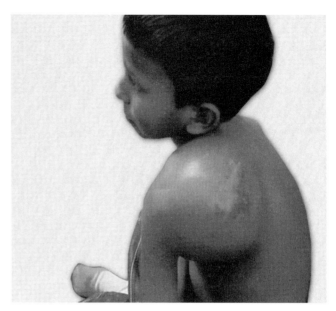

Fig.18.1: Clinical photograph of child with scapular Ewing's sarcoma

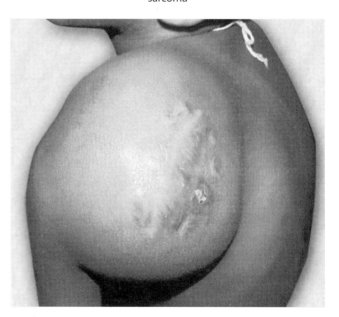

Fig.18.2: Clinical photograph of child with scapular Ewing's sarcoma

ill-defined margins and invasion of the bone, is found in 25% of cases (Figs 18.4 and 18.5). The lesion can transverse the Haversian system after invasion of cortical bone and produce a huge soft-tissue mass outside the bone without any sign of cortical destruction. This occurrence is observed in approximately 50% of Ewing sarcoma. A periosteal reaction is common and it appears as an onion-skin or sunburst pattern, which is a sign of

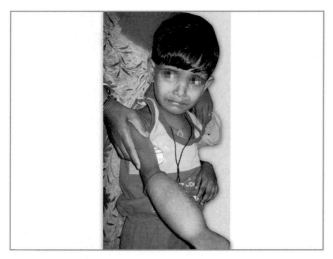

Fig.18.3: Clinical photograph of child with Ewing's sarcoma of forearm

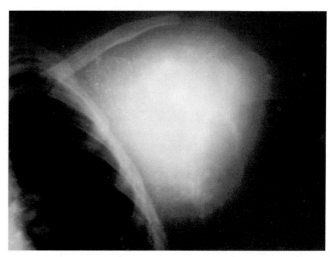

Fig.18.4: X-ray showing destruction of bones in Ewing sarcoma

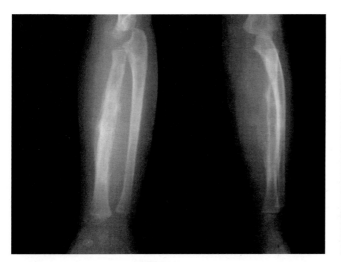

Fig.18.5: X-ray forearm suggestive of Ewing's sarcoma

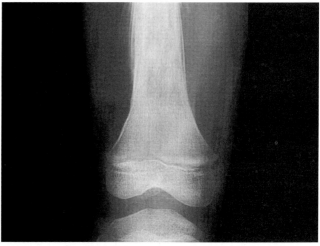

Fig.18.6: X-ray of lower limb showing onion peel appearance suggestive of Ewing's sarcoma

an aggressive pattern (Fig. 18.6). Codman triangles are usually found at the margins of the lesion. It is formed by the rise of the periosteum and central destruction of the periosteal reaction. Rarely, plain radiographs show no changes.

CT and MRI: CT scanning may be revealing the bone destruction that is associated with Ewing sarcoma (Figs 18.7 to 18.10). MRI is most preferred imaging modality to define the stage and to follow-up. Minimum false negative report with both CT-scan and MRI studies is noticed. MRI has an accuracy of approximately 90%.

However, CT scanning cannot differentiate between Ewing sarcoma and osteosarcoma, other bone tumors, osteomyelitis and other conditions. False-positive report is high. MRI is important to elicit soft-tissue encroachment as the ES has low signal intensity on T1-weighted images in comparison to the normal high signal intensity of the bone marrow. On T2-weighted images, the ES is hyperintense in comparison to muscle. The gadolinium based MRI contrast study not so much valuable. The reduced signal intensity is valuable sign of therapeutic effect. However, accuracy 71% has been detected but it

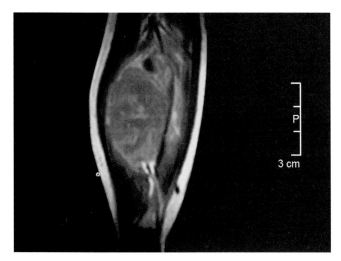

Fig.18.7: MRI forearm sagittal section in Ewing's sarcoma showing bony involvement

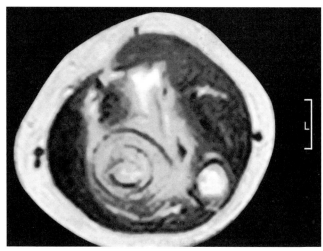

Fig.18.8: MRI coronal section of radius showing onion peel appearance in Ewing's sarcoma

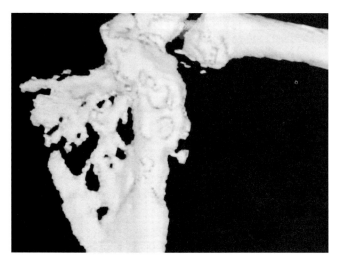

Fig.18.9: 3D MRI of bony destruction of involved bone in Ewing's sarcoma

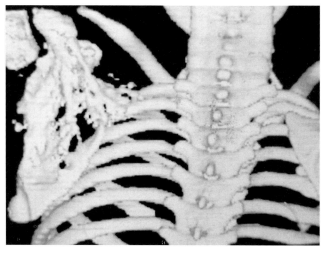

Fig.18.10: 3D MRI of bony destruction of involved bone in Ewing's sarcoma

is controversial. The accuracy of MRI is 90.3% (the positive predictive value plus the negative predictive value). In most patients, MRI is superior to specific information than CT scanning. MRI is the best of choice for staging in Ewing sarcoma.

Ultrasonography (US): US is not only used for follow-up care to delineate the extraosseous portion of the cancer US but also useful for a US guided biopsy of cancer, to exclude metastases in the liver and ES in abdominal and pelvic area.

Nuclear medicine: Static bone scintigraphy to identify the primary tumor of Ewing sarcoma (focal area of increased radionuclide activity). Whole body bone scans to identify the primary lesion and skip lesions and to identify distant metastases during tumor staging.

Three-phase dynamic bone scintigraphy (TPBS) to evaluate treatment effects, with accuracy of 88%. In addition to technetium-99m (^{99m}Tc), other tracers, such as thallium-201 (^{201}Tl), Gallium-67 (^{67}Ga) is used to assess the therapeutic response. Positron emission tomography

(PET) scanning with fluorodeoxyglucose (FDG) is recently used modality. PET scanning with FDG is advocated as the most sensitive modality to identify early changes in cancer metabolism as an effect of therapeutic effects. A low FDG uptake is more commonly found in resistant tumors.

Intervention: The effective treatment of Ewing sarcoma (ES) requires systemic chemotherapy in combination with either surgery or radiation therapy or both for local tumor control. In general, patients receive preoperative chemotherapy prior to instituting local control measures. Postoperative therapy depends on surgical margins and histologic response. In the most of the metastatic diseases reveal a good initial response to preoperative chemotherapy; though, in most of the patients it is only partly controlled or recurs. Lung metastasis as the only metastatic organ shows a better prognosis than bone and/or bone marrow matastasis. Satisfactory local control for metastatic disease, particularly bone metastases, is an important issue.

Chemotherapy for Ewing tumor of bone: Multidrug chemotherapy regimen used for ES and it consists of vincristine, doxorubicin, ifosfamide, and etoposide. United States uses alternate courses of vincristine, cyclophosphamide, and doxorubicin with courses of ifosfamide/etoposide and European protocols generally mixed vincristine, doxorubicin and an alkylating agent with or without etoposide in a single treatment cycle. The time length of primary chemotherapy is from six months to one year.

Local control for Ewing tumor of bone: Surgery complete resection is useful and appropriate locally aggressive tumor. Unresectable cancer can be treated with radiation therapy (RT) alone. The treatment option in the cases of resections with microscopic residual disease is adjuvant RT. Nevertheless, gross total resection with microscopic residua, the role of adjuvant RT is controversial. Surgery is definitive local treatment for suitable patients, who accept the morbidity, but RT is suitable for unresectable disease or the patient does not accept the definitive surgery. Adjuvant RT may be used for residual microscopic disease, inadequate margins, or viable tumor in the resected tissue and margins. Duration of radiation therapy 5–8 weeks. High-dose chemotherapy with hematopoietic stem cell transplant (HSCT).

Rescue for Ewing sarcoma of bone: It is used for high risk of relapse with conventional treatments, bone and/or bone marrow metastases at diagnosis and in clinical trial for patients with pulmonary metastases. It is used for consolidation treatment, in an effort to improve outcome.

Prognosis

For localized disease show 70 to 80% survival when treatment was chemotherapy. Long-term survival for metastatic disease is variable, it is less than 10 to 25–30%.

SUGGESTED READING

1. Arceci RJ, Weinstein HJ. Neoplasia. In: Avery GB, Fletcher MA, MacDonald MG (Eds). Neonatology: Pathophysiology and Management of the Newborn. 4th (Edn) Philadelphia, Pa: JB Lippincott. 1994:1211-28.
2. Bacci G, Balladelli A, Forni C, et al. Ewing's sarcoma family tumours: Differences in clinicopathological characteristics at presentation between localised and metastatic tumours. J Bone Joint Surg Br. 2007;89:1229-33.
3. Bacci G, Ferrari S, Bertoni F, et al. Prognostic factors in nonmetastatic Ewing's sarcoma of bone treated with adjuvant chemotherapy: analysis of 359 patients at the Istituto Ortopedico Rizzoli. J Clin Oncol. 2000;18:4-11.
4. Bernstein M, Kovar H, Paulussen M, et al. "Ewing's sarcoma family of tumors: current management". Oncologist. 2006;11:503-19.
5. Clark JC, Dass CR, Choong PF. A review of clinical and molecular prognostic factors in osteosarcoma. J Cancer Res Clin Oncol. 2008;134:281-97.
6. Dehner LP. Peripheral and central primitive neuroectodermal tumors. A nosologic concept seeking a consensus. Arch Pathol Lab Med. 1986;110:997-1005.
7. Erlemann R, Sciuk J, Bosse A, et al. Response of osteosarcoma and Ewing sarcoma to preoperative chemotherapy: assessment with dynamic and static MR imaging and skeletal scintigraphy. Radiology. 1990;175:791-6.
8. Ewing J. Classics in oncology. Diffuse endothelioma of bone. James Ewing. Proceedings of the New York Pathological Society, 1921. [reprint]. CA Cancer J Clin. 1972;22:95-8.
9. Mankin HJ, Mankin CJ, Simon MA. The hazards of the biopsy, revisited. Members of the Musculoskeletal Tumor Society. J Bone Joint Surg Am. 1996;78:656-63.

10. Marulanda GA, Henderson ER, Johnson DA, Letson GD, Cheong D. Orthopedic surgery options for the treatment of primary osteosarcoma. Cancer Control. 2008;15:13-20.

11. Mateo-Lozano S, Gokhale PC, Soldatenkov VA, Dritschilo A, Tirado OM, Notario V. "Combined transcriptional and translational targeting of EWS/FLI-1 in Ewing's sarcoma". Clin Cancer Res. 2006;12:6781-90.

12. Owen LA, Kowalewski AA, Lessnick SL (2008). "EWS/FLI mediates transcriptional repression via NKX2.2 during oncogenic transformation in Ewing's sarcoma". PLoS ONE 3:e1965. doi:10.1371/journal.pone.0001965. PMID 18414662.

13. Peltier LF. Tumors of bone and soft tissues. Orthopedics: A History and Iconography. San Francisco, Calif: Norman Publishing. 1993:264-91.

14. Ries LAG, Smith MA, Gurney JG, et al. Cancer incidence and survival among children and adolescents: United States SEER program 1975-1995. Bethesda, Md: National Cancer Institute; 1999. NIH Pub No 99–4649. Available at http://seer.cancer.gov/publications/childhood/.

15. Riggi N, Stamenkovic I. The biology of Ewing sarcoma. Cancer Lett. 2007;254:1-10.

16. Rogers LF. Bone tumors and related conditions. In: Juhl JH, Crummy AB, Paul L (Eds). Paul and Juhl's Essentials of Radiologic Imaging. 5th edn. Philadelphia, Pa: Lippincott-Raven. 1987;85-384.

17. Strauss LG, Koomaegi R, Dimitrakopoulou-Strauss A. Dynamic positron emission tomography (PET) with 18F-deoxyglucose (FDG) in bone tumors: correlation of quantitative PET and gene expression [abstract]. J Nucl Med. 2001;42:33P.

18. Vander Griend RA. Osteosarcoma and its variants. Orthop Clin North Am. 1996;27:575-81.

19. Verrill MW, Judson IR, Harmer CL, et al. Ewing's sarcoma and primitive neuroectodermal tumor in adults: are they different from Ewing's sarcoma and primitive neuroectodermal tumor in children? J Clin Oncol. 1997;15:2611-21.

20. Weis LD. Common malignant bone tumors: osteosarcoma. In: Simon MA, Springfield D (Eds). Surgery for Bone and Soft-tissue Tumors. Philadelphia, Pa: Lippincott-Raven; 1998:265-74. Link MP, Eilber F. Osteosarcoma. In: Pizzo PA, Poplack DG (eds). Principles and Practice of Pediatric Oncology. 3rd edn. Philadelphia, Pa: Lippincott-Raven. 1997:889-920.

Sumantra Sarkar

INTRODUCTION

Neonatal neoplasms are a special group of tumors having unique distinguishing features. Histologically, they are same as the tumors that occur in older children or in adults but vary in their incidence, presentation, biology, course and treatment response. For example, stage IV S neuroblastoma, a good response tumor in older children, may be rapidly fatal and constitute an oncologic emergency in the neonates. On the other hand, many tumors behave in a less aggressive fashion at this age than in the older child. The incidence of neonatal tumor is estimated to be 1.7 to 3.6 per 1,00,000 live births and it is 2% of all childhood tumors. The wide spectrum of neoplasms consists of neuroblastoma, germ cell tumors, renal tumors, sarcoma, CNS tumors, retinoblastoma, hepatoblastoma and congenital leukemias. Neuroblastoma is the most common neonatal malignancy followed by leukemias. But considering all tumors including the benign ones teratoma ranks first.

ETIOLOGY

Definite etiology is most of the times uncertain. Some are inheritable. Maternal tumor may metastasize through placenta. One review literature in 2001 has shown 68 cases of placental involvement with 14 cases of neonatal affection (melanoma 7 and leukemia 7). External environmental factors like parental exposure to X rays, metals, chemicals like hair dyes and drugs used to treat infertility are also reported to be risk factors.

CLINICAL FEATURES

Lump or mass in any location particularly in the head neck region, abdominal or thoracic cavity or sacrococcygeal areas are usual presentation (Table 19.1). Non-specific sepsis like features such as poor feeding, vomiting, and lethargy may be at times misleading. Congenital anomalies like VSD, limb or fusion defect, imperforate anus, meningocele as well as Down's syndrome and Fanconi's anemia are rare associations of neonatal malignancy.

DISCUSSION OF INDIVIDUAL TUMORS

Teratomas

These are due to abnormal development of pluripotent germ cells or embryonal cells. Gonadal tumors are germ

Table 19.1: Common neonatal tumors with their anatomical locations

Head neck region	Neuroblastoma, rhabdomyosarcoma, fibrosarcoma
Thoracic cavity	Neuroblastoma, rhabdomyosarcoma, teratoma
Abdominal cavity	Neuroblastoma, teratoma
Sacrococcygeal area	Teratoma, rhabdomyosarcomas
Kidney	Mesoblastic nephroma, Wilms' sarcoma
Liver	Hepatoblastoma
Extremities	Congenital fibrosarcoma, rhabdomyosarcoma
Pelvic/genital region	Neuroblastoma, teratoma, sarcoma
Skin	Neuroblastoma, congenital leukemias
Bone marrow	Leukemias, disseminated neuro/ retinoblastoma

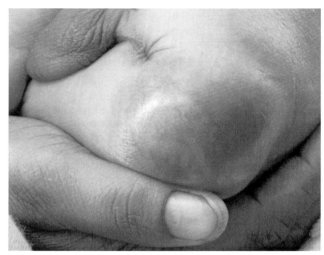

Fig. 19.1: Clinical photograph of infant with sacrococcygeal teratoma

cells derived. Sacrococcygeal and cervical teratomas derived from embryonal cells (Fig. 19.1). The incidence is 1 in 40,000 births. These midline tumors contain bone, tooth, hair, limbs or other organs. Mature, encapsulated tumors are benign and more frequent in females; while immature teratomas are typically malignant with male preponderance. They may arise from brain, neck, tongue, nose, mediastinum, etc. Teratomas are considered congenital tumors as they are thought to be present since or before birth. Antenatal USG can detect teratomas projecting into amniotic fluid. MRI is more informative. In the case of large sacrococcygeal teratomas, a significant portion of the fetal blood is redirected toward the teratoma (steal syndrome) causing heart failure or hydrops fetalis.

Diagnosis is based on histology. Regardless of its origin, teratomas are classified by a cancer staging system. The classification (Gonzalez-Crussi) is—grade 0 or mature (benign); grade 1 or immature, probably benign; grade 2 or immature, possibly malignant; and grade 3 or frankly malignant. A "benign" grade 0 teratoma may have malignant potential. Apparently benign grade 1 immature teratoma with much higher risk requires adequate follow-up.

Depending on which tissue (s) it contains, a teratoma may secrete a variety of substances. Alpha-fetoprotein (AFP) is secreted from the yolk sac element. This is a marker for recurrence or treatment efficacy but not used for initial diagnosis. β hCG, thyroxine are also secreted.

The treatment of choice is complete surgical removal. Mature ones are easily resectable. Surgery may not be possible for very large, complex or inaccessible tumors especially which are firmly attached to deep structures. For malignant teratomas, usually, surgery is followed by chemotherapy. Surgically inaccessible or very complex tumors are likely to be malignant (due to late discovery and/or treatment). Chemotherapy may be the first option here. Adequate follow-up requires close observation, scanning (USG, MRI, or CT), and measurement of AFP and/or β hCG.

Neuroblastoma

This is the commonest malignancy in neonatal age group. This neuroendocrine tumor originates from neural crest element of the sympathetic nervous system. The tumor usually present as a mass arising from adrenal glands or nerve tissues in the neck, chest, abdomen, or pelvis. Presentation with metastases is found in half of the cases. Anemia may result from marrow infiltration. Rarely, primary location may be unidentifiable.

A rare germline mutation in the anaplastic lymphoma kinase (ALK) gene may explain the origin of familial neuroblastoma. Occupational chemicals exposer, smoking, alcohol, drugs used during pregnancy, atopy and exposure to infection early in life, use of hormones and fertility drugs, and maternal use of hair dye are the proposed risk factors.

Histology is confirmatory for the diagnosis. The tumor cells are small, round and blue, with rosette patterns (Homer-Wright pseudo-rosettes). Immunohistochemical stains are used to differentiate neuroblastomas from rhabdomyosarcoma, lymphoma, Ewing's and Wilms' tumor. 90% of cases of neuroblastoma have elevated levels of catecholamines dopamine, homovanillic acid (HVA), and/or vanillylmandelic acid (VMA) in the urine or blood. The MIBG scan (meta-iodobenzylguanidine), also detect 90 to 95% of all neuroblastomas.

According to anatomical site, the International Neuroblastoma Staging System" (INSS) (1986), revised in 1988, classified neuroblastoma as in Table 19.2:

Although international agreement on staging (INSS) has been used, the need for an international consensus on **risk assignment** has also been recognized. The new

Table 19.2: Classification of neuroblastoma

Localized tumor confined to the area of origin	*Stage 1*
Unilateral tumor with incomplete gross resection; identifiable ipsilateral and contralateral lymph node negative for tumor.	*Stage 2A*
Unilateral tumor with complete or incomplete gross resection; with ipsilateral lymph node positive; identifiable contralateral lymph node negative	*Stage 2B*
Tumor infiltrating across midline with or without regional lymph node involvement; or unilateral tumor with contralateral lymph node involvement; or midline tumor with bilateral lymph node involvement	*Stage 3*
Dissemination of tumor to distant lymph nodes, bone marrow, bone, liver, or other organs except as defined by Stage 4S	*Stage 4*
Age < 1 year with localized primary tumor as defined in Stage 1 or 2, with dissemination limited to liver, skin or bone marrow (less than 10 percent of nucleated bone marrow cells are tumors)	*Stage 4s*

Table 19.3: Treatment options for different risk groups

Low-risk patients	Observation or surgery alone
Intermediate risk	Surgery and chemotherapy
High risk	Intensive chemotherapy, surgery, radiation, bone marrow/stem cell transplant, biological-based therapy with 13-cis-retinoic acid (isotretinoin or accutane) Antibody therapy– cytokines GM-CSF and IL-2.

International Neuroblastoma Risk Group Staging System (INRGSS):

Stage L1: Localized disease without image-defined risk factors

Stage L2: Localized disease with image-defined risk factors

Stage M: Metastatic disease

Stage MS: Metastatic disease "special" where MS is equivalent to stage 4S

Biologic and genetic criteria that include the age of the patient, extent of disease spread, microscopic appearance, and genetic features including DNA ploidy and N-myc oncogene amplification (N-myc regulates microRNAs) stratified into low, intermediate, and high-risk disease. Low-risk disease is most common in infants and highly curable, whereas high-risk disease is difficult to cure even with the most intensive multi-modal therapies available. The different treatment options for different risk groups are shown in Table 19.3.

Combination chemotherapy is highly effective. Common agents for induction and for stem cell transplant conditioning are platinum compounds (cisplatin, carboplatin), alkylating agents (cyclophasphamide, ifosfamide, melphalan), topoisomerase II inhibitor (etoposide), anthracycline antibiotics (doxorubicin) and vinca alkaloids (vincristine). For recurrent disease, topoisomerase I inhibitors (topotecan and irinotecan) are effective.

Excellent prognosis is reported with cure rates above 90% for low risk and 70–90% for intermediate risk disease. Cure rate is only about 30% for high-risk cases. High-risk nonresponders of frontline treatment are labeled refractory. The refractoriness may be due to the protein p53. Irinotecan, topotecan, temozolomide and cyclophosphamide are effective in refractory and recurrent neuroblastoma. Survivors of intermediate and high-risk groups often experience hearing loss. Growth failure, learning problem, thyroid disorder and secondary cancers are also reported. A study in November 2009 in mice shows that activating the tumor suppressor p53 with a new drug, nutlin-3, may slow tumor growth.

Renal Tumors

Commonest renal tumor in this age group is mesoblastic nephroma. The median age at diagnosis is 2 months with a definite male preponderance. Perirenal extension is very common without distant metastasis. Histologically bundles of spindles cells resembling fibroblast or smooth muscle is characteristic. Radical nephrectomy is the best treatment option with least chances of recurrence.

Though uncommon, 15 cases Wilm's tumors are reported in the neonatal age group with favorable histology. Abnormalities in the 11th chromosome are also detected. About 64% patients have nephroblastomatosis. Treatment guidelines are same as in case of older children with radical nephrectomy followed by chemotherapy with VCR, actinomycin D, doxorubicin, cyclophosphamide. Prognosis depends on the size of the tumor, stage of the disease and histopathological features.

Soft Tissue Sarcomas

Based on histological picture, clinical behavior, and treatment response, three types are being described: a) Rhabdomyosarcoma, b) Congenital fibrosarcoma, and c) Others.

Rhabdomyosarcoma

It is a very rare tumor accounting for 0.5% of all rhabdomyosarcomas of childhood. Caudal distribution (sacrococcygeal region, around the bladder, rectum, vagina) is more commonly (50%) reported than the cranial distribution. Trunk and limbs are also involved. Histologically, these are small round cell tumor and may show embryonic histology. Surgery followed by chemotherapy with or without radiotherapy is offered in all cases except in case of inoperability due to greater extension of the disease, poor accessibility or late diagnosis. In these cases neo-adjuvant chemotherapy involving doxorubicin, cyclophosphamide/ifosfamide, actinomycin D with appropriate dosage modification is given. According to International Rhabdomyosarcoma Study Group, survival is same as that observed in the older children. Tumor site is an important factor and caudal tumors have got better prognosis than the tumors of other areas.

Congenital Fibrosarcoma

It is a locally malignant tumor and distant metastasis is unusual. It commonly involves the extremities (60 –70%). Histologically, it is a spindle cell tumor with characteristic herring bone pattern having parallel arrays of interweaving fascicles in densely packed tumor cells. Surgery is the treatment of choice with excellent outcome but chemotherapy may be needed for preoperative reduction of the tumor size.

Other Tumors

These are retinoblastoma, hepatoblastoma, CNS tumors, histiocytosis, etc. Treatment guidelines are same as that of older children with necessary modifications.

Congenital Leukemia (CL)

Congenital leukemia (CL) is a term applied to leukemia diagnosed at birth or within the first month of life. It is an exceedingly rare disease; with reported incidence between 4.3 and 8.6 per million live births. The majority CL are myeloid in origin unlike pediatric leukemias which are usually lymphoid. Familial incidence is extremely rare. Congenital leukemia is also reported in association with certain syndromes namely Down's, Turner , Klippel-Feil and Ellis-van Creveld and other congenital anomalies.

CL may be evident at birth with hepatosplenomegaly, petechiae and ecchymosis. One fourth patients have specific cutaneous infiltrates (leukemia cutis) felt as firm blue or red nodules (Blueberry Muffin). In infants in whom the disease develops within the first month (not at birth), the symptoms are ill-defined with low-grade fever, diarrhea, hepatomegaly and poor gain weight which is very similar to sepsis.

Diagnosis depends on cellular morphology, immunophenotype and chromosomal studies. Congenital ALL is characterized by a higher WBC count and a higher incidence of MLL rearrangements and CD10-negative B-lineage ALL compared to older infants. FAB classification based on cell morphology reveals that monocytic variety is the most frequent subtype in neonatal acute nonlymphocytic leukemia. The commonest genetic abnormality found to be t(11;19) translocation followed by t (9;11) translocation.

Diagnostic Criteria

a. Disease presentation at or shortly after birth (<30 days)
b. Proliferation of immature white cells
c. Infiltration of the cells into extra hematopoietic tissues
d. Absence of any other condition that mimics congenital leukemia.

Differential Diagnosis

a. Sepsis
b. Intrauterine infections (TORCH)
c. Hemolytic disease of the newborn (HDN)
d. Neuroblastoma, and
e. Transient myeloproliferation syndrome associated with Down's syndrome.

Prognosis

CL is an aggressive disease causing rapid downhill with death from secondary infections and hemorrhage. In

ALL, the treatment outcome is significantly poorer in infants younger than 1 year at diagnosis (23% disease-free survival compared with 70% for older children) and may be even lower in newborns. Success of remission induction in congenital AML is almost same as in older children using combination chemotherapy. However, rare cases of CL with spontaneous remission have been described, most of which were associated with Down's syndrome or mosaicism for trisomy.

Bad Prognostic Factors

Bad prognostic factors are:
Leukocytosis, massive organomegaly, CNS involvement, thrombocytopenia, hypogammaglobulinemia, DIC and remission not achieved by 2 weeks.

At the end, it can be concluded that malignancies in the neonatal age group creates a challenging scenario regarding the diagnosis, management and follow up. Proper histological identification of the tumor tissue is of utmost importance before making the decision for the treatment. Management also requires knowledge of the biology of the neonatal development, pharmacology of their drug handling, the higher frequency of acute chemotoxicity and long-term treatment related morbidity. Though the treatment is an uphill task in reality but the results are extremely encouraging if a dedicated multidisciplinary team effort and an appropriate infrastructure is available.

SUGGESTED READING

1. "Neuroblastoma Treatment - National Cancer Institute". http://www.cancer.gov/cancertopics/pdq/treatment/neuroblastoma/HealthProfessional/page3#Section_17. Retrieved, 2008;07-30.
2. Bajwa RP, Skinner R, Windebank KP, Reid MM. Demographic study of leukaemia presenting within the first three months of life in the northern health region of England. J Clin Pathol. 2004;57:186-8.
3. Brodeur GM, Castleberry RP. Neuroblastoma. In: Pizzo PA, Poplack DG. Principles and practice of pediatric oncology, 3rd edn. 1997;761-97.
4. Brodeur GM, Seeger RC, Barrett A, et al. "International criteria for diagnosis, staging, and response to treatment in patients with neuroblastoma". J Clin Oncol. 1988;6:1874-81.
5. Cohn SL, London WB, Monclair T, Matthay KK, Ambros PF, Pearson AD, for the INRG Working Group (2007). "Update on the development of the international neuroblastoma risk group (INRG) classification schema" (abstract). Journal of Clinical Oncology ASCO Annual Meeting Proceedings Part 1, 2007;25(18S).
6. Halperin EC. Neonatal neoplasms. Int J Rad Oncol Phys. 2000;47:171-8.
7. Heerema-McKenney A, Harrison MR, Bratton B, Farrell J, Zaloudek C. Congenital teratoma: A clinicopathologic study of 22 fetal and neonatal tumors. Am J Surg Pathol. 2005;29:29-38.
8. Isaacs H Jr. Fetal and neonatal leukemia. J Pediatr Hematol Oncol. 2003;25:348-61.
9. Lobe TE, Wiener ES, Hays DM, et al. Neonatal rhabdomyosarcoma: The IRS experience. J Ped Surg. 1994;29:1167-70.
10. Maris JM, Hogarty MD, Bagatell R, Cohn SL. "Neuroblastoma". Lancet. 2007;369(9579):2106-20.
11. Nathan O: Congenital leukemia. In: Haematology of Infancy and Childhood. 3rd edn. Philadelphia: WB Saunders. 1987;1052-3.
12. Neonatal soft tissue sarcomas. The influence of pathology on treatment and survival. J Ped Surg. 1995;30:1038-41.
13. Parikh P, Kanbinde S in Ch 23 "Solid tumors in the neonatal period" In: Textbook of Neonatal Hematology –Oncolgy. Lokeshwar MR, Dutta AK, Sachdeva A (Eds). 1st edition. 2003;206-11.
14. Parkes SE, Muir KR, Southern L, et al. Neonatal tumors: A thirty-year population based study. Med Pediatr Oncol. 1994;22:309.
15. Perek D, Brozyna A, Dembowska-Baginska B, Stypinska M, Sojka M, Bacewicz L, Polnik D, Kalicinski P. Tumours in newborns and infants up to three months of life. One institution experience. 2006;10(3 Pt 1):711-23.
16. Resnick KS, Brod BB. Leukemia cutis in congenital leukemia: Analysis and review of the world literature with report of an additional case. Arch Dermatol. 1993;129:1301-6.
17. Thomas D, Lankin MD, Alan S Gamis. Neonatal Oncology. 16:385.

20 Adolescent Oncology

Nibedita Chatterjee, Dipankar Gupta, Goutam Mukherjee

The variety of cancer distribution is unique during the 15–24 year age interval, and infrequently been related to environmental carcinogens, an inherited predisposing cause, or a family cancer syndrome. Cancer cases that fall in this age group have the lowest rate of coverage of health insurance and quintessential delays in diagnosis. Their psychosocial needs are quite unique and generally much less attended. In spite of an intrinsically equal ability to tolerate chemotherapy, older adolescents and young adults frequently receive lower dose intensities than do younger patients, and at times, much less than in older patients. Whereas the 15- to 24-year age group once had a better overall survival rate than either younger or older patients, a relative lack of progress has resulted in the majority of cancers in the age group having a worse overall survival rate than in younger patients, and several of these having a worse prognosis than in older patients. Against this background, young adults with cancer have unique survival challenges, medically, psychosocially, and economically, that are now beginning to be recognized.

The most common cancers among the 15- to 19-year olds are Hodgkin's disease (16%), germ cell tumors (15%), CNS tumors (10%), non-Hodgkin's lymphoma (NHL) (8%), thyroid cancer (7%), malignant melanoma (7%), and acute lymphocytic leukemia (6%) (Figs 20.1 to 20.4). This pattern is very much different from the pattern in younger and older persons. Many of the common malignancies in children younger than 5 years of age are virtually absent in the 15- to 19-year olds including the embryonal malignancies of Wilm's tumor, medulloblastoma, neuroblastoma, hepatoblastoma, ependymoma, and retinoblastoma. Similarly, those

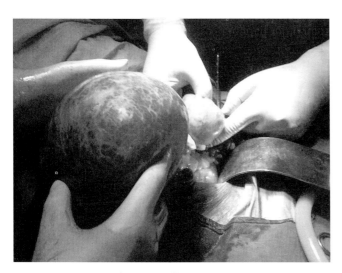
Fig. 20.1: Yolk sac tumor

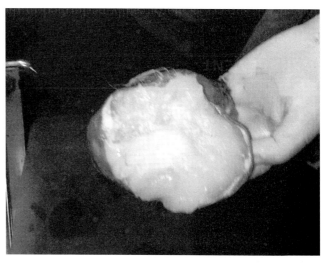
Fig. 20.2: Dermoid cyst

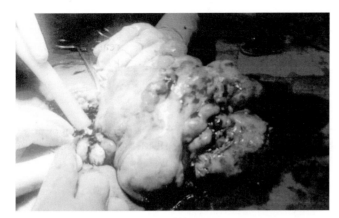

Fig. 20.3: Endodermal sinus tumor

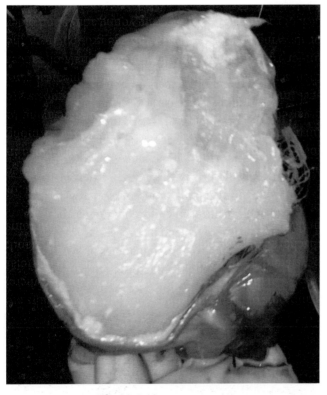

Fig. 20.4: Mature teratoma

Osteosarcoma, Ewing's sarcoma, gonadal germ cell tumors and Hodgkin's cancer peaks in incidence during the adolescent and young adult interval. Fewer than 1% of epithelial ovarian cancers occur before the age of 20 years, with two thirds of ovarian malignancies in such patients being germ cell tumors. In the first two decades of life almost 70% of ovarian tumors are of germ cell tumors and one third of these are malignant. The two sarcomas peak during the 15- to 19-year interval and the latter two cancers during the 20- to 29-year age range. The soft tissue sarcoma that occurs in 15- to 19-years old is clinically distinct from that of the young patients. Rhabdomyosarcoma predominates among the sarcomas of childhood, and account for more than 60% of the soft tissue sarcomas in children younger than 5 years of age. In 15- to 19- year old, rhabdomyosarcoma accounts for only 25% of the soft tissue sarcomas. Non-rhabdomyosarcomas soft tissue sarcomas account for 75% of the soft tissue sarcomas. These include synovial sarcoma, liposarcoma, malignant fibrous histiocytoma and malignant peripheral nerve sheath tumors.

Leukemias and lymphomas are also distributed quite differently than in young children. ALL declines with age from the 0- to 5-year age group upwards, such as 15- to 19-year age. ALL accounts for only 6% of the cancers as contrast to the 30% level in children younger than 15 years. In 15- to 24-year olds, NHL is more common than ALL and steadily increases with age, but the subtype specification changes with age from a predominance of lymphoblastic and Burkitt's lymphoma during the early childhood to a predominance of diffuse large cell lymphomas during adolescence and early adulthood. AML is nearly as common as ALL in 15-to 19-year old and more common than ALL in 20-to 29-year olds. Chronic myelogenous leukemia increases steadily with age from birth onwards, but it is not as common as either ALL or AML during the 15-year to 24-year range.

Gender incidence of tumors is equal in the age group of 15 to 19 years as contrast to a 20% higher rate in boys younger than 15 years of age. The gender difference is ALL, in which males are more than twice likely to get the disease. The gender difference is most unique in thyroid carcinoma, with females being ten times more likely to get the disease. Females are also 50% more likely to be diagnosed with melanoma and approximately 15% more

cancers that predominate in adults, such as carcinoma of the breast, and gastrointestinal and genitourinary tracts, are uncommon in the adolescents.

At least six of the common malignancies in the 15- to 19-year olds increased in incidence between 1973 and 1995. NHL and testicular carcinoma underwent the greatest increases over this interval, each averaging more than 2% per year for 24 years. ALL osteosarcoma and germ cell tumors and gonadal tumors showed similar increments.

likely to sustain Hodgkin's disease. Males are twice as likely to have NHL or Ewing's sarcoma, 50% more likely to develop osteosarcoma, and 20 to 30% more likely to have brain tumors or NHL.

ETIOLOGY

Similar as in younger patients, little information is known with regards to the cause of cancer in adolescents and young adults. Few of the cancers in adolescents and young adults have been attributed to environmental or inherited factors. Most cases of clear cell adenocarcinoma of the vagina or cervix in adolescent females were found to be caused by diethylstilbestrol (DES) taken prenatally by their mothers in an attempt to prevent spontaneous abortion. Radiation induced cancer may occur in adolescents and young adults, in most cases when the radiation exposure occurred during early childhood. Many of the adolescents and young adult cancers that have been linked to etiologic factors are second malignant neoplasms in patients who were treated with chemotherapy or radiotherapy, or both for a previous cancer. Dermatologic cancers, sarcoma, liver cancers and lymphoma occur with higher frequency in patients with inherited conditions like ataxia telangiectasia, Li-Fraumeni syndrome, neurofibromatosis, Fanconi's syndrome, hereditary dysplastic nevus syndrome, xeroderma pigmentosa, nevoid basal cell carcinoma, and Turner's syndrome.

Given the duration of exposure to potential environmental carcinogens is directly proportional to age, older adolescents and young adults should be more likely to develop tobacco, sunlight or diet related cancers than younger persons. Nevertheless, there is very little substantial evidence that the cancers in the 15- to 29-year olds are substantially related to these new environmental factors, which is not the similar case with cancer in the adults. It appears to take considerably longer than one or two decades in most persons for the environmental related cancers to become manifested.

SYMPTOMS AND SIGNS

The signs and symptoms differ in adolescent and young adults from the typical for adults and children. Common symptoms of cancer in adolescents and young adults are masses in the neck, testis, abdomen, breast, or elsewhere; persistent fatigue and lethargy; abnormal orificial discharge; change in mole; swelling of lymph gland; unilateral joint swelling; or a neurodeficit or symptoms of increased intracranial pressure.

Because of psychological and social factors in adolescents and young adults, patients in this age range may be at higher risk for a delay in diagnosis, which in turn, may have an impact on cancer survival. Among a variety of explanations for young adults delaying to seek medical care and obtain a correct diagnosis are their sense of invincibility, lack of routine medical care, under-recognition by medical professionals of cancer or its symptoms and signs in the age group. Given the lack of routine care, empowering young adults and older adolescents for self-care and detection is important, particularly learning how to perform self-examination of the skin and, in females, being able to recognize any changes of the breasts.

DIAGNOSTIC IMAGING AND PATHOLOGY CONSIDERATIONS

Many of the procedures for diagnostic imaging, pathologic evaluation, biopsies, and staging have been derived from the more common malignancies in adults, especially from the carcinomas that predominate in patients. Older adolescents and young adults are typically referred to physicians based on the patient's age rather than on the disease. Yet, the workup for cancer is nearly always disease specific and usually not patient-age dependent. Hence, responsibility may be better undertaken by those who specialize in the age group to which the patient is referred. Most appropriate investigations are carried out after proper evaluation of signs and symptoms in relation to common sites of tumors. With very few exceptions, the signs and symptoms of cancer in adolescents are similar to signs and symptoms of the same cancer in older persons, because of the psychological and social factors, patients in this age range may be at higher risk for a delay in diagnosis. Adolescents may present with advanced disease, large masses because they were embarrassed to bring this problem to attention.

MANAGEMENT

Surgery

In general, surgery is more readily performed in the larger patient and anesthesia is quite easier to administer. That young adults are generally healthier than the older patients is a distinct advantage.

Radiation Therapy

The growing and developing tissues in the young and adolescents are more vulnerable to the adverse effects of ionizing radiation. This is particularly true for the CNS, the cardiovascular system, gonads, the connective tissue system, and the musculoskeletal system which all may be irradiated to much higher doses or larger volume or both with less long-term morbidity in the older individuals.

Chemotherapy

For the same chemotherapeutic agents, acute and chronic, are given similar in children, adolescents and adults. Exception for the older patients in the age range is the greater degree of anticipatory vomiting, a somewhat less recovery potential from myeloablative agents, and fewer stem cells in the peripheral blood available for autologous rescue. Adherent therapy regimens, particularly oral chemotherapy is much more problematic than older patients.

Treatment Intensity

On the other hand, the acute toxicities of radiation and chemotherapy are generally less problematic than older patients who have coexisting morbidities, decreased tissue reserve, or are on medications that adversely affect the toxicity profile or treatment efficacy of chemotherapy. Adolescents and young adults better tolerate more intensive therapy than adults because of better organ function, especially marrow reserve. They typically recover more rapidly from myelosuppressive therapy and can tolerate higher dose-intensive regimens without dose delays or modifications required in older patients.

For autologous rescue transplant regimens, they usually have more stem cells available in their peripheral blood than older patients.

PAUCITY OF CLINICAL TRIALS

Cancer patients between age 15 and 35 years have had the lowest proportion of patients accrued to clinical trials. The reasons for the gap include a lack of available trials, lack of informing the young adult patient about clinical trials, inability or reluctance of the patient to participate in the trial, and financial limitations by the patient, family and care provider.

SUGGESTED READING

1. Bleyer A, Albritton K. Cancer in the young adult and adolescent, in Kufe DW, Pollock RE, Weichselbaum RR, et al. (Eds). Holland-Frei: Cancer Medicine. 7th edn. Hamilton, Ontario: BC Decker; 2006;2028-36.
2. Bleyer WA, O'Leary M, Barr R, Ries LAG (Eds). Cancer Epidemiology in Older Adolescents and Young Adults 15 to 29 Years of Age, including SEER Incidence and Survival: 1975-2000. National Cancer Institute, NIH Pub. No. 06–5767. Bethesda, MD: National Cancer Institute; 2006.
3. Franeeschi S, Parazzini F, La Vecchia C, Booth M, et al. Pooled analysis of three European care-control studies of epithelial ovarian cancer: II. Age at menarche and menopause. Int J Cancer. 1991;49:61-5.
4. Goldman S, Stafford C, Weinthal J, et al. Older adolescents vary greatly from children in their route of referral to the pediatric oncologist and national trials [abstract]. Proc Am Soc Clin Oncol. 2000;18:18. Abstract 1766.
5. Lewis IJ. Cancer in adolescence. Br Med Bull. 1996; 52:887-97.
6. Rauck AM, Fremgen AM, Menck HR, et al. Adolescent cancers in the United States: a National Cancer Data Base (NCDB) report. J Pediatr Hematol Oncol. 1999;21:310.
7. Schroeder H, Kjeldahl M, Boeson AM, et al. Prognosis of ALL in 10–20 year old patients in Denmark 1992–2001 [abstract]. Pediatr Blood Cancer. 2005;45:578.

21 Ovarian Germ Cell Tumor

Goutam Mukherjee, Nibedita Chatterjee, Kakoli Chowdhury

INTRODUCTION

Germ cell tumors (GCT) of the ovary are uncommon accounting for 10% of all ovarian cancers but aggressive tumors seen most often in young women or preteen and adolescent girls. Germ cell tumors begin in the reproductive cells, i.e. egg or sperm of the body. Germ cell tumors that originate outside the gonads are also seen.

ETIOLOGY

The primordial germ cells first become evident in the extraembryonic yolk sac by the fourth week of gestation. By the fifth week, the germ cells migrate through the mesentry to the gonadal ridge. This migration appears to be mediated by the c-kit receptor and its ligand and stem cell factor. No factors have been associated with the etiology of GCT, apart from an increased incidence associated with dysgenetic gonads. Some patients with dysgerminomas are associated with constitutional cytogenetic abnormalities involving the entirety or part of the Y chromosome; 46, XY (testicular feminization), gonadal dysgenesis and mixed gonadal dysgenesis (45, X, 46, XY). However, 95% of females with dysgerminomas are cytogenetically normal. In genetic syndromes with a high-risk of cancer, GCTs are found rarely. GCT may be found infrequently in individuals with Li-Fraumeni.

GENETICS AND MOLECULAR BIOLOGY

Ovarian germ cell tumor is a general name that is used to describe several different types of cancer. The genetic biology of ovarian germ cell tumor is complex and is considered separately.

Immature teratoma- heterogeneous in nature—some meiotic stem cell origin, some of mitotic, i.e. early meiotic arrest. Apparently a correlation exists between the histological grade and DNA content. Grades 1 and 2 are diploid whereas Grade 3 tumors are aneuploid. Malignant ovarian germ cell tumors—mostly aneuploid; approximately 75% contain i(12p), 42% and 32% have gains of chromosomes 21 and 1q, respectively, and 25% and 42% have loss of chromosomes 13 and 8, respectively.

Mature teratoma- 95% are karyotypically normal, only 5% showing gains of single whole chromosomes.

EPIDEMIOLOGY

Although 20 to 25% of all benign and malignant ovarian tumors are germ cell origin, only about 3% of these are malignant. In the first two decades of life, approximately two thirds of ovarian tumors are of germ cell origin, of which one third are malignant. GCTs are also seen in the third decades of life but thereafter become rare.

PATHOLOGY

GCTs show numerous histological subtypes. According to WHO classification of ovarian GCT –

- Dysgerminoma
- Yolk sac tumor (endodermal sinus tumor)
- Embryonal carcinoma
- Polyembryoma

- Choriocarcinoma
- Teratoma—immature and mature
  - Monodermal
  - Specialized
  - Struma ovarii
- Carcinoid
- Strumal carcinoid and others.

Teratomas

Teratomas develop from totipotential germ cells and consequently contain all three germ cell layers—ectoderm, mesoderm and endoderm. Teratomas are classified into immature (malignant), mature (dermoid cyst) and monodermal (struma ovarii, carcinoid). Dermoid cysts contain mature tissue, and upon gross examination skin, teeth, bone, hair, sebaceous glands and neural tissue predominate; whilst cartilage, respiratory and intestinal epithelium are also common. They are cystic tumors with a firm capsule. Monodermal teratoma comprise mainly one tissue element. For example, the most common type of monodermal teratoma, struma ovarii, is comprised of at least 50% mature thyroid tissue. Argentaffin cells in dermoid cysts are usually the site of origin for ovarian carcinoid, although this is rare. Immature teratomas account for approximately 20% of all malignant GCT. They are classified as Grade I, II or III if they have 0 or 1, 3 or less, or 4 or more low-power fields (x-40) containing immature neuroepithelium per section, respectively. Immature teratomas are solid tumors containing immature or embryonal tissues. Immature neuroepithelium is the predominant immature tissue found.

Dysgerminoma

Dysgerminomas have a solid, lobulated, tan, flesh-like gross appearance with a smooth surface. Microscopically dysgerminoma cells are round and ovoid, contain abundant cytoplasm, irregularly shaped nuclei, >1 prominent nucleolus. These cells have a propensity to aggregate forming cords and sheets. Lymphocytic and granulocytic infiltration of the fibrous septa is evident.

Endodermal Sinus Tumor (EST)

Gross examination of EST, also known as yolk sac tumor, demonstrates smooth, glistening, hemorrhagic

and necrotic surfaces. Histology reveals a wide range of patterns, i.e. microcystic, endodermal sinus, solid, alveolar-glandular, papillary, macrocystic, hepatoid, primitive endodermal. The classic pattern contains Schiller-Duval bodies, i.e. central capillary surrounded by simple papillae and eosinophilic globules containing AFP. Intracellular and extracellular hyaline droplets, periodic acid-Schiff positive are seen in EST.

Embryonal Carcinoma

Gross examination of embryonal carcinoma reveals a solid, hemorrhagic, necrotic tumor, resembling a larger form of EST. Embryonal glands, gland-like clefts and syncytiotrophoblastic giant cells are present microscopically.

Choriocarcinoma

Choriocarcinoma is a rare solid, hemorrhagic tumor, composed of malignant cytotropohoblast and syncytiotrophoblast. Non-gestational and gestational choriocarcinoma have identical histologies.

Mixed Germ Cell Tumor

As the name suggests, mixed germ cell tumors contain more than one histological type. Dysgerminoma with EST and immature teratomas with EST are frequent combinations.

CLINICAL FEATURES

Ovarian germ cell tumors can be difficult to diagnose early. Often there are no symptoms in the early stages. Because young girls have yet to have a gynecologic examination, the only symptoms may be a swelling or hard distended abdomen without weight gain. Most GCTs are benign and unilateral with the exception of dysgerminomas. Patients usually present at stage I. Abdominal pain or adnexal torsion is the commonest presenting symptom of GCT, however they may be asymptomatic. The mass may cause acute pain due to torsion, rupture or hemorrhage. Patients may also have abdominal distension, vaginal bleeding or fever. Teratomas are usually diagnosed in premenopausal women without presenting symptoms. Complications of mature cystic teratoma, i.e. dermoid cyst include torsion, rupture, infection and hemolytic anemia. Approximately 50% of pre-pubertal girls with non-gestational choriocarcinoma are iso-sexually precocious. Only 1–2% of dermoid cysts become malignant, usually in postmenopausal women. Patients with ESTs frequently present following spontaneous rupture and hemorrhage.

INDIVIDUAL TUMORS

Teratoma

Mature cystic teratoma is the most common ovarian teratoma and most common ovarian germ cell tumor typically occurs during reproductive years. It is cystic tumor with firm capsule, filled with sebaceous material and hair occasionally. Thickened area from which hair and teeth arise is called "Rokitansky's protuberance" composed of mature elements derived from all three germ layers. Ectodermal elements such as skin, hair, sebaceous glands, and mature neural tissue predominate; cartilage, bone, respiratory and intestinal epithelium are common. Complications include torsion, rupture, infection, hemolytic anemia benign neoplasm. Immature teratomas contain elements that resemble tissues derived from the embryo. It is the second most common germ cell malignancy.

Monodermal Teratoma

A teratoma composed predominantly of one tissue element most common type is "struma ovarii", which is mature thyroid tissue. Immature teratoma: occurs in children and young adults usually a unilateral, 10% bilateral, solid tumor similar to mature teratoma but contains immature or embryonal tissues. Immature elements are almost always immature neuroepithelium graded on the basis of the quantity of immature tissue malignant neoplasm hematogenous metastasis to the lungs, liver or brain.

Dysgerminoma

Three to five percent of ovarian malignant tumors, 50% of ovarian GCT most common malignant ovarian germ cell tumor typically occurs in 2nd and 3rd decades. They are most often associated with abnormal gonads, viz. pure or mixed gonadal dysgenesis, testicular feminization

syndrome typically a unilateral, solid, firm to fleshy tumor composed of malignant germ cells, similar to primordial germ cells, admixed with non-neoplastic chronic inflammatory cells. They metastasize commonly by lymphatic spread, hematogenous or direct invasion. Metastasis to contralateral ovary may occur.

ENDODERMAL SINUS TUMOR (EST)

Yolk Sac Tumor

Third most common malignant ovarian germ cell tumor occurs in childhood, adolescence and adult life. It can be pure or a component of a mixed germ cell tumor almost always a unilateral solid or solid and cystic tumor. It displays a wide range of histologic patterns. Classic pattern shows perivascular formations (Schiller-Duval bodies) and eosinophilic globules that contain alpha fetoprotein (AFP). Most common presentations are abdominal pain (80%), asymptomatic pelvic mass associated with elevated serum AFP levels, rarely alpha 1 antitrypsin.

Embryonal Carcinoma

Uncommon ovarian germ cell neoplasm occurs in children and young adults mean age 12 years. It occurs in combination with yolk sac tumor typically unilateral, presents usually with adnexal mass, with precocious pseudo- puberty or irregular bleeding due to estrogen secretion.

Choriocarcinoma

Very rare as a pure ovarian neoplasm or as a component of a mixed germ cell tumor occurs in children and young adults associated with elevated serum hCG levels. Typically a unilateral, solid, hemorrhagic tumor composed of malignant cytotrophoblast and syncytiotrophoblast. Nongestational choriocarcinoma is a highly malignant neoplasm that responds to combination chemotherapy.

Polyembryoma

Extremely rare tumor, which is composed of 'embryoid bodies'. This tumor replicates the structure of early embryonic differentiation. They occur in very young, premenarchical girls with signs of pseudopuberty, raised AFP and hCG.

DIAGNOSIS

Ovarian germ cell tumors can be difficult to diagnose. Often there are no symptoms in the early stages, but tumors may be found during regular gynecologic examinations. Tests that examine the ovaries, pelvic area, blood and ovarian tissue are used to detect and diagnose ovarian germ cell tumor. The following tests and procedures may be helpful.

Pelvic Examination

An exam of the vagina, cervix, uterus, fallopian tubes, ovaries and rectum. The doctor inserts one or two lubricated, gloved fingers of one hand into the vagina and the other hand is placed over the lower abdomen to feel the size, shape and position of the uterus and ovaries. A speculum is also inserted into the vagina and the doctor looks at the vagina and cervix for signs of disease. A Pap test or Pap smear of the cervix is usually done. The doctor inserts a lubricated, gloved finger into the rectum to feel for lumps or abnormal areas.

Laparotomy

A surgical procedure in which an incision is made in the wall of the abdomen to check the inside of the abdomen for signs of disease. Sometimes organs are removed or tissue samples are taken for biopsy.

Lymphangiogram

A procedure used to X-ray the lymph system. A dye is injected into the lymph vessels in the feet. The dye travels upward through the lymph nodes and lymph vessels, and X-rays are taken to see if there are any blockages. This test helps to find out whether cancer has spread to the lymph nodes.

CT scan

A dye may be injected into a vein or swallowed to help the organs or tissues show up more clearly.

Blood Tests

Apart from routine blood tests, tests to measure the levels of alpha fetoprotein (AFP) and human chorionic gonadotropin (HCG) in the blood. AFP and HCG are substances that may be signs of ovarian germ cell tumor when found at increased levels.

Tumor Markers

Many of the GCTs have a marker that shows up in the blood that indicates the tumors presence. Levels of alphafetoprotein (AFP) and human chorionic gonadotropin (HCG) should be obtained as soon as the diagnosis is established. The levels should decrease after surgery, a failure to do so would indicate a remaining tumor. Monitoring these levels can also indicate a recurrence.

Tumor markers are divided into embryonic or cellular. Oncofetal substances associated with embryonic derivatives, e.g. AFP, βhCG. Cellular enzymes, e.g. LDH, placental alkaline phosphatase, alpha 1-antitrypsin, etc.

AFP

Serum protein of early embryo barely detected soon after birth secreted from trophoblastic cells—fetal yolk sac, liver GIT. Half-life is 5–7 days. Normalize after complete surgery. Increased level of AFP is seen in the following non-malignant and malignant conditions like cirrhosis of liver, viral hepatitis pure embryonal CA, teratocarcinoma, yolk sac tumor, mixed GCT, hepatocellular, gastric pancreatic and lung cancers.

βhCG

Secretory product of the placenta barely detected soon after birth. The source is syncytiotrophoblastic cells. Half-life is 24–34 hours. Normalize after 5–8 days complete surgery.

Increased level of βhCG seen in non-malignant-pregnancy, hydatidiform mole. Malignant – choriocarcinoma, embryonal carcinoma (40–60%), lung cancer, breast cancer, hepatocellular carcinoma, multiple myeloma.

TREATMENT

There are different types of treatment for patients with ovarian germ cell tumors. Because the disease principally affects girls and young women, special consideration must be given to preserve the infertility and use of chemotherapy as needed. Three types of standard treatment are used: Surgery, chemotherapy, radiation therapy. Other types of treatment are being tested in clinical trials. These include the following: High-dose chemotherapy with bone marrow transplant.

Surgery

Surgery is the most common treatment of ovarian germ cell tumor. A doctor may take out the cancer using one of the following types of surgery (Figs 21.1 to 21.7):

Unilateral salpingo-oophorectomy: A surgical procedure to remove one ovary and one fallopian tube.

Total hysterectomy: A surgical procedure to remove the uterus, including the cervix.

Tumor debulking: A surgical procedure in which as much of the tumor as possible is removed. Choosing the most appropriate cancer treatment is a decision that ideally involves the patient, family and health care team.

Chemotherapy

The way the chemotherapy is given depends on the type and stage of the cancer being treated.

Combination intravenous chemotherapy for germ cell tumors of the ovary studied by the gynecologic oncology group: BEP; Bleomycin, Etoposide, Cisplatin. PVB; Cisplatin, Vinblastin, Bleomycin. VAC; Vincristrin, Dactinomycin, Cyclophosphamide are used.

Radiation Therapy

The way the radiation therapy is given, depends on the type and stage of the cancer being treated. Certain special type of tumors like dysgerminomas are very sensitive to radiation but loss of fertility is a problem for young women, so radiation showed rarely be used as a first-line treatment. Treatment given after the surgery to increase the chances of a cure is called adjuvant therapy.

Second Look Laparotomy

Following radiation or chemotherapy, a second-look laparotomy is sometimes done. This is similar to the laparotomy that is done to determine the stage of the cancer. During the second-look operation, take samples of lymph nodes and other tissues in the abdomen to see if any cancer is left.

Other types of treatment are being tested in clinical trials. These include the following: High-dose chemotherapy with bone marrow transplant—High-dose chemotherapy with bone marrow transplant is a method of giving very high doses of chemotherapy and replacing blood-forming cells destroyed by the cancer treatment. Stem cells are removed from the bone marrow of the patient or a donor and are frozen and stored. After the chemotherapy is completed, the stored stem cells are thawed and given back to the patient through an infusion. These re-infused stem cells grow into the body's blood cells.

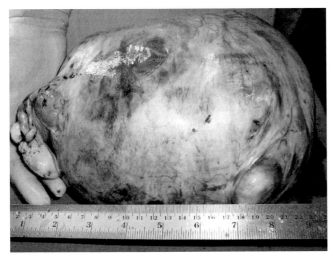

Fig. 21.1: Mucinous cyst ovary

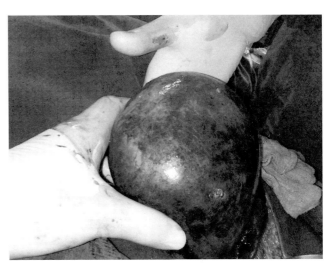

Fig. 21.2: Mucinous cyst twist with gangrene

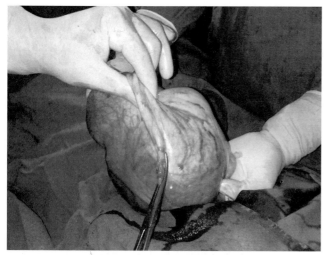

Fig. 21.3: Mucinous cystadenoma

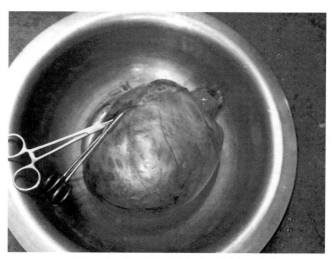

Fig. 21.4: Simple serous cystadenoma

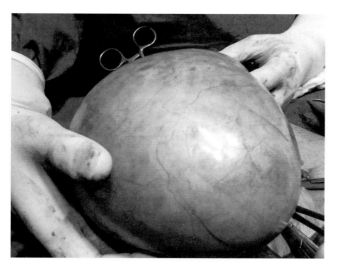

Fig. 21.5: Serous cystadenoma

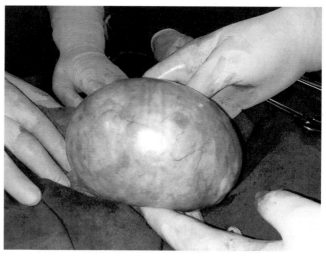

Fig. 21.6: Twisted simple cyst

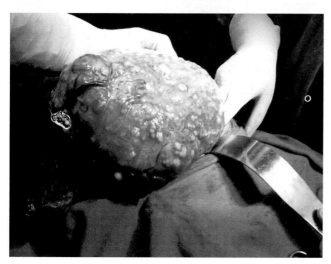

Fig. 21.7: Uterine leiomyosarcoma

New treatment options: Combination chemotherapy is being tested in clinical trials.

TREATMENT OPTIONS BY STAGES

Stage I Ovarian Germ Cell Tumors

Treatment depends on whether the tumor is dysgerminoma or another type of germ cell tumor. Treatment of dysgerminoma may include the following: Unilateral salpingo-oophorectomy. Unilateral salpingo-oophorectomy followed by observation. Unilateral salpingo-oophorectomy followed by radiation therapy. Unilateral salpingo-oophorectomy followed by chemotherapy.

Treatment of other germ cell tumors may be either: unilateral salpingo-oophorectomy followed by careful observation; or unilateral salpingo-oophorectomy, sometimes followed by combination chemotherapy.

Stage II Ovarian Germ Cell Tumors

Treatment of dysgerminoma may be either—hysterectomy and bilateral salpingo-oophorectomy followed by radiation therapy or combination chemotherapy; or unilateral salpingo-oophorectomy followed by chemotherapy.

Treatment of other germ cell tumors may include the following: Unilateral salpingo-oophorectomy followed by combination chemotherapy.

Stage III Ovarian Germ Cell Tumors

Treatment of dysgerminoma may include the following: Hysterectomy and bilateral salpingo-oophorectomy, with removal of as much of the cancer in the pelvis and abdomen as possible. Unilateral salpingo-oophorectomy followed by chemotherapy. Treatment of other germ cell tumors may include the following: Hysterectomy and bilateral salpingo-oophorectomy, with removal of as much of the cancer in the pelvis and abdomen as possible. Chemotherapy will be given before and/or after surgery.

Stage IV Ovarian Germ Cell Tumors

Treatment of dysgerminoma may include the following: Hysterectomy and bilateral salpingo-oophorectomy followed by chemotherapy, with removal of as much of the cancer in the pelvis and abdomen as possible. Unilateral salpingo-oophorectomy followed by chemotherapy. Treatment of other germ cell tumors may include the following: Hysterectomy and bilateral salpingo-oophorectomy, with removal of as much of the cancer in the pelvis and abdomen as possible. Chemotherapy will be given before and/or after surgery.

PROGNOSIS

The prognosis of ovarian GCT is excellent, as most cases are benign. The prognosis and treatment options depend on the following: The type of cancer, the size of the tumor,

the stage of cancer, e.g. whether it affects part of the ovary, involves the whole ovary, or has spread to other places in the body. When malignant they are very aggressive, but the prognosis is still good provided it is treated without delay with surgery and combination chemotherapy. The survival rates for dysgerminomas presenting at early and advanced stages are 95% and >80% respectively. The survival rates for stage I and II ESTs are reported to be 60 to 100%, whereas for those with stage III or IV disease the prognosis is less favorable (50–75%). Survival rates for embryonal carcinoma are slightly higher than those for ESTs. The prognosis of immature teratomas is governed by grade and stage. Grade 1, stage 1 have 100% survival rate, whereas stage III, grade 1 has only a 50% chance of survival. Meanwhile, most patients with mature teratomas show long survival times. The prognosis is better for gestational choriocarcinoma than non-gestational carcinoma (Fig. 21.8). The prognosis for mixed GCT is dictated by the proportion of the more malignant component and the stage.

CONCLUSION

Use of combination chemotherapy after initial surgery has dramatically improved the prognosis for many of these tumors in last few decades. To conclude, that germ cell tumor of the ovary is conspicuously a disease of adolescent period. But the disease must not be allowed

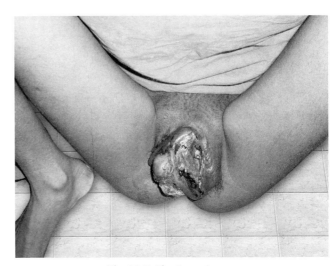

Fig. 21.8: Choriocarcinoma

time in any way lest it may become incurable. Hence, awareness in regard to this disease is important.

SUGGESTED READING

1. Cancer: Principle & Practice of Oncology: Vincent T DeVita (Eds). 7th edition:1390-2.

2. Gershenson DM, Del Junco G, Herson J, Rutledge FN. Endodermal sinus tumor of the ovary: the MD Anderson experience. Obstet Gynaecol. 1983;61: 194-202.

3. Gershenson DM, Del Junco G, Silva EG, et. al. Immature teratoma of the ovary. Obstet Gynaecol. 1986;68:624-9.

4. Hoffner L, Deka R, Chakravarti A. Cytogenetics and origins of pediatric germ cell tomors. Cancer Genet Cytogenet. 1994;74:54.

5. Jacobs AJ, Newland JR, Green RK. Pure choriocarcinoma of the ovary. Obstet Gynaecol Surv. 1982;37:603-9.

6. Kurman RJ, Norris HJ. Germ cell tumors of the ovary. Hum Pathol. 1978;1:291.

7. Loehrer PJ, Elson P, Johnson DH, et al. A randomized trial of Cisplatin plus etoposide with or without bleomycin in favorable prognosis disseminated germ cell tumors: an ECOG study. Proc AM Soc Clin Oncol. 1991;10:540.

8. Principle and practice of pediatric oncology: Philip A Pizzo, David G Poplack(Eds): 4th edn 2001.

9. Riopel M, Spellerberg A, Griffin CA, et al. Genetic analysis of germ cell tumors by comparative genomic hybridization. Cancer Res. 1998;58:3105.

10. Scully Re, Young RH, Clement PB. Germ cell tumors: general features and primitive forms. In: Tumors of the ovary and maldeveloped gonads, fallopian tubes and broad ligament. Washington DC: Armed Forces Institute of Pathology, 1998;239-66.

11. Silver SA, Wiley JM, Perlman EJ. DNA ploidy analysis of pediatric germ cell tumors. Mod Pathol. 1994;7:951.

12. Strohmeyer T, Rees D, Press M, et al. Expression of c-kit proto-oncogene and its ligand stem cell factor in normal and malignant human testicular tissue. J Urol. 1995;153:511.

22 Breast Cancer

Diptendra Sarkar, Subhayan Mandal, Nibedita Chatterjee, Rakesh Mondal

Breast malignancies in adolescent female are relatively uncommon. Only 0.2% of patients with breast carcinoma are younger than 25 years.

1. Primary carcinoma of the breasts of adolescents consists of only few case reports. Therefore, when considering an adolescent with a breast mass, it is important to keep in mind the very low incidence of breast cancer in this population.

2. Risk factors for breast carcinoma include chest radiation and chronic anovulation as per adult based studies. Even if the risk is increased with unopposed estrogen, this issue remains unresolved. The latency period for breast cancer after unopposed estrogen is 15-20 years, so presentation during adolescent is not likely. Protective effect of progestin added to estrogen therapy may be applicable to young patients to reduce risk of endometrial or breast carcinoma later in life.

In the child or adolescent with breast carcinoma, the lesion tends to present as an asymptomatic nodule adjacent to but discrete from the nipple. Because of their rarity, the natural history of the breast carcinomas in adolescent is not well defined. Malignant cystosarcoma phyllodes tumors have been reported very rarely in adolescent. Although these neoplasms are usually benign, they can be malignant and can disseminate via hematogenous spread to the lungs. The biological behavior of these tumors cannot be predicted from its histological appearance. These tumors are treated with surgery with or without radiation and chemotherapy.

Malignancies of the breast in adolescent are more likely to be something other than carcinoma and mostly are secondary metastases tumors. They include rhabdomyosarcoma, lymphoma, neuroblastoma, acute leukemia and other primary malignant neoplasms which have been reported.

Intraductal papilloma or papillomatosis of the breast is rare in young persons. Although it is a benign condition, it can be pre-malignant, and patients should be followed carefully for malignant transformation. The variant of juvenile papillomatosis has been reported to be linked with a high risk of breast carcinoma in the patient's family.

Although breast cancer is rare in adolescents, it should influence the evaluation and management of the breast mass and education of the population regarding routine self-examination of the breast. At present, there are no data sufficient to establish the validity of teaching breast self-examination of adolescent females, so in United States both WHO and Canadian task force do not recommend teaching women younger than 20 years to do breast self-examination.

EPIDEMIOLOGY AND RISK FACTORS

1. Breast cancer demographic profile between 1975 to 2000 shows an increase in incidence with increase in age with an average incidence in per million of 1.3, 12.1 and 81.1 in age groups of 15 to 19 years, 20 to 24 years, and 25 to 29 years respectively. In each age group, however, no variation of annual incidence has been demonstrated over the same time period. Overall breast cancer in < 30 years age group

female constitute only 1% of all the reported cases irrespective of all age groups.

African/American blacks between 10 to 30 years of age group have been reported to have higher incidence of breast carcinoma than white non-hispanic women of similar age group.

Due to lower rate of incidence of breast cancer in adolescent and young adults; few epidemiological studies have done with the focus in this age group.

2. Risk factors for development of breast cancer include:
   - Age
   - Reproductive history
   - Personal or family history [specifically 1st and 2nd degree relatives]
   - Environmental exposure to carcinogen
   - Young women with germline mutations of
     - BRCA1/BRCA2
     - P53 (Li-Fraumeni syndrome)
     - Mutations consistent with Muir syndrome
     - PTEN (Cowden syndrome)
   - Breast tissue density
   - Unopposed circulating estrogen
   - Increased cytochrome P_{450} IA2 function
   - Unique group of survivors of Hodgkin's lymphoma who received
     - Radiation to chest/mantle with or without alkylating agent based therapy
   - Effect of some unidentified growth factors.

Peculiarity of Breast Cancer in Adolescent

- Often tend to be more aggressive histologically
- More likelihood of positive metastatic deposits in lymph nodes (microscopic)
- About 5% adolescent breast cancers are hereditary variety
- More incidence of negative hormone receptor status
- Relative preponderance of infiltrating ductal histology mostly < 30 years [British study]
- High grade and vascular invasion [French study]

- Relatively poor prognosis overall
  - Survival rate on 5 years basis poor in age group < 30 years for all types except localized disease
  - Though benefit of modern therapeutic armamentarium noted in respect to 5 years survival rate and mortality in > 35 years age groups, these remain unchanged for < 30 years age group.

SUGGESTED READING

1. Canadian task force on periodic health examination; The periodic health examination; 1998 update; Can Med Assoc J., 1988;138:617-26.
2. Coulam C, Annegers J, Kranz J. Chronic anovulation syndrome and associated neoplasia. Obstet Gynecol 1983;61:403-7.
3. Daniel WA, Mathews MD. Tumors of the breast in adolescent females; Pediatrics. 1968;41:743.
4. Dupont WD, Page DL. Menopausal estrogen replacement therapy and breast cancer; JAMA. 1991; 265:1985-90.
5. Haagensen CD. Diseases of the breasts. 2nd edn; Philadelphia; WB Saunders, 1971.
6. Hulka BS. Hormone replacement and the risk of breast cancer. CA. 1990;40:289-96.
7. Ivins JC, Taylor WF, Wold LE. Elective whole lung irradiation in osteo-sarcoma treatment; Appearance of bilateral breast cancer in two long-term survivors; Skeletal Radiol. 1987;16:133.
8. Korenman SG. The endocrinology of breast cancer. Cancer. 1980;46:876-8.
9. Rosen PP, Kimmel M. Juvenile papillomatosis of the breast; A follow up study of 41 patients having biopsies before 1979. Am J Clin Pathol. 1990;93:599-603.
10. Steinberg KK, Thacker SB, Smith SJ, et al. A meta-analysis of the effect of estrogen replacement therapy on the risk of breast cancer. JAMA. 1991;265:1990-5.
11. World Health Organization: Self-examination in the early detection of breast cancer; A report on a consultation on self-examination in breast cancer early detection programmes; Geneva, WHO;1983.

Miscellaneous Neoplastic Disorders in Children (Hepatoblastoma/Retinoblastoma/ Germ Cell Tumors)

Rakesh Mondal, Jayanta Dasgupta, Jayanta Ghosh

HEPATOBLASTOMA

Hepatoblastoma is a malignant tumor of the liver which usually occurs in young children. This is different from hepatocellular carcinoma which usually occurs in adults and occasionally in older children. About 10–15 children develop hepatoblastoma in the UK each year. The average age at diagnosis is one year and most cases occur before two years of age. Hepatoblastoma is not associated with previous hepatitis, unlike hepatocellular carcinoma. Usually, there are no associated genetic factors. There may be an increased risk of hepatoblastoma in children who have a family history of familial polyposis coli, or if the child has a condition called Beckwith-Wiedemann syndrome.

Signs and Symptoms

Hepatoblastoma usually presents as a lump in the abdomen. Other symptoms may include: Poor appetite, weight loss, lethargy, fever, vomiting, and jaundice.

Investigations

Apart from the routine hemogram and chest X-ray, USG and CT scan should be done to know the position, size and extent of spread of the tumor. Biopsy is required for the confirmation of the diagnosis. Hepatoblastoma usually produces a protein called alpha-fetoprotein (AFP), which is released into the bloodstream. This is usually referred to as a tumor marker and is used to monitor response to treatment.

Staging

Staging is a measure of how far the tumor has spread. For treatment purposes, there are 2 groups of hepatoblastoma.

Standard-risk is when the tumor is confined to the liver and involves at most 3 segments of the liver. High risk is when the tumor involves all 4 segments of the liver and/ or the tumor has spread outside of the liver.

Treatment

The treatment modalities are chemotherapy, surgery or occasionally liver transplantation depending on the risk group. Cisplatin, cyclophosphamide, VP-16, etc. are commonly used as chemotherapy to shrink the tumor-size. Surgery is carried out by the specialized liver surgeons.

Prognosis

The prognosis depends on the risk group of the tumor, but many children with hepatoblastoma are cured.

RETINOBLASTOMA

Retinoblastoma is a rare cancer originating from the retina. The retina is a thin layer of nerve tissue that coats the back of the eye and enables the eye to see. Retinoblastoma is a malignant tumor composed of retinoblasts in the retina. Retinoblasts develop from a single cell during the early development of an infant in the womb. During gestation and early life, these cells are able to divide and multiply. This is the process that helps make enough cells to populate the retina. As children age, their cells undergo a process called differentiation and become mature rods and cones. The cells are no longer able to divide and multiply, which is why retinoblastoma occurs very rarely after the age of 5 years.

Children may be born with retinoblastoma, but the disease is rarely diagnosed at birth.

A mutation in the both copies (one from each parent) of the retinoblastoma gene (RBI) may be responsible for the tumor. What precisely triggers this change or mutation is not known.

Retinoblastoma can spread to lymph nodes, bone, bone marrow and occasionally to the central nervous system. Children may be cured if the treatment is started before the spread beyond the eye. A major goal of treatment in children with retinoblastoma is preserving vision. Great strides have been made in treating retinoblastoma in recent years; many children retain their vision and more than 95 percent of children with retinoblastoma can be cured.

Incidence

About 300 children are diagnosed with retinoblastoma in the United States each year. The disease occurs most often in children under 4 years old, and accounts for 2.8 percent of all cancers in children ages 0 to 14 years old. The average age of children with retinoblastoma is 18 months — and boys and girls are affected equally. About 60 percent of children with retinoblastoma develop a single tumor in one eye only (unilateral). There is no increased risk of additional tumors later in life. When retinoblastoma affects both eyes (bilateral), it is considered a genetic condition. Rarely, the genetic form occurs only in one eye. The genetic form of the disease occurs in the youngest children rarely beyond 1 year old and increases the child's risk of developing another cancer later in life. The risk of additional tumors is higher in children who receive radiation therapy to the orbit to preserve vision or to other parts of the body where the tumor has spread.

Hereditary Retinoblastoma

Some children, 40 percent of patients with retinoblastoma are born with a change in one copy of the RB1 gene in every cell in the body, including the cells in the retina. If the second copy of the gene undergoes a change, a retinoblastoma tumor can develop. That's because every cell already has the first copy of RB1 mutated — making it relatively easy for more than one cell to undergo a change in the second copy or the gene. These children may have more than one tumor, and they usually have both eyes affected. Most children (80

percent) with the genetic form do not have a parent with retinoblastoma. The change in the gene occurred in either the ovum or the sperm of one parent before conception. Even if the child has the genetic form, if neither parent has the tumor there is less than a 1% chance that retinoblastoma will occur in another child in family.

Children with the genetic form may also develop tumors in other parts of their body, such as the pineal gland in the brain. The pineal gland develops from cells that sense light and are similar to retinoblasts. As is the case with retinoblastoma, when these cells become mature and can no longer divide and multiply, they are much less likely to become cancer cells.

Nonhereditary Retinoblastoma

Most children with retinoblastoma do not have the genetic form. They are not born with the RB1 gene mutated in every cell of the body. They develop a tumor in only one eye because both RB1 genes in a single retinoblast have undergone the mutation. If neither parent has had retinoblastoma and the child is over 2 years of age at diagnosis, the probability of having the genetic form is very small. If eye tumor tissue is available for study, there is a blood test that can be done to determine whether a child with a unilateral tumor is one of the 10 percent of children with a tumor in only one eye who has the genetic form.

The Signs and Symptoms of Retinoblastoma

Sometimes children with retinoblastoma do not show any of the following signs or symptoms. Often, doctors find retinoblastoma on a routine well-baby examination. Most often, however, parents notice symptoms such as:

- White (leukocoria) or red pupil instead of the normal black
- Misaligned eyes (strabismus) looking toward the ear or nose (Fig. 23.1)
- Reddened, painful eye
- Enlarged pupil
- Different-colored irises
- Poor vision.

Diagnosis of Retinoblastoma

The diagnosis of retinoblastoma is made by examining the eyes. If a newborn has a family history of retinoblastoma,

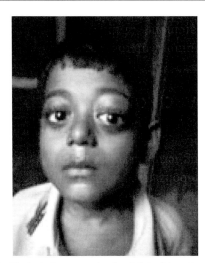

Fig. 23.1: Clinical photograph of a child with retinoblastoma showing bilateral proptosis and misaligned eyes

the baby should be examined shortly after birth by an oph-thalmologist specialized in cancers of the eye. If a white pupil or strabismus (crossed-eyes) is noticed by a parent or pediatrician, the child should be referred to an ophthal-mologist familiar with the treatment of retinoblastoma. The doctor will do a thorough examination to check the retina for a tumor. Depending on the age of the child, either a local or general is used during the eye examination. The ophthalmologist will make a drawing or take a photograph of the tumors in the eyes to provide a record for future examinations and treatments, and may use additional tests to confirm or detect tumors. These tests may include:

Imaging tests: Ultrasound—This test looks for tumors in the child's eye. Computerized tomography (CT or CAT) scan—Sometimes, a special dye (a contrast medium) is injected into a vein to provide better detail. A CT scan helps to find cancer outside of the eye. Magnetic reso-nance imaging (MRI)—MRI uses electromagnetic waves to create computer-generated pictures of the brain and spinal column. MRIs may create more detailed pictures than CT scans and provide the specialist with a picture of the inside of the eye and the brain.

Additional tests: Children who are diagnosed with retin-oblastoma will require a complete physical examination and, if there are any additional symptoms or abnormal findings, may also undergo additional tests to determine if the cancer has spread elsewhere in the body. Children with retinoblastoma taking certain chemotherapy drugs

may have their hearing tested (audiology test) to make sure the drugs are not causing hearing loss.

Staging: After a retinoblastoma has been detected, the doctor will determine the extent of disease in the eye and if the disease has spread (metasized) outside the eye. Staging categories include: The Reese-Ellsworth stages of retinoblastoma include:

Stage I—either one or more tumors that are less than 4 disc diameters (DD) in size and located at or behind the equator.

Stage II—either one or more tumors that are 4 to 10 DD in size located at or behind the equator.

Stage III—any lesion in front of the equator or any tumor(s) larger than 10 DD.

Stage IV—multiple tumors with some or all greater than 10 DD in size or any lesions that extend beyond the back of the eye.

Stage V—very large tumors involving more than half of the retina and have spread to other sites in the body.

Intraocular: This means that cancer occurs in one or both eyes, but has not spread into surrounding tissues or other parts of the body.

Recurrent: The cancer that recurred in the eye or con-tinued to grow after it has been treated.

Extraocular: The cancer has spread to tissues around the eye or to other parts of the body.

Treatment

The goal of treatment is to prevent tumor cells from growing and spreading, and to preserve vision.

Standard treatment for retinoblastoma has changed over the years. A decade ago, treatment options included enucleation (removal of the involved eye) or radiation. When only one eye is involved, enucleation is usually the treatment of choice. Children adjust very well to the loss of one eye, and their vision does not suffer a great deal. However, if a child is very young, there is a risk that a tumor will develop in the other eye, so the goal in these children is to remove as much of the tumor as possible while preserving vision.

Small tumors can often be treated successfully using local measures, including:

Cryotherapy: Extreme cold may be used to destroy cancer cells. The procedure is done in the operating room. The child is discharged the same day after recovering from anesthesia.

Photocoagulation (laser therapy): Laser light may be used to destroy blood vessels that supply nutrients to the tumor. The procedure is done in the operating room. The child is discharged the same day after recovering from anesthesia.

Plaque radiotherapy: A radioactive device is implanted in the affected eye with a specific dose of radiation directly applied to the tumor.

Radiation therapy: Radiation therapy has been the treatment of choice for children with bilateral disease. However, radiation may produce damage to the retina many years after it has been given. That damage can result in loss of vision. Radiation when given to very young children also results in decreased growth of the bone surrounding the orbit. It can also increase the risk of second non-retinoblastoma cancers many years after treatment.

Chemotherapy: In case of very large tumor chemotherapy is required to reduce the size of the tumor. Cyclophosphamide, doxorubicin, cisplatin, etc. are used.

Prognosis

The extent of the disease, the size and location of the tumor, presence or absence of metastasis, the tumor's response to therapy, the age and overall health of the child, the child's tolerance of specific medications, procedures are the determinants of prognosis.

GERM CELL TUMORS

About 90 percent of all germ cell tumors are gonadal, which means they develop within the ovaries and testes (Fig. 23.2). The remaining 10 percent are extragonadal, which means they develop somewhere outside the gonads, usually the chest, lower back, and head. Germ cell tumors can be benign or malignant.

Germ cell tumors are seen during childhood. Extragonadal germ cell tumors account for approximately 3% of all childhood cancers.

Etiology

Research has shown that extragonadal germ cells. Tumors are caused by problems that occur during fetal development. The germ cells normally move from the yolk sac into the embryo and grow within the developing gonads. The common sites for extra-gonadal germ cell tumors are mediastinum, pre-sacral, area, pineal gland, etc.

Signs and Symptoms

The symptoms of a germ cell tumor depend upon its location. Malignant tumors in the mediastinum, which is around midchest, near the lungs, can cause chest pain, breathing problems, cough, and fever. Germ cell tumors in the presacral area, just above the buttocks, are seen more often in infants or young children. Malignant presacral tumors can cause difficulty with walking, urinating, or having bowel movements. They may be felt as a mass just above the buttocks or in the lower abdominal area. Presacral germ cell tumors in children younger than 6 months are almost always benign. However, around 65% of presacral germ cell tumors in children older than 6 months are malignant. Malignant germ cell tumors in the pineal area, put pressure on the brain or block the flow of cerebrospinal fluid. This causes symptoms that can include problems with balance, lethargy, nausea, vomiting, headache, memory loss, double vision, problems looking upward, and uncontrolled eye movements. Gonadal germ cell tumors can produce hormones that induce precocious puberty.

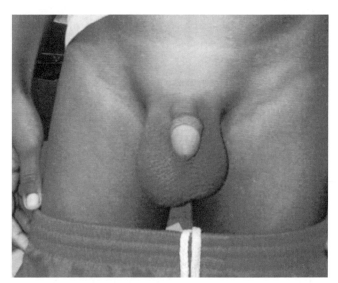

Fig. 23.2: Clinical photograph showing enlargement of right testes following testicular germ cell tumor

Diagnosis

Proper medical history followed by detailed examination including rectal and pelvic area are required. Neurological examination is mandatory for detection of pineal tumors. Diagnostic modalities include chest X-ray, CT scan and MRI of the involved area, bone scan, and histopathological examination for confirmation. With most germ cell tumors, blood tests show high levels of alpha-fetoprotein (AFP), which is produced by the liver, and beta-human chorionic gonadotropin (beta-hCG), a hormone that is produced during pregnancy, but also occurs in people with certain types of cancer. These substances may also be found in the spinal fluid of patients with pineal tumors.

Benign germ cell tumors are called teratomas, and are divided into mature teratomas, immature teratomas, and teratomas that include some malignant germ cell components. Cancers that contain malignant germ cell tumors include embryonal carcinoma, germinoma, choriocarcinoma, and endodermal sinus, or yolk sac tumor.

Treatment

Treatment depends upon the type of germ cell tumor and its location. The first step in treatment is to surgically remove the tumor as much as possible. Infants and children with benign germ cell tumors can usually be treated successfully with surgery. Older children with malignant germ cell tumors, especially those in the presacral region above the buttocks, may first be treated with chemotherapy. Then, the tumor is surgically removed.

Chemotherapy has also been used successfully in infants with endodermal sinus tumors. After treatment, continue to monitor child's alpha-fetoprotein (AFP) and beta-human chorionic gonadotropin (beta-hCG) levels to make sure the tumor has been completely removed. If the child has a rare type of malignant germ cell tumor, experimental treatment programs can be tried. It is important to keep in mind that, today, malignant germ cell tumors in children have a higher cure rate than they did in the past. Chemotherapeutic drugs used are cyclophosphamide, doxorubicin VP-16, etc.

SUGGESTED READING

1. Bosl GJ, et al. Testicular germ-cell cancer. N Engl J Med. 1997;337:242.
2. International germ cell cancer consensus group: International Germ Cell Consensus Classification: A prognostic factor-based staging system for metastatic germ cell cancers. J Clin Oncol. 1997;15:594.
3. Rao AA, Naheedy JH, Chen JY, Robbins SL, Ramkumar HL. A clinical update and radiologic review of pediatric orbital and ocular tumors. J Oncol. 2013;975908. doi: 10.1155/2013/975908. Epub 2013 Mar 12.
4. Rodriguez-Galindo C, Krailo M, Frazier L, Chintagumpala M, Amatruda J, Katzenstein H, et al. COG Rare Tumors Disease Committee. Children's Oncology Group's 2013 blueprint for research: rare tumors. Pediatr Blood Cancer. 2013;60:1016-21.
5. Voute PA, et al (Eds). Cancer in children: clinical management 5th ed. OUP, 2005.

24 Rare Carcinomas in Pediatric Oncology

Rakesh Mondal

Some carcinomas occur in children rarely. Most of them are the counterpart of adult type carcinomas. They are overall very aggressive and had poor prognosis. The list may include:

i. Hepatocellular carcinoma
ii. Adenocarcinoma of the colon and rectum
iii. Renal cell carcinoma
iv. Thymoma
v. Nasopharyngeal carcinoma
vi. Thyroid tumors
vii. Basal cell carcinoma
viii. Melanoma.

HEPATOCELLULAR CARCINOMA

Hepatocellular carcinoma occurs mostly in older children and often is associated with hepatitis B or C infection. Important predisposing factors are hereditary tyrosinemia, galactosemia, glycogen storage disease, α1-antitrypsin deficiency, and biliary cirrhosis, aflatoxin B contamination, etc. Hepatocellular carcinoma usually presents as a multicentric, invasive tumor consisting of large pleomorphic cells with a lack of underlying cirrhosis. The fibrolamellar variant of hepatocellular carcinoma occurs more often in adolescent and young adult patients. Hepatocellular carcinoma usually presents as a hepatic mass, abdominal distention, and symptoms of anorexia, weight loss, and abdominal pain. The AFP level is elevated in most of the children with hepatocellular carcinoma. Evidence of hepatitis B and C infection usually is found. Diagnostic imaging should include plain radiographs and ultrasonography of the abdomen to characterize the hepatic mass. Ultrasonography can differentiate malignant hepatic masses from benign vascular lesions. CT or MRI is an accurate method of defining the extent of intrahepatic tumor involvement and the potential for surgical resection. Because of the multicentric origin of hepatocellular carcinoma, complete resection of this tumor is accomplished in only 30–40% of cases. Chemotherapy, including cisplatin, doxorubicin, etoposide, and 5-fluorouracil, has shown some activity against this tumor. Other techniques used are chemoembolization and liver transplantation. Few of them are long-term survivors with all sorts of advanced management.

ADENOCARCINOMA OF THE COLON AND RECTUM

Epithelial tumors of the digestive tract are rare in children. Carcinoma of the colon without any known predisposing factors is rarest entity. Several childhood conditions predispose to development of gastrointestinal adenocarcinoma, for example, familial adenomatous polyposis, hereditary nonpolyposis colon carcinoma (HNPCC), Peutz-Jeghers syndrome, juvenile polyposis, ulcerative colitis, Crohn disease, and disorders associated with chromosomal fragility, etc. The usual site is the colon, but gastric and intestinal lesions are rarely reported (Figs 24.1 to 24.6). Diagnosis is made based on family history, endoscopic findings, with symptomatology of gastrointestinal bleeding, or obstruction. Presenting symptoms include bloody stools or melena, abdominal pain, weight loss, and changes in bowel patterns. Signs are often inconclusive resulting in a delay in diagnosis and advanced disease. The tumors are relatively undifferentiated and highly malignant. Mutations in the APC gene, leading to FAP and DNA mismatch repair are most commonly associated with colorectal carcinoma in children. Diagnosis of HNPCC should be suspected in the presence of family history of early onset colon carcinoma and should be confirmed by genetic analysis. There is a male predominance in children. Hereditary nonpolyposis colon cancer (HNPCC), an autosomal dominant disorder, may present with early-onset colon cancer as well as a predisposition to cancers in other tissues. The majority of pediatric tumors produce mucin. Treatment consists of surgical resection when possible, with chemotherapy for unresectable tumors. The treatment of colorectal carcinoma is primarily surgical. Prognosis is related to stage of disease. It is important to obtain a complete family history and provide effective genetic screening and counseling to their families to identify at-risk family members.

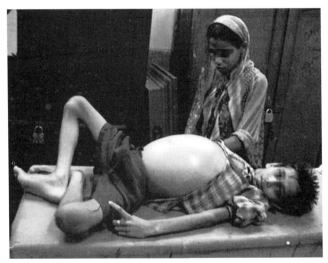

Fig. 24.1: Clinical photograph of a child with huge ascites and emaciation following rare adenocarcinoma of intestine

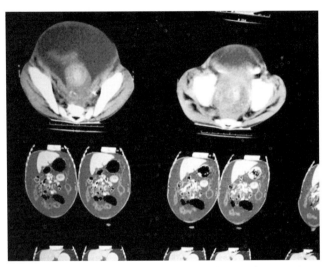

Fig. 24.2: CT scan of abdomen and pelvis showing huge ascites and intestinal mass in adenocarcioma

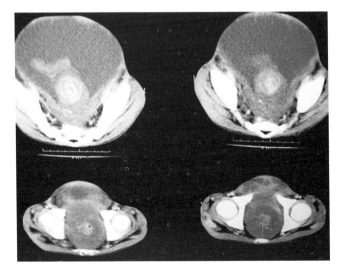

Fig. 24.3: CT scan of abdomen and pelvis showing huge ascites in adenocarcioma of intestine

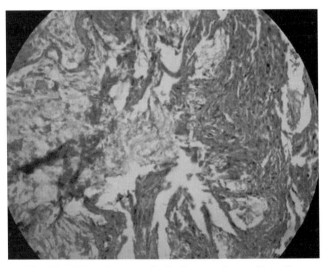

Fig. 24.4: Microphotograph of adenocarcioma of intestine
(For color version, see Plate 4)

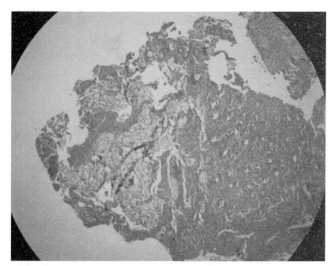

Fig. 24.5: Microphotograph of adenocarcioma of intestine
(For color version, see Plate 4)

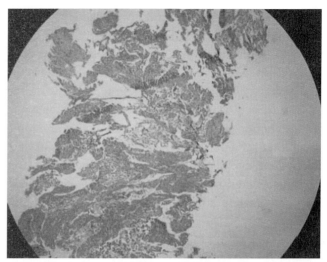

Fig. 24.6: Microphotograph of adenocarcioma of intestine
(For color version, see Plate 4)

RENAL CELL CARCINOMA

Renal cell carcinoma is rare in the first decades of life. It usually presents as an abdominal mass and/ or hematuria. Complete resection may achieve cure. Adjuvant treatment with interferon and 5-fluorouracil has been recommended. Renal medullary carcinoma is a rare, highly aggressive tumor associated with sickle cell trait, presenting with hematuria and a flank mass. The prognosis is poor.

THYMIC TUMORS AND THYMOMA

The thymus is developed from the third and fourth pharyngeal pouches and is located in the anterior mediastinum. The thymus is composed of epithelial, stromal cells and lymphoid cells. Thymus is an important organ for differentiation of T cells. It is organized into functional regions, the cortex and the medulla. It appears that the primitive bone marrow progenitors enter the thymus at the cortico-medullary junction and migrate first through the cortex toward the periphery of the gland and then toward the medulla. The lymphoid cell within the thymus develops lymphoma or T cell lymphoblastic lymphoma. Rarely B cells in the thymus developed B cell lymphoma. Other rare tumors that can arise from thymus are germ cell tumors and carcinoid tumors, etc. Thymoma developed from epithelial cells

of the thymus. Thymomas are uncommon in children. About 40–50% of patients are asymptomatic, masses are detected incidentally on routine chest radiographs. When symptomatic, patients may have cough, chest pain, dyspnea, fever, wheezing, fatigue, weight loss, night sweats, anorexia or with superior vena cava syndrome (Fig 24.7). A majority of patients with thymoma have systemic autoimmune illness like myasthenia gravis, pure red cell aplasia, hypogammaglobulinemia, polymyositis, systemic lupus erythematosus, thyroiditis, Sjögren's syndrome, ulcerative colitis, pernicious anemia, Addison's disease, scleroderma, and panhypopituitarism, etc. An initial mediastinoscopy or limited thoracotomy with tissue biopsy is mostly required for confirmation of the diagnosis. Fine-needle aspiration is poor at distinguishing between lymphomas and thymomas. Once a diagnosis of thymoma is defined, subsequent staging is generally done at surgery. MRI is important diagnostic tool in the staging of posterior mediastinal tumors (Fig 24.8). The staging system for thymoma was developed by Masaoka et al. It is an anatomic system in which the stage is increased based on the degree of invasiveness. The French Study Group on Thymic Tumors has modifications to the Masaoka scheme. In their system, stage I tumors are divided into A and B based on whether the surgeon suspects adhesions to adjacent structures; stage III tumors are divided into A and B based upon whether disease was subtotally

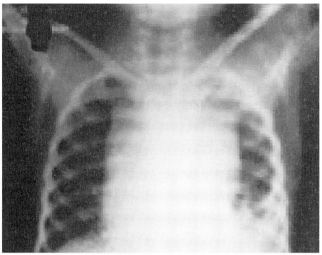

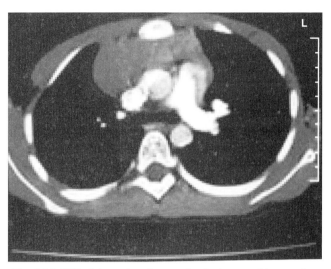

Fig. 24.7: X-ray chest showing mediastinal mass with superior vena caval syndrome following thymoma

Fig. 24.8: MRI of chest showing mediastinal mass with superior vena caval syndrome following thymoma

resected or only biopsied. Thymomas are epithelial tumors have a variable percentage of lymphocytes within the tumor. The epithelial component of the tumor may consist primarily of round or oval cells derived mainly from the cortex or spindle-shaped cells derived mainly from the medulla. Most of A, AB and B1 tumors are localized. Thymic carcinomas are invasive and carry a poor prognosis. Treatment is determined by the stage of disease. For patients with encapsulated tumors and stage I disease, complete resection is sufficient to cure majority of patients. For patients with stage II disease, complete resection is usually followed by postoperative radiation therapy to the site of the primary tumor. For patients with stage III and IV disease, the use of neoadjuvant chemotherapy followed by radical surgery, radiation therapy, and additional consolidation chemotherapy is given. Induction chemotherapy given includes cyclophosphamide, doxorubicin, cisplatin. This multimodality approach produces a 5-year survival 50% in patients with advanced-stage disease.

NASOPHARYNGEAL CARCINOMA

Nasopharyngeal carcinoma is rare in the pediatric population, but is one of the most common nasopharyngeal tumors in pediatric patients primarily in adolescents. It occurs in males twice as often as in females. In the pediatric population the tumors are more commonly of undifferentiated histology and associated with Epstein-Barr Virus (EBV) infection. Most pediatric patients present with advanced disease manifesting as cervical lymphadenopathy. Epistaxis, trismus, and cranial nerve deficits may be seen. The diagnosis is established from biopsy of the nasopharynx or cervical lymph nodes. In most cases the lactate dehydrogenase level is elevated. CT or MRI evaluation of the head and neck is performed to determine the extent of disease. Treatment consists of combination of chemotherapy and irradiation. Cisplatin-based chemotherapy is given before or concurrent with irradiation. The outcome depends on the extent of disease. The use on intensity-modulated radiation therapy (IMRT) has improved local control and survival.

THYROID TUMORS

Most thyroid cancers occur among adolescents. The greatest risk factor for thyroid cancer is prior radiation exposure, especially following head and neck irradiation. Thyroid cancer accounts for about 10% of second malignancies among cancer survivors, especially survivors of Hodgkin lymphoma, due to treatment not only with radiation but also with alkylating agents. Almost all are differentiated carcinomas (papillary or follicular). Medullary thyroid carcinoma (MTC) may occur in familial cases, especially with multiple endocrine neoplasia (MEN type 2). In MEN type 2a, MTC usually occurs in older children and may be associated with pheochromocytoma and parathyroid hyperplasia. MEN type 2b is associated with onset of MTC at early age. Other findings of MEN 2b include mucosal neuromas and marfanoid habitus. MEN type 2 is associated with mutations in the RET proto-oncogene. Patients present with a thyroid mass and/or cervical lymphadenopathy; symptoms related to abnormal hormone levels are rare. About 20% of thyroid nodules in young children are malignant, compared with about 10% in adults. Fine-needle aspiration (FNA) cytology commonly used to assess thyroid. Evaluation should include determination of thyroid hormone levels, thyroid scan, chest radiography, and CT of the chest, etc. Total thyroidectomy for disease confined to one lobe has been controversial in pediatrics owing to good prognosis and the risk of complications such as hypoparathyroidism. However, total or near-total thyroidectomy reduces the risk of local recurrence. Treatment with iodine 131 is used to eradicate residual disease. The patient will subsequently require lifelong thyroid hormone replacement therapy.

BASAL CELL CARCINOMA

Basal cell carcinoma is rare in children in the absence of a predisposing condition, such as nevoid basal cell carcinoma syndrome, xeroderma pigmentosum, arsenic intake, or exposure to irradiation. The lesions are smooth, pearly, pink, telangiectatic papules that enlarge slowly and may bleed or ulcerate. Sites of predilection are the face, scalp, and upper back. The differential diagnosis includes pyogenic granuloma, nevocellular nevus, epidermal inclusion cyst, closed comedo, dermatofibroma, and adnexal tumor. Depending on the site of occurrence and associated disease of the host, electrodesiccation and curettage or simple excision is usually curative. Nevoid basal cell carcinoma syndrome is an autosomal dominant syndrome with an incidence of 1 in 60,000. Consequently, the syndrome includes a wide spectrum of defects involving the skin, eyes, central nervous and

endocrine systems and bones. The predominant features are early onset basal cell carcinomas and mandibular cysts. A majority of those in whom a basal cell carcinoma develops before adolescence have this syndrome. The facies of patients with this syndrome are characterized by temporoparietal bossing, prominent supraorbital ridges, a broad nasal root, ocular hypertelorism and prognathism. Osseous defects such as anomalous rib development, spina bifida, kyphoscoliosis, and brachymetacarpalism may occur. Some males have hypogonadism, with absent or undescended testes. Kidney malformations have also been reported. Neurologic manifestations include calcification of the falx, seizures, mental retardation, partial agenesis of the corpus callosum, hydrocephalus, and nerve deafness. Treatment of these patients requires team of specialists according to individual clinical problems. Basal cell carcinomas should not be treated with irradiation. Most of the basal cell carcinomas have a clinically benign course, and it is often impossible to remove all of them. Oral retinoids are helpful in preventing the development of new tumors in some patients.

MELANOMA

Although sun exposure is a well-known risk factor for melanoma in adults, its role in pediatric melanoma is less clear. Pediatricians should counsel patients regarding avoidance of sun exposure to decrease the risk of later development of melanoma. Patients with fair skin and a family history of melanoma are at particularly high risk. Known risk factors for children are giant hairy nevus (> 20 cm), dysplastic nevus syndrome, and xeroderma pigmentosum. Findings of a rapidly enlarging nevus that is dark, has changed colors, has irregular borders, or bleeds easily can transform into melanoma. The primary treatment is local excision with lymph node mapping and sentinel node biopsy for most of them except superficial melanomas. If the sentinel node is positive, a formal lymph node dissection is recommended. High-dose adjuvant interferon has shown some efficacy in the treatment of melanoma, while chemotherapy in combination with biologic agents and vaccine therapy has been used for treatment as recent advances.

SUGGESTED READING

1. Ayan I, Kaytan E, Ayan N. Childhood nasopharyngeal carcinoma: From biology to treatment. Lancet Oncol. 2003;4:13-21.
2. Grady WM. Genetic testing for high-risk colon cancer patients. Gastroenterology. 2003;124:1574-94.
3. Hung W, Sarlis NJ. Current controversies in the management of pediatric patients with well-differentiated nonmedullary thyroid cancer: A review. Thyroid. 2002;12:683-702.
4. Jennifer Couzin. In Their Prime, and Dying of Cancer, Science. 2007;317:1160-2.
5. Machens A, Holzhausen HJ, Thanh PN, et al. Malignant progression from C-cell hyperplasia to medullary thyroid carcinoma in 167 carriers of RET germline mutations. Surgery. 2003;134:425-31.
6. Marcos I, Borrego S, Urioste M, et al. Mutations in the DNA mismatch repair gene MLH1 associated with early onset colon cancer. J Pediatr. 2006;148:837-9.
7. Mones JM, Ackerman AB. Melanomas in prepubescent children: Review comprehensively, critique historically, criteria diagnostically, and course biologically. Am J Dermatopathol. 2003;25:223-38.
8. Pappo AS. Melanoma in children and adolescents. Eur J Cancer. 2003;39:2651-61.
9. Robert M Kliegman, Richard E Behrman, Hal B Jenson, Bonita F Stanton. Nelson Textbook of Pediatrics, 18th Edn; Philadelphia. Saunders Elsevier.
10. Sherman SI. Thyroid carcinoma. Lancet 2003;361:501-10.
11. Szinnai G, Meier C, Komminoth P, et al. Review of multiple endocrine neoplasia type 2A in children: Therapeutic results of early thyroidectomy and prognostic value of codon analysis. Pediatrics. 2003;111:e132-9.
12. Tsao SW, Lo KW, Huang DP. Nasopharyngeal carcinoma. In: Tselis A, Jenson HB (eds). Epstein-Barr Virus, New York, Taylor and Francis. 2006:273-95.
13. Virchow's node: Rare presentation of childhood hepatocellular carcinoma. Indian J Pediatr. 2012;72:177-8.

Opportunistic Infection in Pediatric Oncology

Rakesh Mondal

Opportunistic infection is a common problem in pediatric oncology patients. It depends upon underlying immunocompromised state. Defective B cell, phagocyte cells and complements predispose the patient to serious bacterial infection by encapsulated organism. Defective T cell state enhances infection with intracellular pathogens and chronic viral and fungal infection. Detailed evaluation in a child with cancer who is receiving chemotherapy is essential for management. They are as follows:

PATHOGENS

Viral

The main pathogens are:
a. CMV – Cytomegalovirus
b. Herpes – Herpes group of virus
c. EBV – Epstein-Barr virus

Bacterial

a. Serious bacterial infection
b. Mycobacteria
c. Atypical mycobacteria
d. Gram-positive cocci
   – *Staphylococcus epidermidis*
   – *Staphylococcus aureus*
   – *Viridans streptococcus*
   – *Enterococcus faecalis*
   – *Streptococcus pneumoniae*
e. Gram-negative bacilli
   – *Escherichia coli*
   – *Klebsiella spp.*
   – *Pseudomonas aeruginosa*
   – *Non-aeruginosa Pseudomonas spp.*
   – *Enterobacter spp.*
   – *Serratia spp.*
   – *Acinetobacter spp.*
   – *Citrobacter spp.*
f. Gram-positive bacilli
   – Diphtheroids

Fungal

a. *Candida albicans* and non-albicans
b. *Pneumocystis jiroveci*
c. *Cryptococcosis*
d. *Aspergillus*

Protozoan

a. Cryptosporidiosis
b. *Toxoplasmosis gondii*
c. *Isospora belli*

COMMON OPPORTUNISTIC INFECTION ENCOUNTERED

A. ***Pneumocystis carinii (Jiroveci pneumonia):*** It is one of the common opportunistic infections in a child with febrile neutropenia. Presentation is non-specific which requires high degree of suspicion for diagnosis. It presents with fever, tachypnea, dyspnea, cough, unexplained weight loss, retrosternal chest pain, etc. Extra pulmonary manifestations are rare but it may involve any part including ear, eye, GIT, spleen, liver, etc. Chest X-ray shows bilateral diffuse parenchymal infiltrate or ground glass or reticulogranular pattern. Hypoxemia in blood gas analysis is an important clue. Diagnosis is confirmed by demonstration of organism in pulmonary tissue. The sample is collected by saline nebulization induced sputum in older child, bronchoalveolar lavage and fibreoptic bronchoscopy and transbronchial biopsy. The specimen are stained with toluidine blue, giemsa, etc. Currently PCR based diagnosis is available in some centers. Treatment option includes: i) Trimethoprim and sulphamethoxazole combination (15-20) mg/kg/day TMP 6 hrly for 21 days along with corticosteroids in presence of hypoxemias. ii) Pentamidine isothionate 4 mg/kg/day OD IV over one hour are the alternative when previous drugs are not effective, iii) Atovaquone, clindamycin, primaquine are also tried in some cases. Prophylaxis is given with trimethoprim and sulphamethoxazole combination 5 mg/kg/day TMP during induction period in most of the pediatric oncology centers.

B. **Cryptosporidiosis:** It is a protozoan species that mainly causes enteric illness. The common strains are *C. hominis, C. parvum, C. meliagricles,* etc. the clinical features include frequent bloody diarrhea, persistent diarrhea, abdominal cramps, vomiting, anorexia, poor weight gain. It can also have complication like acalculous cholecystitis, sclerosing cholangitis, pneumonia, etc. Stool examinations revealing acid-fast oocysts are diagnostic. The management is done with adequate hydration, correction of electrolyte balance and specific anti-protozoan therapy with nitazoxanide (100–200 mg day), paromomycin (25-35 mg/kg/day), azithromycin (10 mg/kg/day), etc. Oral hyperimmune bovine colostrum are effective in some children.

C. *Mycobacterium tuberculosis:* Most common opportunistic infection in India in general. All age groups may be affected. Diagnosis is difficult in pediatric population because of non-specific symptoms in most of the times. They manifest with fever, hepato-splenomegaly, failure to weight gain, etc. Mantoux test > 5 mm indurations in presence of immunocompromised state is suggestive. Chest X-ray delineates paratracheal adenopathy. Isolation of AFB though diagnostic is difficult in most of the cases. Treatment is started with four drugs ATD including INH, rifampicin, pyrizinamide, ethambutol followed by maintenance. Many studies recommend prolong therapy, in these cases nine months for pulmonary disese and twelve months for extra pulmonary diseases in view of treatment failure in presence of severe immunosuppression.

D. **Mycobacterium avium complex (MAC):** This is common atypical mycobacterial infection in children with immunosuppressive state. It manifests with fever, malaise, night sweat, weight loss, diarrhea, abdominal pain, etc. Chest X-ray reveals bilateral lower lobe infiltrates. Isolation of organism from blood or bone marrow is diagnostic. Clarithromycin or azithromycin combined with ATD are used for treatment.

E. **Candidiasis:** The most common fungal infection among neutropenic patients are caused by candida species. It may manifest with oral thrush, candida esophagitis, fungal sepsis, etc. The symptoms vary according to the site of involvement; like esophageal candidiasis presents with dysphagia, odynophagia, retrosternal pain, etc. It is diagnosed by smear with KOH preparation and fungal blood culture. Barium swallow studies showed cobble stone appearance. Endoscopy revealed white patches in mucosa. Oropharyngeal candidiasis is managed with topical application of nystatin or clotrimazole. Esophageal candidiasis is managed with parenteral fluconazole 6 mg/kg/day for two weeks or amphotericin B in resistant cases. Invasive candidiasis is managed with amphotericin B along with flucytosine.

F. **Cryptococcosis:** It is another pathogen related to immunocompromised state. It manifests mainly with meningoencephalitis. Presenting symptoms are fever, headache, photophobia, altered mental status, seizure, meningism of insidious onset. It can have symptoms of recurrent fever, unexplained cough, cutaneous lesion, etc. Investigation requires chest X-ray, radio-imaging studies along with CSF examination. CSF examination is to be done with for detection of cryptococcus even with antigen assays. It is managed with amphotericin B and flucytosine in combination for initial two weeks of therapy followed by maintenance of imidazole group of drugs for eight weeks.

G. **Cytomegalovirus:** It is one of the common viral infections encountered during BMT. It may present with fever, pneumonia, hepatitis, etc. It is diagnosed with DNA PCR studies from the clinical specimen along with ancillary investigations like chest X-ray, etc. It is treated with IV ganciclovir 5 mg/kg/dose twice-daily infusion for at least two weeks. Foscarnet is alternative drugs for resistant cases.

H. **Herpes simplex:** It can cause devastating cuteneous, ocular, CNS and disseminated lesion in immunocompromised hosts. It is diagnosed by clinical appearance of vesicles and ulcers and supported by isolation of virus in culture; sometimes Tzanck smear may also help. It is managed with acyclovir 10 mg/kg/dose 8 hourly for two weeks.

SUGGESTED READING

1. Green M, Michaels MG: Infections in solid organ transplant recipients. In: Long SS, Pickering L, Prober C (eds): Principles and Practice of Pediatric Infectious Disease. New York, Churchill Livingstone. 1997.

2. Hughes WT, Armstrong D, Bodey GP, et al: 2002 guidelines for the use of antimicrobial agents in neutropenic patients with cancer. Clin Infect Dis. 2002;34:730-51.

3. Paul M, et al: Empirical antibiotic monotherapy for febrile neutropenia: Systematic review and meta-analysis of randomized controlled trials. J Antimicrob Chemother. 2006;57:176.

26 Immunization and Antibiotic Policy in Pediatric Oncology

Jaydeep Chowdhury

The children who are suffering from various malignancies are immunocompromised. Their vaccinations or their treatment with antibiotics is a challenge. Over the years, the numbers of such children are increasing specially as of late the cancer chemo- and radiotherapy has been substantially intensified in children suffering from malignancies. As acute leukemia is the most common childhood malignancy, so this discussion mostly refers to acute leukemia in children.

IMMUNIZATION IN CHILDREN WITH MALIGNANCIES

General Principles

Many children with malignancies receive corticosteroids. Children receiving oral corticosteroids in high doses, e.g. prednisolone 1–2 mg/kg/day for more than 14 days should not receive live virus vaccines until the steroid has been discontinued for at least one month. Killed vaccines are safe but may be incompletely effective in such situations.

Children on low dose steroid or on inhaled or topical therapy can receive all age appropriate vaccines, children on chemotherapy or radiotherapy should avoid all live vaccines during treatment and for at least 3 months after stopping therapy.

Live Vaccines

Measles vaccine—Measles infection which is quite common has high mortality in patients with cancer. Even there may be loss of immunity in children treated for leukemia previously vaccinated against measles.

Immunization with live, attenuated vaccine is contraindicated because of risk of severe side-effects in cancer patients undergoing chemotherapy. Immunization with live vaccines like measles might be considered in cancer patients not receiving active chemotherapy in epidemiologic situations when the risk for measles is increased.

Varicella vaccine—Varicella infection is associated with high mortality in children with cancer (Fig. 26.1). The existing vaccine is live, attenuated and based on Oka strain. The vaccine has been shown to be safe and effective in children with leukemia who are in remission. The frequency of side-effects from the vaccine is low

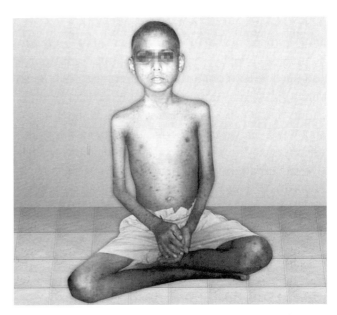

Fig. 26.1: Clinical photograph of a child with Hodgkin's disease developed disseminated chickenpox during chemotherapy

and breakthrough vaccine disease can usually be treated effectively with acyclovir. The risk of herpes zoster after vaccination is lower, compared to that in patients who had natural varicella disease.

Household exposure to varicella is associated with more extensive disease in secondary cases. Healthy seronegative family members may be immunized when the child with cancer is undergoing intensive therapy and a live vaccine cannot be given.

Oral polio vaccine – The oral polio vaccine can induce paralytic disease in immunocompromised patients and should not be used for immunization against poliomyelitis.

Other live vaccines – There is limited data on immunization with BCG, mumps, measles and rubella vaccines in cancer patients. These vaccines are not recommended during active cancer therapy.

Killed Vaccines

DPT vaccines – The protection against diphtheria, tetanus and pertussis is low in cancer patients undergoing chemotherapy. The loss of specific immunity is related to the intensity of given chemotherapy. Most children respond well to vaccination after chemotherapy for malignancies. For major/contaminated wounds tetanus immunoglobulin is to be given along with toxoid even if 3 or more doses of TT were given previously.

Inactivated poliovirus vaccine – As the protection against poliovirus is low in immunocompromised patients and oral polio vaccine cannot be used, inactivated poliovirus vaccine should be used for immunization of the patients with cancer. The poliovirus vaccine strain might be transferred from the healthy family members, so the use of inactivated vaccine when relatives are immunized is recommended.

Hepatitis B virus vaccine – Hepatitis B virus infection is a major cause of morbidity and mortality, more so in immunocompromised patients. Immunization of patients against hepatitis B virus is indicated in countries like India where the prevalence of hepatitis B virus is high. Higher doses and more number of doses are required and antibody titres are to be checked regularly.

Hemophilus influenzae type B (Hib) vaccine–Children with leukemia are at a greater risk for Hib infection compared to normal children. Immunization with conjugated Hib vaccine is indicated in children with cancer, preferably early during anticancer therapy.

Pneumococcal vaccine – Pneumococci are important causes of infection in patients with hematological malignancies. Lymphoma patients with poor antibody responses to polysaccharide vaccine have an increased risk for severe pneumococcal infections. So the vaccines which are able to induce better immune responses such as the conjugate pneumococcal vaccines are preferred. Immunization of patients with hematological malignancies including lymphoma against pneumococcal infections is recommended as early as possible after diagnosis and before chemotherapy and/or radiotherapy is initiated.

Influenza vaccine – The mortality and morbidity of influenza vary in different types of cancer patients. The most severe consequences occur in acute leukemia patients undergoing induction chemotherapy. Influenza vaccination with inactivated vaccine is recommended in immunocompromised patients. Two doses might give a better immune response.

Meningococcal vaccine – Vaccination should also be considered against meningococcal infections.

Household Contact Vaccination

Household and other close contacts of immunocompromised patients should receive all age appropriate vaccines except transmissible vaccine, such as live oral poliovirus vaccine. Varicella and influenza vaccine must be given them to reduce the transmission to immuno-compromised.

There are no effective vaccines available against several infections which are of great importance in these patients such as CMV, adenovirus and aspergillus infections.

Infection in Children with Malignancies

Children suffering from various malignancies are at increased risk of infection. Besides bloodstream and other invasive infections, they suffer frequently from skin and soft-tissue infection. As they are caused by a wide range of pathogens and are often part of a widely disseminated infection, they frequently pose a very difficult clinical problem.

Infection prevention is of utmost importance in children suffering from malignancies. When infections develop, it is critical to establish a specific etiologic diagnosis as very often the infection is nosocomial and is caused by pathogens with increased antibiotic resistance. Even the skin lesions, no matter how small and trivial should be carefully evaluated. The gross appearance of any skin lesion is frequently altered by decreased inflammatory response. It is very important to thoroughly investigate any infection. Blood culture should always be done.

The current treatment protocols for cancer patients are very intense. Even though several arms of the immune system can be affected, neutropenia is the major abnormality. Neutropenia is defined as an absolute count < 1500 cells/mm^3 and major risk of infection occurs when the count decreases to < 500 cells/mm^3. During these episodes the patients are at increased risk of developing potentially fatal invasive infections. Antibiotic therapy should be initiated on the basis of important clinical parameters identified and the most likely offending pathogens.

Causative Organisms

Few years back the Gram-negative organisms were the leading cause of infection in neutropenic patients. Over the years, with the use of antibiotics to cover the Gram-negative organisms, Gram-positive organisms have become the predominant cause of infections, currently accounting for more than 60–70% of isolates. In some centers, Gram-negative infections have become common probably due to misuse of vancomycin.

The common Gram-positive organisms are coagulase negative staphylococci, *Staphylococcus aureus*, *Streptococcus viridans*, *S. pneumoniae*, enterococci and sometimes bacillus and corynebacterium species. The frequent Gram-negative organisms isolated are *E. coli*, *Klebsiella*, *Pseudomonas* species and sometimes *Proteus* species, *Acinetobacter*. Anaerobic organisms seen are bacteroides and fusobacterium. The common fungal infections encountered are *Candida albicans* followed by *Aspergillus fumigatus*.

Initial Antibiotic Therapy

Febrile neutropenia in cancer patients is one of the indications of empirical antibiotic therapy as bloodstream infections in these patients can be rapid and fatal. The following are the three options for initial antibiotic therapy:

i. *Single antibiotic therapy without vancomycin*—The single antibiotic used should cover Gram-negative infection including *Pseudomonas*. The options are ceftazidime, cefepime, carbapenem or piperacillin-tazobactam. Aminoglycosides and quinolones should not be used as a single drug.

ii. *Two-drug combination without vancomycin*—It is preferred in complicated cases and to achieve better coverage and reduce drug resistance. The options are ciprofloxacin, amoxicillin-clauvulinic acid or aminoglycoside.

iii. *Vancomycin plus 1 or 2 drugs*—Vancomycin is not recommended as the first line drug except the following situations, such as catheter induced sepsis, complicated patients with high-fever and hypotension, culture showing infection with drug resistant Gram-positive organism, a patient known to be colonized with such an organism in the past. Vancomycin should be used in combination with other first line drugs. Linezolid is equally effective as vancomycin.

Antibiotic Therapy in Initial 5–7 Days

The culture report is expected after 48–72 hours. If the culture report is positive, the antibiotics should be adjusted still keeping broad spectrum coverage. Usually, it takes 3–5 days for response to the first line of antibiotics. In the mean time, if the patient deteriorates one may have to add or change the antibiotics even before 72 hours. If vancomycin is started initially and the organism shows sensitivity to other drugs, vancomycin should be stopped.

Occasionally, the situation may be such that culture is negative but the patient is still febrile on day 3 after initial antibiotics. It may be a case of delayed response as some patients may take up to 5 days for response. The presence of an organ infection and abscess somewhere or sub-optimal dose of antibiotics has to be ruled out. The possibility of a non-bacterial infection, drug resistant organism or fungal infection should be considered.

Duration of Antibiotics

When the patient is afebrile by 3–5 days, clinically stable without any complications, no organism is isolated on culture and absolute neutrophil count is above 100 cells/cu mm of blood, one can switch to oral antibiotics (cefixime or amoxiclav) and should continue 7 days. If the patient is afebrile but absolute neutrophil count continues to be low, one should ideally continue antibiotics till the neutrophil count is normal. But even in such situations, antibiotics can be stopped after 5–7 days. Clinically stable patients with unknown etiology whose neutropenia persists even after 2 weeks antibiotics may be stopped.

Infections occur in children with cancer even without neutropenia, usually these are viral etiology. *P. carinii* can cause pneumonitis regardless of neutrophil count. Co-trimoxazole prophylaxis is an effective preventive strategy.

It is utmost important to use antimicrobials judiciously in any children, more so in children who are suffering from malignancies. Globally antibiotic resistance is spreading like wildfire, and when the multiple drug resistant organisms attack these immunocompromised children they are at greater risk. Though infection cannot be completely prevented in children who have defects in one or more arms of their immune system, but some measures can decrease the risk of infection and make treatment fruitful.

SUGGESTED READING

1. Gershon A, Steinberg S. Persistence of immunity to varicella in children with leukemia immunized with live attenuated varicella vaccine. N Engl J Med. 1989;320:892-7.
2. Green M, Michael MG. Infections in immunocompromised persons. In: Behrman RE, Kliegman RM, Jenson HB (Eds). Nelson Textbook of Pediatrics. 18th edn, Philadelphia: Saunders 2007;1100-07.
3. Ljungman P. Vaccination in the immunocompromised host. In: Plotkin SA, Orenstein WA, Offit PA, eds. Vaccines. 5th edn. Philadelphia: Saunders Elsevier 2008;1403-16.
4. Prevention and control of influenza: recommendations of Advisory Committee on Immunization Practices (ACIP). MMWR 1999;48:1-28.
5. Shah NK, Lokeshwar MR. Antimicrobial therapy in febrile neutropenia. In: Shah NK, Singhal T (eds). IAP Specialty Series on Rational Antimicrobial Practice in Pediatrics. 1st edn, Mumbai: Indian Academy of Pediatrics 2007;221-33.
6. Singhal T, Amdekar YK, Agarwal RK (Eds). IAP guide book on immunization. Edition 2009, New Delhi, Jaypee Brothers Medical Publishers (P) Ltd. 2009;99-101.
7. Stevens DL, Bisno AL, Chambers HF, et al. Practice guidelines for the diagnosis and management of skin and soft-tissue infections. Clinical Infect Dis. 2005;41: 1373-406.

Rakesh Mondal

Blood products are prepared from collected whole blood or apheresis. Donated whole blood is separated as required into several components. Blood components are transfused selectively depending on the need of an individual patient and the underlying disease.

Besides providing patients what they need blood component transfusion ensures optimal utilization and minimize the risk of transfusion related complication.

Blood components are:

Standard
- Whole blood
- Packed RBC
- FFP
- Platelet
- Cryoprecipitate.

Specialized
- Saline washed RBC
- Frozen red cell
- Leukodepleted product
- Irradiated product
- Granulocyte
- Lymphocyte.

WHOLE BLOOD

Whole blood is used when a patient requires both replacements of circulatory volume and to enhance oxygen carrying capacity.

INDICATIONS

1. Acute massive blood loss (> 25% of estimated blood volume).

2. Hyperleukocytosis, i.e. white blood cell count >100 × 10^9/L in acute leukemia.

PACKED RED BLOOD CELL

RBCs are most frequently transfused blood component, are given to increase the oxygen carrying capacity of the blood.

GUIDELINES FOR PEDIATRIC RED BLOOD CELL TRANSFUSION

Children and Adolescent

- Acute blood loss > 25% of estimated blood volume
- Hemoglobin < 8.0 gm/dl in preoperative period, symptomatic chronic anemia, marrow failure
- Hemoglobin < 12.0 gm/dl and severe cardiopulmonary disease.

Infants within the First 4 Months of Life

- Hemoglobin < 13.0 gm/dl and severe pulmonary disease and severe cardiac disease
- Hemoglobin < 10.0 gm/dl and moderate pulmonary disease and major surgery
- Hemoglobin < 8.0 gm/dl and symptomatic anemia.

Factors other than hemoglobin concentration to be considered in the decision to transfuse RBC includes:

- The patients' symptoms, signs and functional capacity
- Presence of cardiorespiratory, vascular, CNS disease
- The cause and anticipated course of anemia
- Alternative therapies, such as recombinant human erythropoietic therapy.

FRESH FROZEN PLASMA

Immediately following collection from normal donor plasma contents approximately 1 unit/ml of each coagulation factor. Plasma frozen within 8 hours of donation contains at least. 7 IU /ml of factor VIII. It can be stored for 12 months at temperature – 18°C or colder.

FFP contains stable coagulation factor, plasma protein, fibrinogen, anti-thrombin, albumin as well as protein C and S.
Guideline for pediatric FFP transfusion:
1. Replacement of coagulation factor in liver disease, deficiency of vitamin K dependent factors (II, VII, IX, X), DIC, overdoses of oral anticoagulants, cardiopulmonary bypass, massive transfusion.
2. Specific deficiencies of factor V, VIII, XI.
3. Replacement of hemostatic factors when specific concentrate preparation are not available. Example: Hemophilia A and B, deficiency of factor VII, X, fibrinogen and prothrombin, von Willebrand's disease, anti-thrombin III deficiency.
4. In situation where certain plasma constituents are lacking: Example
   • Fibronectin in septicemia
   • C1-Esterase in hereditary angioneurotic edema
   • Hereditary protein C, protein S deficiency.

PLATELET

The usual platelet bags contain 5.5×10^{10} platelet/unit, about 50 ml plasma, trace to 0.5 ml of RBC, and varying numbers of leukocytes upto 10^8/unit. It can be stored upto 5 days at 20–24°C in shaker.
Guidelines for pediatric platelet transfusion
1. Children and adolescent, platelet count ($\times 10^9$/L)
   • PLTs < 50 and bleeding and invasive procedure
   • PLTs < 20 and marrow failure with hemorrhagic risk factor
   • PLTs at any count but with platelet dysfunction plus bleeding or invasive procedure.
2. Infants with first 4 months of life, PLTs count ($\times 10^9$/L)
   • PLTs < 100 and bleeding and clinically unstable
   • PLTs < 50 and invasive procedure
   • PLTs < 20 and clinically stable.

Cryoprecipitate
Cryoprecipitate is the precipitate formed when FFP is thawed at 4°C. It is refrozen within 1 hour in 10 to 15 ml of donor plasma and stored at – 18°C or less for a period up to 1 year.

One unit contains 80–100 units of factor VIII, 100–250 mg of fibrinogen, 40–70% of VwF, 30% factor XIII. Cryoprecipitate is used in:
• von Willebrand's disease and mild hemophilia A
• Dysfibrinogenemia, hypofibrinogenemia, con-sumptive coagulopathy
• Congenital factor XIII deficiency.

OTHERS GRANULOCYTE TRANSFUSION

The use of granulocyte transfusion has remained limited in clinical practice, largely due to the availability of newer antibiotics and use of agents like IVIG , G-CSF, other recombinant cytokines and immune modulating agents.
1. Children and adolescent
   • Neutrophil of $< 0.5 \times 10^9$/L and bacterial infection unresponsive to appropriate antimicrobial therapy
   • Qualitative neutrophil defect and infection unresponsive to antimicrobial therapy.
2. Infants within the first 4 months of life
   • Neutrophil of $< 3.0 \times 10^9$/L (1st week of life) or $< 1.0 \times 10^9$/L (thereafter).
   • Fulminant bacterial infection.

Albumin

Albumin preparations are available in concentration of 5% and 20% plasma protein fraction (PPF) has approximately 85% albumin. The rest being betaglobulin.
It may be used to replace plasma proteins in:
• Burns, extensive surgery, hemorrhagic shock when awaiting blood
• Hypoproteinemia associated with massive anasarca.

Normal and Specific Immunoglobulins (Ig)

Normal immunoglobulins are obtained by fractionation of plasma. Specific Ig are separated from plasma from donors who possess a high tighter of specific antibodies.

The indications for use are:

a. Specific
   i. Prevention and treatment of disease such as hepatitis, rubella, varicella—zoster, tetanus, measles, rabies and diphtheria, etc.
   ii. Prevention of sensitization in Rh (D) negative women by administering anti-D.

b. Normal
   i. Replacement therapy in deficiency syndrome
   ii. Treatment of immune disorders such as immunothrombocytopenic purpura
   iii. Prophylaxis and treatment of neonatal sepsis
   iv. Kawasaki disease and other immune mediate disease.

Transfusion Reaction may Result from Immune and Nonimmune Mechanism

Immune mediated reactions are often due to pre-formed donor or recipient antibody, however, cellular element may also cause adverse effect.

Nonimmune causes of reactions are due to chemical and physical properties of the stored blood component and its additives.

Infectious complications of transfusion have become less frequent.

Potential problem following massive transfusion:
- Platelet depletion
- Coagulation factor depletion
- Increase blood oxygen affinity
- Hypocalcemia, Hypercalcemia
- Hypothermia
- Acidosis
- Hyperglycemia
- Respiratory distress syndrome.

Immue Mediated Reaction

Acute hemolytic reaction: Immune mediated hemolysis occurs when the recipient has preformed antibodies that lyses donor erythrocytes. The ABO isoagglupinins are responsible for the majority of the reactions, although alloantibodies directed against other RBC antigen, i.e. Rh, Kell and Duffy may result in hemolysis.

Delayed hemolytic and serologic transfusion reaction: This reaction occurs due to alloantibody that binds donor RBCs. The alloantibody is detectable 1 to 2 weeks following the transfusion and post-transfusion DAT assay becomes positive due to circulating donor antibody and complement.

Febrile non-hemolytic transfusion reaction: This is most common reaction associated with the transfusion of cellular blood components. Antibody directed against donor leukocyte and HLA antigens may mediate these reactions.

Allergic reactions: Urticarial reactions are related to plasma proteins found in transfused components releated to IgE.

Anaphylactic reactions: It may occur with a few milliliters of blood component. Patient who is deficient may be sensitize to this IgA class and are risk for anaphylactic reactions.

Graft versus host disease:
- Transfusion related GVHD is mediated by donor T-lymphocytes that recognized host HLA antigen as foreign body and mount an immune reaction
- GIVHD can also occur when blood components that contain viable T-lymphocytes are transfused to immunodeficient or to immunocompetent recipients who share HLA antigen with the donor that is family donor.

Transfusion related lung injury: This uncommon reaction results from the transfusion of donor plasma that contains high tighter anti-HLA antibodies that bind recipient leukocytes. The leukocytes aggregate in the pulmonary vasculature, release mediators that increase capillary permeability.

Post-transfusion purpura: The reaction present as thrombocytopenia 7 to 10 days after platelets transfusion and occurs predominantly in women. Platelets specific antibodies are found in the recipient serum and the most frequent recognized antigen is HPA-1a [(Human platelet antigen (a)] found on the platelets glycoprotein III a receptor.

Alloimmunization: A recipient may become allommunized to a number of antigens on cellular blood elements and plasma proteins.

Non-immune Meditated Reaction

Fluid overload: Blood components are excellent volume expander and transfusion may quickly lead to volume overload.

Hypothermia: Refrigerated (4°C) on frozen (–18 degree C or decrease) blood component can result in hypothermia when rapidly infused. Cardiac arrhythmias can result from exposing the sinoatrial node to cold fluid.

Electrolyte toxicity:

- RBC leakage during storage increases the concentration of potassium in the unit
- Citrate, commonly used to anticoagulate blood components, chelates calcium and thereby inhibits the coagulation cascade.
- **Iron overload:** Each unit of RBCs contains 200 – 250 mg of iron. Symptom and sign of iron overload are found affecting endocrine, hepatic, cardiac function after 100 units of RBC transfused.
- **Hypotensive reactions:** Transient hypotension may be noted among transfused patient who take ACE inhibitors. Since blood products contain bradykinin that is normally degraded by ACE, patient on ACE inhibitors may have increased bradykinin levels that cause hypotension.

INFECTIOUS COMPLICATIONS

Viral Infections

Hepatitis C virus, hepatitis B virus, hepatitis G virus, and human immunodeficiency virus type I, cytomegalovirus, human T lymph tropic virus (HTLV) type I, parvovirus B-19.

Bacterial Contamination

Most bacteria do not grow well at cold temperature, thus RBCs and FFP are not common sources of bacterial contamination. However, some Gram-negative bacteria notably *Yersinia* and *Pseudomonas* species can grow at 1–6°C.

Platelet concentrates which are stored as room temperature are more likely to be contaminated with skin contaminants such are Gram-positive organism, including coagulase negative staphylococci.

Symptom and Sign of Transfusion Reaction

Acute hemolytic reaction may present with—

- Hypotension and tachycardia
- Fever and chill

- Hemoglobinemia and hemoglobinuria
- Chest and flank pain
- Discomfort at the transfusion site
- Acute renal failure.

Anaphylactic reaction

- Difficult breathing, respiratory arrest may occur
- Cough and bronchospasm
- Nausea and vomiting
- Hypotension
- Shock
- Loss of consciousness.

Graft versus host disease

- Fever, diarrhea
- Cutaneous eruption
- Liver function abnormality
- Marrow aplasia
- Pancytopenia.

Transfusion related lung injury

- Symptoms of respiratory compromise
- Sign of non-cardiogenic pulmonary edema
- Bilateral interstitial infiltrate on chest X-ray.

Alloimmunization

- Women of child bearing age who are sensitized to certain RBC antigen are at risk of bearing a fetus with hemolytic disease of newborn.

Electrolyte toxicity

- Hypocalcemia manifested by circumoral numbness or tingling sensation of finger and toe.

Infectious complication sequelae

- Infection may be asymptomatic or lead to chronic active hepatitis, cirrhosis, liver failure
- HTLV 1 associated with adult T cell leukemia or lymphoma and tropical spastic paraparesis
- Parvovirus B 19 shows tropism for erythroid precursors and inhibits both erythrocytes production and maturation
- Bacterial contamination causes fever, chill, septic shock and DIC.

Preventive Measures for Transfusion Reaction

The study of red blood cell antigen and antibody forms the foundation of transfusion medicine. Other cellular elements and plasma protein are also antigenic and can result in alloimmunization. The first blood group antigen system recognized in 1900 was ABO, the most important in transfusion medicine. The major blood group of this system A, B, AB and O. Rh system is the 2nd most important blood group system in pretransfusion testing. Other antigens are: Lewis system carbohydrate antigen system kell protein, Duffy antigen, Kidd antigen. Pretransfusion testing of a potentials recipient consists of the type screen, the forward type determine the ABO Rh phenotype of the recipients RBC by using antisera directed against A, B and D antigen. The "Reverse Type" detects isoagglutinins in the patients' serum and should correlate with ABO phenotype on "Forward Type".

Crossmatching is ordered when there is a high probability that patient requires a packed RBC transfusion. Blood selected for crossmatching must be ABO compatible and lack antigen for which the patient has alloantibodies. In case of Rh-patient every attempt must be made to provide Rh-blood components to prevent alloimmunization to the D antigen.

Others

a. Nucleic acid amplification test (NAT)
   NAT identifies circulating viral genes in the window period before antibodies develop and are available for HIV, Hepatitis C.
b. Transfusion associated cytomegalovirus (CMV) can be eliminated by transferring leukocyte depleted blood product or by selecting blood from donor who are seronegative for antibody to CMV or using both.
c. Vaccination of individuals who require long-term transfusion therapy can prevent Hepatitis B virus infection.
d. To avoid transfusion associated graft verses host disease, directed donation by family member should be discouraged. The blood products from family member should always be irradiated by exposing blood bag to ionizing radiation at a dose of 1500 CGY.
   To avoid GVHD identify the patient at risk of transfusion induced GVHD

- Bone marrow transplant recipients
- Recipients of cellular blood products from 1st degree relatives
- Neonatal exchange transfusion, especially after intrauterine transfusion.

e. To prevent allo-immunization use leukocyte reduced cellular components.
f. To avoid allergic reaction cellular component can be washed to remove residual plasma for extremely sensitized patient.
g. To prevent hypothermia use of an in line warmer is preferred.
h. Neonates and patient in renal failure are at risk for hyperkalemia. To avoid this complication use relatively fresh RBCs (< 7 days of storage).
i. Autologous RBC transfusion may be another alternative. For autologous transfusion, blood is collected a few weeks before the procedure.
j. Avoid errors at the patient's bed side, such as mislabeling the sample or mismatch transfusion.
k. Avoid clerical errors in blood bank.

Management

Management of acute hemolytic transfusion reaction.

- When acute hemolysis is suspected the transfusion must be stopped immediately
- Intravenous access maintained
- Treatment is largely supportive:
  - Infusion of normal saline to maintain adequate urine output
  - Furosemide
  - Dopamine to enhance renal cortical perfusion
  - Dialysis may be required if acute tubular necrosis develops.
- The laboratory evaluation for the hemolysis includes the measurement of
  - Serum haptoglobulin
  - Lactate dehydrogenase
  - Indirect bilirubin levels
  - Other coagulation studies including prothrombin time and partial thromboplastin time.
- Reaction reported to the blood bank and a correctly labeled post-transfusion blood sample and

any untransfused blood should be sent to the blood bank.

Further investigation at the blood bank includes:

– Examination of the pre-and post-transfusion sample for hemolysis and repeat typing of patient sample

– Direct antiglobulin test (DAT), sometimes called the direct Coomb's test at the post-transfusion sample, DAT detects the presence of antibody or complements bound to RBC

– Checking all clerical records for error.

- GVHD is highly resistant to treatment. Immunosuppressive therapy including glucocorticoids, cyclosporine, antithymocyte globulin and ablative therapy followed by allergeneic bone marrow transplantation.

- In case of post-transfusion purpura platelet transfusion should be avoided as it may worsen thrombocytopenia. Intravenous immunoglobulin may be needed.

- To avoid allergic reaction cellular components can be washed to remove residual plasma for the extremely sensitized patient

– Premedicated with antihistamine

- If hypocalcemia then injection calcium must be given through a separate intravenous line

- In case of iron overload desferoxamine and other chelating agents are available

- Febrile non-hemolytic transfusion reaction

– Premedication with acetaminophen or other antipyretic agent

- Anaphylactic reaction

– Stopping transfusion

– Maintaining vascular access

– Administering epinephrine (0.5 to 1.0 ml at 1:1000 dilution)

– Glucocorticoid may be required in severe cases.

Alternatives to Transfusion

- Oxygen carrying blood substitutes such as perfluorocarbons and aggregated hemoglobin solutions are presently in various stages of clinical trial

- Granulocyte and granulocyte macrophage colony stimulating factor are clinically useful to hastier leukocyte recovery in patients with leukopenia related to high dose chemotherapy

- Erythropoietin stimulates erythrocyte production in patients with anemia at chromic renal failure and other condition, thus, avoiding or reducing the need for transfusion

- Thrombopoietin, a cytokine that promotes megakaryocyte proliferation and maturation, is being tested for its ability to reduce the need for platelet transfusion.

SUGGESTED READING

1. Anderson KC, NESS pm (Eds). Scientific basis at transfusion medicine, implication for clinical practice. Philadelphia, Saunders, 1999.

2. Arendt A, Carmean J, Koch E, et al. Fatal bacterial infection associated with platelet transfusion. United States, 2004. MMWR 2005;57:168.

3. Blajchman MA, Vamvakan EC. The continuing risk of transfusion—transmitted infection. N Engl J Med. 2006:355:1303-5.

4. Bolton – Maggs PHB, Marphy MF. Blood transfusion. Arch Dis Child. 2004;89:4-7.

5. Busch MP, Kleinman SH, Nemo GJ. Current and emerging infectious risk of blood transfusions. JAMA. 2003;289:959-62.

6. Eskinazi AE, Bernstein ML, Gordon JB. Hematologic disorder in the pediatric intensive care unit. In: Rogers MC (Ed).Textbook of pediatric intensive care. Baltimore: William and Wilkins; 1996;1395-431.

7. Jeffery S, Dzieezkowski, Kennneth C. Anderson, et al. Transfusion biology and theraphy. Harrison's principles of internal medicine 2001;114:733-8.

8. Menitove JE, et al. The technical manual 18th edn. Arlingto VA, American Association of Blood Bank, 1997.

9. OP Ghai, Pyush Gupta, VK Paul, et al. Blood transfusion. Ghai essential pediatrics. 2004;27(12):669-70.

10. RK Marwaha, Sudeshna Mitra, Deepak Bansal, et al. Transfusion medicine and component theraphy in pediatrics. IAP Textbook of Pediatrics. 2006;14:675-82.

11. Ronald G. Strauss, et al. Blood component transfusion. Nelson Textbook of Pediatrics, 2007;470:2055-60.

12. Schreiber GB, et al. The risk of transfusion—transmitted viral infection. N Engl J Med. 1996;334:1685.

28 Corticosteroid in Childhood Cancer

Abhisekh Roy, Rakesh Mondal

INTRODUCTION

Corticosteroids are steroid hormones synthesized by the adrenal cortex. Its primary biological functions are stress response, inflammatory response, metabolism regulator (Glucocorticoids) and electrolyte balance (Mineralocorticoids). Its biosynthesis is a long pathway starting with cholesterol. Progesterone is also produced in the same pathway.

CLASSIFICATION

Corticosteroids are also synthesized artificially, which are used as drugs in various conditions. Synthetic corticosteroids are broadly classified into four groups called Coopman classification, which is as follows:

Group A: Hydrocortisone Type

Hydrocortisone, hydrocortisone acetate, prednisone, prednisolone, methylprednisolone, cortisone acetate, tixocortol pivalate, etc.

Group B: Acetonides

Triamcinolone acetonide, triamcinolone alcohol, budesonide, mometasone, desonide fluocinonide, fluocinolone acetonide, amcinonide and halcinonide.

Group C: Betamethasone Type

Betamethasone, betamethasone sodium phosphate, dexamethasone, dexamethasone sodium phosphate and fluocortolone.

Group D: Esters

Group D1 – Halogenated (less labile)

Betamethasone dipropionate, betamethasone valerate, hydrocortisone-17-valerate, clobetasone-17-butyrate, clobetasol-17-propionate, alclometasone dipropionate, prednicarbate, fluocortolone caproate, fluocortolone pivalate and fluprednidene acetate.

Group D2 – Labile

Hydrocortisone-17-butyrate, 17-aceponate, 17-buteprate and prednicarbate.

MODES OF ACTION AND INDICATIONS IN VARIOUS PEDIATRIC CANCERS

Corticosteroids are nowadays widely used in pediatric malignancies. Due to its broad spectrum of action, it is included in regimens of hematologic malignancies as well as solid tumors. Prednisolone, hydrocortisone and dexamethasone are most commonly administered. Various indications of corticosteroids according to its different modes of actions are as follows:

Induction chemotherapy: Hydrocortisone/Dexamethasone/Prednisolone are used in induction of chemotherapy in various ALL treatment regimes like UKALL2003, CCG and POG ALL, BFM 90, HKALL protocols. Here, the role is rapid reduction in the number of leukemic cells.

Adjuvant therapy: Prednisolone is used as an adjuvant drug in StanfordV, BEACOPP, MOPP regimen for Hodgkin lymphoma and CHOP regimen for non-Hodgkin lymphoma, etc.

Tumorlysis: Various studies have postulated tumor lysis property of dexamethasone. The probable mechanisms are change in cell-to-cell interaction, decrease in malignant potency and prevention of entry of water-soluble cytotoxic mediators due to reduced membrane permeability.

Lymholysis: When glucocorticoids are used in CNS lymphoma there is shrinkage of mass size by lympholytic action. Glucocorticoid causes apoptosis of lymphoma cells by bcl-2 proto-oncogenes attention.

Prevent neuropathy: Prednisolone is used with vincristine for induction of remission in acute lymphoblastic leukemia. Here, prednisolone prevents peripheral neuropathy, which is a side effect of vincristine.

Prevent adhesion: In CNS directed therapies, intrathecal methotrexate and hydrocortisone are administered simultaneously. This prevents adhesion from acute chemical arachnoiditis caused by methotrexate.

Reduction of edema and raised intracranial pressure: Glucocorticoid imparts cell membrane stability, reduces vascular permeability and prevents the entry of sodium and water inside the cell. This mechanism helps to prevent peritumoral edema and increased intracranial pressure. So it is used in solid tumors of brain and spinal cord.

Antiemetic: Glucocorticoids reduces permeability of blood brain barrier to anti-cancer drugs and reduces nausea and vomiting, which is a common adverse drug reaction of all chemotherapeutics. However, steroids should be prescribed only after conventional anti-emetics have failed.

Antiallergic: Hypersensitivity reactions are very frequently encountered during chemotherapy and blood product transfusion. Prophylactic IV hydrocortisone prevents such situations.

Analgesic: Intense headache due to intracranial tumor can be reduced by IV dexamethasone, which cuts down the cerebral edema.

Replacement treatment: There can be suppression of the hypothalamic-pituitary-adrenal axis by tumors occurring along the pathway. Prior use of corticosteroids prevents this crisis.

Prevents radiotherapy complications: Brainstem tumors requiring radiotherapy often develops peritumoral edema. Administration of glucocorticoids during radiotherapy, prevents such complications.

Preparation for neurosurgery: By reducing peritumoral edema and intracranial pressure in case of CNS tumors, patient is prepared for neurosurgical operative procedure to improve the resection success rate.

ADVERSE DRUG REACTIONS

Corticosteroids when used for a considerable period can result into some side effects like:

a. Gastritis: To prevent this, an antacid should be prescribed along with corticosteroids for long-term use.
b. Osteoporosis: Oral calcium supplementation and periodic X-ray evaluation, bone mineral density should be done.
c. Avascular necrosis: Most common presenting feature is joint pain.
d. Linear growth suppression is a well-known complication.
e. Psychosis: Though rare, but should be suspected if there is change of behavior.
f. Hypertension: Regular blood pressure monitoring is essential.
g. Hypertrichosis is seen in some patients.
h. Cataract: Regular ophthalmologic check-up or follow-up should be done.
i. Weight gain: BMI monitoring should be done regularly.
j. Voracious appetite: Commonly seen soon after starting oral prednisolone.
k. Iatrogenic Cushing syndrome is seen in patients taking long-term prednisolone.
l. Spinal epidural lipomatosis: A new onset back pain is the initial presenting symptom. Whenever suspected, spinal MRI should be done at the earliest. Drug dose modification and surgical decompression is done depending upon severity of lesion.
m. Adrenal insufficiency is noted when sudden withdrawal is tried inadvertently.

RECENT UPDATES

a. Several studies conducted abroad have shown that dexamethasone is more effective than prednisolone both in induction as well as later phases of chemotherapy. Use of dexamethasone gives better event free survival (EFS), has less chance of relapse and better long-term follow-up results than prednisolone. Other RCTs found that there is no significant change in outcome on using appropriate the drug doses.

b. However, some other studies found that dexamethasone is not only more toxic, but also increases chance of infection, osteonecrosis and causes more short-term growth suppression than prednisolone.

c. Recently, methyl prednisolone is being used in treatment of refractory hypercalcemia in acute lymphoblastic leukemia where other means have failed.

d. Trials on use of oral deflazacort instead of prednisolone in maintenance phase of acute lymphoblastic leukemia needs to be studied.

TITBITS

1. Never stop steroid without consulting the physician.
2. A record of chemotherapy and steroid intake should be maintained and should be produced during follow-up.
3. If one or multiple doses of steroid are missed, consultation should be done with the physician about the next dose to prevent complication.

SUGGESTED READING

1. Ahmed SF, Tucker P, Mushtaq T, et al.: Short-term effects on linear growth and bone turnover in children randomized to receive prednisolone or dexamethasone. Clin Endocrinol (Oxf). 2002;57:185-91.

2. Asselin BL, Whitin JC, Coppola DJ, et al. Comparative pharmacokinetic studies of three asparaginase preparations. J Clin Oncol. 1993;11:1780-6.

3. Belgaumi AF, Al-Bakrah M, Al-Mahr M, et al. Dexamethasone-associated toxicity during induction chemotherapy for childhood acute lymphoblastic leukemia is augmented by concurrent use of daunomycin. Cancer. 2003;97:2898-903.

4. Coopman S, Degreef H, Dooms-Goossens A. Identification of cross-reaction patterns in allergic contact dermatitis from topical corticosteroids. Br J Dermatol. 1989;121:27-34.

5. Eisenberg HM, Barlow CF, Lorenzo AV. Effect of dexamethasome on altered brain vascular permeability. Arch Neurol. 1970;23:18-22.

6. Foot ABM, Hayes C. Audit of guidelines for effective control of chemotherapy and radiotherapy induced emesis. Arch Dis Child. 1994;71:475-80.

7. Freshney RI. Effects of glucocorticoids on glioma cells in culture. Minireview on cancer research. Experimental Cell Biology. 1984;52:286-92.

8. Glucocorticoid Treatment of Primary CNS Lymphoma. Michael Weller. Journal of neuro-oncology;Volume 43, Number 3:237-23.

9. Hurwitz CA, Silverman LB, Schorin MA, et al. Substituting dexamethasone for prednisone complicates remission induction in children with acute lymphoblastic leukemia. Cancer. 2000;88:1964-9.

10. Igarashi S, Manabe A, Ohara A, et al. No advantage of dexamethasone over prednisolone for the outcome of standard- and intermediate-risk childhood acute lymphoblastic leukemia in the Tokyo Children's Cancer Study Group L95-14 protocol. J Clin Oncol. 2005;23: 6489-98.

11. Maciunas RJ, Mericle RA, Sneed CL, et al. Determination of the lethal dose of dexamethasome for early passage in vitro human gliblastoma cell cultures. Neurosurgery. 1993; 33:485-8.

12. Mattano LA Jr, Sather HN, Trigg ME, et al. Osteonecrosis as a complication of treating acute lymphoblastic leukemia in children: a report from the Children's Cancer Group. J Clin Oncol. 2000;18:3262-72.

13. McNeer JL, Nachman JB: The optimal use of steroids in paediatric acute lymphoblastic leukaemia: no easy answers. Br J Haematol. 2010;149:638-52.

14. Mealy J, Chen TT, Schanz GP. The effects of dexamethasome and methylprednisolone on cell cultures of human glioblastoma. J Neurosurg. 1971;34:324-34.

15. Miller JD, Leech P. Effects of mannitol and steroid therapy on intracranial volume-pressure relationships in patients. J Neurosurg. 1975;42:274-81.

16. Mitchell CD, Richards SM, Kinsey SE, et al. Benefit of dexamethasone compared with prednisolone for childhood acute lymphoblastic leukaemia: results of the UK Medical Research Council ALL97 randomized trial. Br J Haematol. 2005;129:734-45.

17. Shapiro WR, Posner JB. Corticosteroid hormones; effects in an experimental brain tumour. Arch Neurol. 1974;30:217-21.

18. Sherbert GV, Lakshmi MS, Haddah S. Does dexamethasome inhibit the growth of human gliomas? J Neurosurg. 1977;47:864-70.

19. Zager RF, Frisby SA, Oliverio VT. Cellular transport and antitumor action of methotrexate with several drugs. Proceedings of the American Academy of Cancer Research. 1972;13:33.

20. Ünal Ş, Durmaz E, Erkoçoğlu M, Bayrakçı B, Bircan Ö, Alikaşifoğlu A, Çetin M. The rapid correction of hypercalcemia at presentation of acute lymphoblastic leukemia using high-dose methylprednisolone. Turk J Pediatr. 2008;50:171-5.

29 Nuclear Medicine Practices in Pediatric Oncology

Rakesh Mondal, Sumantra Sarkar

In recent years, the contribution of nuclear medicine has been of increasing interest to pediatric oncology, particularly in imaging for diagnosis, staging and follow-up, assessment of as well as in radionuclide therapy. Nuclear medicine studies in children require special considerations regarding the performance of the procedure and the attitude of the staff. In tumor imaging the trend has been to use more or less specific tumor-seeking radiopharmaceuticals. A great number of these agents are available, exploiting various metabolic and biological properties of individual tumors. Parallel to these developments radionuclide therapy becomes more widely used.

A list of tumor seeking radiopharmaceuticals, which are currently available for diagnosis and therapy are given below.

OBJECTIVE

Imaging

Radiopharmaceutical

a. 67Ga-citrate:
   Lymphoma
b. 201Tl-chloride :
   Differentiated thyroid ca.
   Lymphoma
   Osteosarcoma
   Brain tumors
   Rhabdomyosarcoma
c. 99mTc-sestamibi:
   Lymphoma
d. 99mTc-tetrofosmin:
   Lymphoma
e. 99mTc-diphosphonate:
   Osteosarcoma
f. 99mTc-pentavalent DMSA:
   Medullary thyroid ca.
   (MEN II syndromes)
g. 123I/131I-MIBG:
   Neuroblastoma
   Pheochromocytoma
   Ganglioneuroma
h. 111 In-pentetreotide:
   Neuroendocrine tumors
   Lymphoma
i. 99mTc-HIDA derivatives:
   Hepatoblastoma
j. 111In-antimyosin Fab:
   Rhabdomyosarcoma
k. Radiolabeled antibodies:
   Neuroblastoma

Positron Emission Tomography (PET)

Radiopharmaceuticals

- 18F-deoxyglucose
  - Lymphoma
  - Neuroblastoma
- 124I-MIBG
  - Neuroblastoma
- 124I-3F8 antibodies
  - Neuroblastoma

- 11C-hydroxyephedrine
  - Neuroblastoma
  - Pheochromocytoma

Therapy

Radiopharmaceutical

a. 131I-iodide:
   Differentiated thyroid ca.
b. 131I-MIBG:
   Neuroblastoma
c. 125I-MIBG:
   Neuroblastoma
d. 131I-3F8 antibodies:
   Neuroblastoma
e. 131I-Rose Bengal:
   Hepatoblastoma
f. 131I-antiferritin antibodies:
   Hepatoblastoma
g. 89Sr-chloride:
   Osteosarcoma
h. 186Re-HEDP:
   Osteosarcoma
i. 153Sm-EDTMP:
   Osteosarcoma
j. 131I-anti-CD20 antibodies:
   Lymphoma
k. 90Y-anti-CD20 antibodies:
   Lymphoma

DIAGNOSTICS

Lymphoma

This common childhood malignancy occurs as Hodgkin's disease or non-Hodgkin lymphoma of the B-cell- or T-cell type. The diagnosis is based on histopathology of lymph nodes, bone marrow, cerebrospinal fluid, etc. Anatomical diagnostic imaging is done by X-ray, ultrasonography of the abdomen, CT-scan of chest or abdomen and MRI. Nuclear medicine provides functional imaging, i.e. bone scintigraphy and tumor imaging with scintigraphy/SPECT/PET using 67Ga-citrate, 201Tl-chloride, 99mTc-sestamibi, 111 In-pentetreotide and 18F-FDG. 67Ga-citrate has been used for decades in the detection and staging of lymphomas. 67Ga-SPECT is better than planar scintigraphy. More recently, it is also used for early recognition of response to chemotherapy or radiotherapy: failure of a positive 67Ga-scan to convert to negative is associated with a poor prognosis. In follow up 67Ga-scintigraphy is better than CT-scan in differentiating residual tumor from fibrosis. 201Tl-chloride scintigraphy and emission tomography and positron emission tomography (PET) using 18F-deoxyglucose can also be used for this purpose. More recently 99mTc-sestamibi and 99mTc-tetrofosmin have been used for imaging lymphoma.

Rhabdomyosarcoma

Eight percent of pediatric malignancies are rhabdomyosarcomas. The primary location is most frequently in the head and neck area (36%) and the genitourinary tract (25%). The diagnosis is confirmed by a biopsy with immunohistochemical staining of the myosin, which is characteristic for this tumor and forms the basis for radioimmunoscintigraphy.

Treatment consists of preoperative chemotherapy or radiotherapy, followed by surgery of the primary tumor and regional lymph nodes and postoperative chemotherapy. A specific tracers, e.g. 67Ga-citrate, 201Tl-chloride and 18F-deoxyglucose (PET), can be used to image rhabdomyosarcoma. Specific targeting of rhabdomyosarcoma is provided by radioimmunoscintigraphy using 111In antimyosin Fab fragments [29], however this radiopharmaceutical is no longer commercially available.

Neuroblastoma

Neuroblastoma is a malignant tumor of the sympathetic nervous system, occurring most frequently in early childhood. 50% of patients are younger than 2 years and the disease is rare after the age of 14. The site of the primary tumor varies: 70% of all tumors originate in the retroperitoneal region. Out of these 30% arise in the adrenal gland and 10% in the abdominal sympathetic chain, and 8% occur in the cervical, 17% in the thoracic and 5% in the pelvic sympathetic chain. The diagnosis is suspected on clinical symptomatology, which varies with the site and size of the tumor and the amount of catecholamines, and is confirmed by increased levels of catecholamines and metabolites in urine and by MIBG scintigraphy. Specific targeting of neuroblastoma may be achieved either via the metabolic route (MIBG), via receptor binding (peptides) or via the immunological route (antibodies). Potential pitfalls in MIBG scintigraphy in neuroblastoma are abnormalities which are located in or close to normal structures that normally take up MIBG, hyperplasia of the residual adrenal gland after contralateral adrenalectomy, hydronephrosis, activity in the reservoir of an administration system or in intravenous lines or in drains, inadequate blockade of the thyroid, and uptake in benign or malignant tumors other than neuroblastoma can concentrate MIBGAs. MIBG SPECT may be helpful in those situations. PET using 18F-deoxyglucose (FDG) has a lower sensitivity than MIBG-scintigraphy.

Ewing Sarcoma

The principle bone tumors in children are osteosarcoma and Ewing sarcoma. The peak incidence is between 10 and 20 years of age. The etiological factors include rapid growth, trauma, radiation and previous chemotherapy. Patients generally present with bone pain, swelling of bone with or without functional impairment. The distribution of the sites of the primary tumor is different for both tumor types. Relevant diagnostic procedures are X-ray, CT, MRI, bone scintigraphy and SPECT, alkaline phosphatase and LDH for Ewing sarcoma. The diagnosis is confirmed by histology and immunocytochemistry.

Ewing sarcoma is treated by radiotherapy or surgical resection of an expendable bone and chemotherapy. Bone scintigraphy is highly sensitive to detect Ewing sarcoma and bone metastases. In differentiated osteosarcoma, bone scintigraphy/SPECT using 99mTc-diphosphonate may visualize not only the primary bone tumor and its skeletal metastases with great intensity and 100% sensitivity, but also the extraosseous metastases in the majority of cases. SPECT can be helpful to distinguish extraosseous from skeletal metastases, particularly in the thorax and pelvis. To study the effect of preoperative chemotherapy in osteosarcoma also Thallium-201 scintigraphy has been used with success.

Miscellaneous

Liver tumors are rare in children and the incidence and distribution of tumor types vary with geography. The most frequent type is hepatoblastoma, which usually presents with abdominal distension, palpable mass or hepatomegaly. Serum assays of α-fetoprotein, produced by the tumor, serve as a tumor marker. Treatment is by surgery and chemotherapy; inoperable or recurrent tumors may also be treated by hepatic arterial embolization and intra-arterial radionuclide therapy. 67Ga-citrate scintigraphy and SPECT may be used for tumor imaging. Some hepatoblastomas have capability to take up hepatobiliary agents, such as 99mTc-HIDA derivatives, and tumor retention of these agents may be demonstrated by hepatobiliary scintigraphy. Apart from tumor imaging, scintigraphy of organs, e.g. of bone, bone marrow, thyroid lungs, kidneys, brain, liver/spleen and lymphnodes, is also widely used in pediatric oncology. Scintigraphy using 99mTc-labeled autologous erythrocytes may be helpful to differentiate hemangioma from other.

THERAPEUTICS

As an oncological treatment modality, radionuclide therapy combines the advantages of being systemic, like chemotherapy, with that of delivering local radiation to tumors, like radiotherapy. It also provides excellent palliation, as it is associated with limited side effects and few late effects. However, problem lies at the need of isolation of patients and storage of radioactive waste, high cost of the newer therapeutic agents, etc. Multiple mechanisms for targeting radionuclides to tumors exists in children. The common indications are differentiated thyroid carcinoma, neuroblastoma, osteosarcoma, painful skeletal metastases, lymphoma, etc. Contraindications are severe myelosuppression and renal function disorders, etc. Special considerations apply for the treatment of children with radionuclides. They must be instructed about issues of radiation protection: to wear disposable gown, gloves and shoes and carry a pocket dose-meter, when entering the isolation room; to restrict the time of exposure, keep as much distance as feasible, how to handle any radioactive waste, etc. Child and parents should be made aware, that items which become contaminated may have to be stored for radioactive decay. Potential hazards are acute radiation effects, like nausea, vomiting, sialoadenitis or temporary swelling of tumor localizations; or side effects due to the targeting agent, e.g. allergic reactions, response to antibodies, vasoactive reaction to MIBG, etc. Potential long-term effects are xerostomia, induction of leukemia or other malignancies.

Lymphoma

Currently, radioimmunotherapy of recurrent lymphoma is not practiced in children. Several protocols are undergoing clinical investigation: either immunotherapy using unlabeled anti-CD20 antibodies, or radioimmunotherapy with nonmyeloablative doses of 131I- or 90Y-labeled anti CD20, etc. The reported objective response rates of radioimmunotherapy are quite good.

Neuroblastoma

Pooled results of major centers indicate an objective response rate of 51% . Most patients had stage IV, progressive and intensely pretreated disease and were only treated with 131I-MIBG when other treatment modalities had failed. Both the 131I-MIBG therapy and the isolation are generally well tolerated by children. For patients with recurrent and progressive disease after conventional treatment 131I-MIBG therapy is probably the best palliative treatment, as its invasiveness and toxicity compare favorably with that of chemotherapy and external beam radiotherapy. The therapeutic effect of 131I-MIBG may be increased by combining it with chemotherapy and/or total body irradiation. More recently, 131I-MIBG therapy has been integrated in the treatment protocol as the initial therapy instead of preoperative combination chemotherapy in children presenting with advanced disease/inoperable neuroblastoma. The objective is to reduce the tumor volume, enabling adequate surgical resection and to avoid toxicity New developments in radioimmunotherapy of neuroblastoma include the use of chimeric antibodies, such as chCE7 and ch14.18.

Thyroid Carcinoma

Radioiodine therapy is indicated in children with differentiated thyroid carcinoma, for ablation of thyroid remnants either after near total thyroidectomy or for treatment of tumor recurrence or metastases. Improved survival rates and objective response has been documented when therapy was given to metastatic thyroid carcinoma. In children with recurrent or metastatic medullary therapy carcinoma, radionuclide therapy may also be considered.

Monitoring

Nuclear medicine is applied to monitor the function of organs at risk during treatment in pediatric oncology, in particular cardiac, pulmonary, renal and salivary function. 111In-antimyosin antibodies monitor Anthracycline- or radiation-induced cardiomyopathy. Pulmonary ventilation and perfusion studies and 111In-pentetreotide scintigraphy are used to detect radiation lesions to the lungs. Renography with 99mTc-DTPA or 99mTc-MAG3 and renal uptake studies using 99mTc-DMSA can monitor radiation nephropathy and renal side effects of cisplatin treatment. Radiation lesions to the salivary glands can be monitored by measuring salivary gland 99mTc-pertechnetate studies.

SUGGESTED READING

1. Chatal JF, Hoefnagel CA. Radionuclide therapy. Lancet. 1999;354:931-5.
2. Chatal JF, Mahé M. Therapeutic use of radiolabelled antibodies. In: Murray IPC, Ell PJ (Eds). Nuclear medicine in clinical diagnosis and treatment. 2nd edition. Churchill Livingstone, Edinburgh. 1998;1101-14.
3. Connolly LP, Drubach LA, Treves TS. Applications of nuclear medicine in pediatric oncology. Clin Nucl Med. 2002;27:117-25.
4. Hoefnagel CA, de Kraker J. Childhood neoplasia. In: Murray IPC, Ell PJ (Eds). Nuclear medicine in clinical diagnosis and treatment. 2nd edition. Churchill Livingstone, London, 1998;1001-14.
5. Hoefnagel CA, Kraker JD: Nuclear medicine in pediatric oncology: Nuclear Medicine Review. 2004;7:69-75.
6. Hoefnagel CA, Lewington VJ. MIBG therapy. In: Murray IPC, Ell PJ (Eds). Nuclear medicine in clinical diagnosis and treatment, 2nd edition. Churchill Livingstone, Edinburgh. 1998;1067-81.
7. Ryad R, et al. Role of Tc-99m SESTAMIBI in Assessment of Treatment Response to Chemotherapy in Bone Sarcomas; Journal of the Egyptian Nat. Cancer Inst. 2001;13:27-33.
8. Shulkin BL. PET imaging in pediatric oncology. Pediatr Radiol. 2004;34:199-204.

30 Radio Imaging in Pediatric Oncology

Tapan Dhibar, Rakesh Mondal

INTRODUCTION

The oncology imaging guidelines are nearly the same for both the pediatric population and the adult population. For pediatric patients suspected or confirmed to have a malignancy, pediatric oncology consultation without delay is a must. Confirmation of malignancy by biopsy should proceed promptly. Excess delay in obtaining tissue confirmation of disease while awaiting imaging is not appropriate. Pediatric oncology patients enrolled or treated according to current Pediatric Oncology Group (POG) protocols should have imaging obtained in accordance with POG protocols. Imaging obtained in accordance with such protocols should not be denied as being investigational.

IMAGING TESTS APPLIED TO PEDIATRIC ONCOLOGY

Chest X-ray: This is to look for metastasis in the lungs, rarely seen in children bone radiographs to look for cancer in the bones.

Ultrasound: Ultrasonography uses sound waves to produce images of internal organs and to distinguish benign conditions from malignant tumors. This is often the first imaging study to be done if a tumor is appreciated in the abdomen because it is painless and noninvasive. But it is not conclusive in most of the situations.

CT/CAT scan: CT scan uses X-rays to create cross-sectional pictures of the tumor. Often, dye will be placed through an intravenous into the child's veins to help make the pictures more clear. CT scanning without contrast is helpful in determining the density of tumor nodules, which is measured in Hounsefeld Units (HUs). Adrenal nodules with densities above 10–25 HUs ordinarily are seen with pheochromocytoma, excluding adrenal adenomas and lipomas. A mass with a low density of <10 HU on noncontrast CT is not likely a pheochromocytoma. For CT scanning with intravenous contrast enhancement, non-ionic contrast is preferred, because it is unlikely to induce hypertensive crisis.

MRI: An MRI scan uses radiowaves and strong magnets rather than X-rays to create pictures of the tumor. MRI gives more detailed images than CT and ultrasound. MRI scanning can be helpful, particularly for imaging bone and hepatic metastases, given most sarcomas and blastomas display increased signal intensity on T2-weighted imaging. MRI is also preferred for children and pregnant women, due to lack of radiation exposure. These different scanning techniques can be considered complementary to each other, with no single imaging modality being 100% sensitive and specific for any particular type of childhood tumors.

MIBG: MIBG is a compound similar to the hormone norepinephrine which is found specifically in sympathetic nervous tissue. MIBG can be labeled with radioactive iodine allowing it to then be visualized with scintigraphy. Thus, MIBG scans can show "hot spots" throughout the body where tumor is located.

99mTc bone scans: They are often done in conjunction with MIBG scans to look for bone lesions. It is an additional test to look for metastases.

Additional test: Intravenous pyelography, HRCT, etc. may be required in specific situation if needed.

Positron emission tomography (PET): It is the most sensitive scanning technique for imaging of pediatric malignancies. PET scanning dramatically displays metastatic tumor burden and the response to therapy. PET scanning with 18F-deoxyglucose (18FDG) works on account of the fact that deoxyglucose is absorbed into cells by a glucose transporter and accumulates in the cells because it cannot enter glycolytic pathways. An estimated 90% of pheochromocytomas metastases have affirmed for 18FDG. However, 18FDG PET is non-specific and may detect other tumors and has increased uptake in areas of increased glucose absorption, such as the brain, inflammation, muscle activity, or bone marrow after G-CSF stimulation. 18F-dopamine PET scanning is both highly sensitive and specific for primary pheochromocytomas and metastases. Although both 18F-dopamine and 131I MIBG are transported into cells by an amine uptake-1 mechanism, 18F-dopamine is more actively transported into neurosecretory vesicles, where it is stored, whereas 131I MIBG may leave the cell. Therefore, 18F-dopamine PET scanning is more sensitive than even 123I MIBG SPECT scanning. 18F-dopamine PET scanning is more selective than 18FDG-PET. However, 18FDG PET scanning may underestimate the number of metastases in patients with advanced metastases and a high tumor burden. False-positives may occur with 18FDG PET, such as gallbladder visualization. Disadvantages of PET scanning include its high cost and radiation exposure. Both 18FDG and 18F-dopamine PET scanning can be combined with CT scanning to produce extraordinarily accurate anatomic imaging. Combined PET/CT fusion imaging is currently the state-of-the-art for accurately detecting and quantifying most of the childhood tumors. For oncologic applications, the skull base to mid-femur procedure code for PET is usually the most appropriate procedure to order.

IMAGING IN DIFFERENT TUMORS

Leukemia

While most leukemia patients do not require advanced imaging, brain MRI with and without contrast can be performed in high-risk patients, patients exhibiting central nervous system (CNS) symptoms of CNS leukemia, and in patients found to have obvious positive CNS cytology.

Lymphomas

Imaging for pediatric lymphomas are similar to the adult oncology guidelines, except imaging after each 2 cycles of chemotherapy is generally allowed. Imaging is initially required for staging. Repeat imaging following chemotherapy is done by contrast CT of those areas which were previously positive in PET/CT many centers do not follow this routinely in pediatric population due to radiation exposure.

Neuroblastoma

Abdominal and pelvic CT or MRI, contrast as requested, with chest X-ray is indicated for the initial evaluation of any child with a palpable abdominal mass. Neuroblastoma should be in the differential diagnosis for young children who present with adrenal tumors. Follow-up chest CT or MRI, contrast as requested, can be performed for any suspected abnormality on above studies. Both CT and MRI may be necessary to fully evaluate patients with neuroblastoma. Radiological imaging included a chest X-ray, and abdomino-pelvic VSG or a CT scan, a bone scan and 131I MIBG scintigraphy or 99mTc bone scan. MIBG or bone scan is the standard staging study to assess the possibility of skeletal disease in most of the cases. MRI of skeleton or central nervous system (CNS) is not routinely indicated in the absence of signs or symptoms of disease in those systems. Re-staging studies can be repeated every 3 to 6 months post-therapy.

Wilms' Tumor

Abdominal and pelvic CT or MRI, contrast as requested, with chest X-ray is indicated for the initial evaluation of any child with a palpable abdominal mass. CT chest can be performed upon verification of Wilms' tumor. Brain MRI with or without contrast may be performed if the patient has the unusual variants of rhabdoid histology and clear cell sarcoma. Re-staging studies may be repeated every 3 to 6 months post-therapy. Pelvic imaging is unnecessary for patients who have had no previous pelvic involvement.

Pediatric Rhabdomyosarcomas

They should be imaged according to institutional protocol. Ultrasound is generally performed initially, followed by CT or PET.

Germ Cell Tumors

Testicular and ovarian germ cell tumor in the children will require abdominal CT and/or MRI to define the lesion and its extent.

Osseous Ewing's Sarcoma

Chest MRI and chest CT may both be indicated to evaluate the chest wall Ewing's sarcoma and rule out lung metastases.

Breast Mass

Chest X-ray and chest CT can be performed to evaluate a breast mass in the pediatric population, as tumor like lymphoma or rhabdomyosarcoma may look alike.

SUGGESTED READING

1. Beierwaltes WH. Clinical applications of 131I MIBG. JL. Quinn Ill. Memorial Essay. In: Hoffer RB (Ed). Yearbook of Nuclear Medicine. Yearbook Medical Publishers, Chicago 1987;17-34.
2. Fitzgerald PA, Goldsby RE, Huberty JP; Malignant pheochromocytomas and paragangliomas: A phase II study of therapy with high-dose 131I-metaiodobenzylguanidine (131I-MIBG): Ann. NY Acad. Sci. 2006;1073:465-90.
3. Gelfand MJ, Hoefnagel CA. Imaging with tumour specific radiopharmaceuticals. In: Pediatric Nuclear Imaging. Miller and Gelfand (Eds). WB Saunders Co. 1994;11:309-20.
4. Ilias I & K Pacak. Anatomical and functional imaging of metastatic pheochromocytoma. Ann. NY Acad. Sci. 2004;1018:495-504.
5. Miller RW, Young Jr JL, Novakovic B. Childhood cancer. Cancer. 1995;75:395.
6. Mukherjee JJ, et al. Pheochromocytoma: Effect of nonionic contrast medium in CT on circulating catecholamine levels. Radiology. 1997;202:227-31.
7. Shapiro B, et al. Iodine-131 metaiodobenzylguanidine for the locating of suspected pheochromocytoma: Experience in 400 cases. J Nucl. Med. 1985;26:576-85.
8. Swanson DP, Carey JE, Brown LE. Human absorbed dose calculations for 131I and 131I-MIBG. A potential myocardial and adrenal medullary imaging agents. In: Proceedings of the 3rd international radiopharmaceutical Dosimetry Symposium. Health and Human Services Publications FDA 81-81-66, Rockville, Maryland. 1981;213-24.
9. Voute PA, De Kraker J, Hoefnagel CA. Tumours of the sympathetic nervous system: Neuroblastoma, ganglioneuroma and phaeochromocytoma. In: Voute PA, Barrett A, Lemerle J (Eds). Cancer in children: Clinical management. Springer, Berlin. 1992;226-43.

31 Radiation in Pediatric Oncology

Kakoli Chowdhury, Anup Majumdar

In developing countries like ours, malignancy is an uncommon disease of childhood in respect to disease like malnutrition, gastroenteritis and other infective diseases. But the subspecialty, i.e. pediatric oncology, has its own importance due to its various aspects. The declaration of diagnosis is not only a difficult task, alteration of growth and development by different treatment modalities is a crucial problem.

Radiotherapy along with chemotherapy has come up in a big way in the cancer care of children since late fifties. It is an indispensible part of multidisciplinary cancer care. The use of preoperative or adjuvant radiotherapy has brought changes in the surgical principles, i.e. a shift towards organ preserving surgery. In radiotherapeutic management for pediatric tumors, we have to pay more attention to confinement of higher dose to the target volume than for adult tumors, in order that the risk of untoward normal tissue complications dose not increase, such as growth retardation. With the advent of megavoltage teleradiotherapy and improvement in pediatric anesthetic techniques radiation of pediatric patient become more precise and the risk of unnecessary morbidity has been reduced significantly. The current approaches to match this purpose are perioperative brachytherapy, IMRT and fractionated stereotactic radiotherapy (F-SRT), etc.

ROLE OF RT IN TREATMENT OF PEDIATRIC CANCER

Radiation is one of the most common treatments for cancer. A child who receives radiation therapy is treated with a stream of high-energy particles or waves that destroy or damage cancer cells. Many types of childhood cancer are treated with radiation in conjunction with chemotherapy or surgery.

The therapeutic doses of radiation in childhood cancers are 20% less than adult tumor dose. Weekly tumor dose is reduced to 850–900cGy in childhood cancer as compared to conventional 10 Gy in five fractions per week.

The vital sensitive structures should be shielded from direct exposure whenever possible, especially the growing epiphyseal ends, gonads, liver, thyroid, spinal cord, pituitary, etc. In the irradiation of long bones a preplanned lymphatic corridor is designed to prevent distal edema. Inclusion of radiation field to molar teeth area can lead to maldevelopement later.

The developmental changes are marked at a dose beyond 45–50 Gy. The doses of radiation are more fractionated in order to decrease the late morbidity.

Role in Individual Malignancy

CNS Tumors

CNS tumors account for nearly 20% of all malignancies of childhood. Although surgery is clearly the most important modality for the majority of children with CNS tumors, radiotherapy also plays a vital role. Recent developments in radiotherapy treatment planning and delivery offer considerable opportunities for therapeutic gain as a consequence of improved targeting. It is particularly beneficial for children with CNS tumors who have a relatively high probability of long-term survival and are at risk for development of long-term sequelae. A multidisciplinary team is required for CNS tumor irradiation. Although radiotherapy is an important modality, quality of survival is frequently compromised by long-term neuropsychological sequelae. A number of strategies have been devised in attempt to minimize it.

- No radiotherapy for low-grade astrocytoma
- Delay to radiotherapy for young children (e.g. 3 to 8 years age) by the use of chemotherapy
- Use of focal rather than extended-field radiotherapy when evidence suggests that extended field (whole brain, craniospinal) radiation dose not influence survival (e.g. ependymoma)
- Improved immobilization techniques allow to reduce margins around GTV/CTV (rigid casts or stereotactic frame)
- Image based treatment planning for greater sparing of normal brain tissue—CT, MRI or CT/MRI-PET fusion
- Newer radiation modalities (e.g. proton beam allows greater sparing of normal brain tissue)
- Reduction of the dose of radiotherapy in craniospinal radiotherapy for medulloblastoma
- Use of smaller dose per fraction sizes of 1.5 Gy each day for patients with radiosensitive tumors such as germinoma or the use of hyperfractionated (HFRT) radiotherapy.

Current treatment protocols almost conform to ICRU definitions. Thus a typical dose fractionation regimen is 54 Gy in 30 daily fractions of 1.8 Gy, which carries a very low-risk of radionecrosis. When treating a spinal cord tumor it is conventional to use a lower total dose (e.g. 50.4 Gy). HFRT may be a useful tool in situations where dose escalation cannot be achieved safely using conventional fractionation. But it is now considered important to maintain the interfraction interval at 6 hours or more because of slow repair of normal CNS tissue.

Children usually recover relatively quickly from the acute effects of radiation such as nausea, vomiting, fatigue, headache, etc. Supportive therapy may be needed during and after radiation. Often, one can get back to their usual routine by 6 weeks to 2 months following completion of therapy. Other predictable effects of treatment include hormonal deficits, especially growth hormone deficit secondary to inclusion of the hypothalamopituitary axis and primary hypothyroidism. Patients should be monitored closely in follow-up, and treatment should be instituted as appropriate.

Wilms' Tumor

Wilms' tumor (WT) or nephroblastoma is a highly curable neoplasm. The management of WT is a paradigm for successful interdisciplinary treatment of solid tumors of childhood to maximize cure rate and to minimize treatment related complications.

Radiation therapy guidelines used for primary and recurrent WT on (National Wilms' Tumor study) NWTS-5 are shown in Table 31.1.

- **Timing of radiation therapy:** The NWTS has shown that although irradiation dose not need to be given immediately after surgery, a delay of 10 days or more after surgery was associated with a significantly higher abdominal relapse rate, particularly patients with UH tumors.
- **Radiation therapy dose:** From the result of five NWTS, it was decided to treat all abdominal disease with 10 Gy.
- **Radiation therapy volume:** Parallel opposing fields using 4–6 MV photons are preferred. The treatment portals should encompass the tumor bed and the site of the excised kidney with a 2 to 3 cm margin. A tangential abdominal wall shield can be used. Femoral heads and acetabulum must be shielded during whole abdominal irradiation.

Neuroblastoma

Neuroblastoma is the third most common malignancy diagnosed in children. It is the most common cancer diagnosed before the age of 12 months.

CT-assisted simulation and 3-DRT treatment planning have the potential to decrease the volume of normal tissues irradiated and thereby decrease the incidence of late effects. As the WT, the radiation oncologist must be aware of the increase risk of spinal deformity or other skeletal anomalies if symmetric irradiation of bone is not administered.

Radiation therapy portals to a primary tumor site should treat the gross residual tumor remaining after

Table 31.1: Radiation therapy guideline for Wilms' tumor

Tumor stage	Radiation dose
1. Stage I and II FH, Stage I anaplastic	No radiation therapy
2. Stage III FH, Stage IV FH with abdominal Stage III, Stage II–IV anaplastic, Stage I–IV clear cell sarcoma of kidney and rhabdoid tumor kidney	10 Gy to flank plus 10 Gy boost to gross (≥ 3 cm) disease residual after surgery
3. Stage IV (lung metastases)	12 Gy whole-lung irradiation
4. Stage IV (liver metastases)	19.8 Gy to the liver
5. Stage IV (brain metastases)	30.6 Gy to whole brain
6. Stage IV (bone metastases)	25.2 Gy to lesion with a margin of at least 3 cm
7. Relapsed WT FH: Favorable Histology UH: Unfavorable Histology	12.6–18 Gy (< 12 of age) and 21.6 Gy in older children if previous radiation dose is ≤ 10.8 Gy. A boost dose of up to 9 Gy to gross residual after surgery. Total dose including previous irradiation not to exceed 30.6 Gy (< 1 year) and 39.5 Gy in older children.

chemotherapy, with at least a 2 cm margin from the tumor to the block edge. Regional lymph node site should be covered if positive, radiologically or pathologically.

Laboratory data suggest that the neuroblastoma is very radiosensitive and exhibit very little repair capacity between fractions. This makes hyper-fractionated radiation therapy an attractive option because comparable tumoricidal doses can be achieved with minimization of the risk of late effects.

- Radiation dose: May be age dependent
- In infants younger than one year, a dose of 12 Gy is sufficient
- Tumor in children aged 12 to 48 months may require doses of at least 25 Gy
- Children older than 4 years of age frequently develop local failures even with a dose of more than 25 Gy

Intraoperative radiotherapy (IORT) with 7 to 16 Gy (median 10 Gy) to the primary tumor bed was associated with a local control rate of 100% in patients who had gross total resection, whereas IORT was unable to control any patients with gross residual disease. If the likelihood of long survival is small, 5 to 20 Gy in one to five daily fractions can allow rapid palliation.

Ewing's Sarcoma

Ewing's sarcoma is the second most common primary tumor of bone in childhood. Both effective local and systemic therapy are necessary for the cure of Ewing's sarcoma. No definite dose response for Ewing's sarcoma has been reported above 40 Gy. For gross disease, standard treatment would be a total dose of 55.8 Gy at 1.8 Gy per day, with a reduction at 45 Gy. Although traditionally the entire marrow cavity was included in the field for at least part of the treatment, it is now accepted that smaller fields are adequate. But geographic miss should be avoided. Three-dimensional treatment planning is almost essential. The initial field should include the prechemotherapy volume with 2 to 4 cm margin. The boost should be to the residual tumor volume at the time of radiotherapy plus a 2 cm margin. The indications for adjuvant radiotherapy after surgery are not firmly established. It is usually given when tumor is close to or extends to the surgical margin.

The most common complication of radiation is abnormal growth and development of the irradiated tissues. Both cosmetic and functional abnormalities can occur. Dose higher than 20 Gy will prematurely close the irradiated epiphysis, growth deficits in the irradiated extremity and the possibility of a limb-length discrepancy. Another late effect of the tumor and its treatment is permanent weakening of the affected bone. There is also risk of second malignancy at the site of primary lesion most commonly osteosarcoma.

Hodgkin's Disease

The establishment of a curative dose range (33 to 44 Gy) and standardized anatomic treatment fields produced the first cure inpatients with HD. Appreciation of the pattern of the contagious spread in the disease promoted the concept of extended radiation treatment volumes. Though the 5 years disease free survival (DFS) rates is high with extended field radiotherapy, long follow-up began to appreciate the morbidity associated with standard dose irradiation in the prepubertal child. Following the observation of radiation-associated cardiovascular disease and solid-tumor malignancies in aging survivors of childhood HD, advances in radiation technology and diagnostic imaging led to further modifications of radiation therapy permitting involved field treatment approaches and more effective shielding of normal tissues. Treatment with standard dose radiation therapy alone has been abandoned by most pediatric centers because of its strong association with solid tumor carcinogenesis. However, low dose (15 to 25.5 Gy), involved-field radiation remains a critical component of combined modality regimens and salvage therapy for patients with refractory or relapsed disease.

NHL

Childhood NHLs are diffuse, high-grade, and poorly differentiated; extranodal is common and dissemination occurs early and often. Radiation therapy was incorporated into the design of early chemotherapy trials, but with no benefit. Hence, most investigators have abandoned the use of involved-field irradiation in localized, early-staged pediatric NHL. The role of local-field radiation therapy in advanced-stage disease is questionable.

- Local residual disease, after induction chemotherapy or as relapse after a complete remission, most often is managed with local-field irradiation in doses ranging from 30 Gy for the SLL/lymphoblastic to 45 Gy for the large cell histiocytic type.
- Primary NHL of bone—Combined chemotherapy and local irradiation resulted in a dramatic improvement in control of both local and distant disease
- CNS relapse was recognized to be an obstacle to cure in about 30 to 35% of children. Indications for cranial irradiation currently are limited to patients with overt CNS lymphoma at diagnosis or relapse and those with leukemic transformation at diagnosis, based on a high rate of CNS relapse with chemotherapy alone and the proven efficacy of intrathecal methotrexate plus cranial irradiation in this setting. Finally, patients with cranial nerve palsies should be considered for irradiation to the skull base or whole cranium.

Rhabdomyosarcoma

Rhabdomyosarcoma is a highly malignant soft-tissue sarcoma that arises from unsegmented, undifferentiated mesoderm or myotome-derived skeletal muscle. It may occur at any site in the body. Most commonly affected areas are the orbit, 9%; head and neck (excluding parameningeal tumors), 7%; paramingeal, 25%; genitourinary, 31%; and extremities, 13%.

- Radiation therapy has important role in the control of microscopic and gross residual Rhabdomyosarcoma.
- It is essential to evaluate the extent of disease by CT scan or MRI as because the Rhabdomyosarcoma infiltrate tissue plane widely.
- Treatment portals presentation with margin (2 cm) including surgical scar and biopsy tracts are designed to encompass involved region at the time of operation.
- Prophylactic lymph node irradiation is not required in children.
- Dose: For microscopic disease, 40 to 41.4 Gy in 4.5 weeks and for gross residual, 50.4 to 55.8 Gy in 5.5 to 6 weeks is recommended for local control as a part of multimodality therapy.
- To achieve adequate coverage of target and minimum toxicities, 3 DCRT treatment planning techniques are valuable.
- Interstitial brachytherapy may be helpful in primary treatment or boost with advantages of precise shaping of the dose distribution, sharp fall-off of radiation dose and shortening of overall treatment time.
- Time: Earlier irradiation, particularly in high-risk patients, may provide better local control and survival.

LATE EFFECTS OF RADIATION

Stunting

It may be generalized or localized variety. Radiotherapy delivered to the brain as in cerebral gliomas and cranial irradiation in CNS prophylaxis for leukemia and medulloblastoma leads to irradiation of pituitary gland. It results in decrease in growth hormone and thyroid stimulating hormone which leads to generalized decrease in somatic development. Irradiation of thyroid may lead to features of cretinism due to hypothyroid. Final height deficit (after spinal irradiation) estimated to be 9 cm for child irradiated at 1st year 7 cm at 5th year, and 5.5 cm at 10 years of age following radiotherapy.

Radiotherapy exposure to the orbit in patients with retinoblastomas leads to underdevelopment of the socket. In extremity sarcoma, there may be local stunting of the limb. In Hodgkin's disease, Wilms' tumor—there may be scoliosis due to inclusion of hemivertebra in the field.

Intellectual and Neuropsychiatric Defect

In association with intrathecal chemotherapy, radiation causes demineralizing leukoencephalopathy, microangiopathy, and somnolence syndrome and also causes decrease in the IQ. There is about 20% decrease in IQ score in patients who received cranial radiotherapy.

Individual Visceral Morbidity

Radiotherapy to the chest in form of mantle field radiation or thoracic irradiation always includes the breasts and leads to maldevelopment of the affected breast in females. Thoracic irradiation can lead to extensive fibrothorax, chronic obstructive airway disease and kyphoscoliosis. There may be maldevelopment of the muscle mass.

Second Malignancy

The development of a second malignancy is a life-time risk in childhood cancer. Second malignancies are the stochastic effects of the radiation. Low doses radiation is the more carcinogenic than the high doses. The overall risk is highest among children treated for retinoblastoma, Hodgkin's Disease, Ewing's sarcoma and rhabdomyosarcoma. The risk increases with combination of chemotherapy and radiotherapy. Second malignancy may be in the radiation field, but-off field radiation is also not uncommon.

CONCLUSION

Radiation therapy is a highly effective treatment modality for many pediatric malignancies. However, in pediatric patients the use of radiation therapy demands attention in both the overall benefits and indications for the use of this treatment and the potential long-term toxicities peculiar to the growing child.

Before drawing any conclusion, we should say, as you all know, such a matter can never be concluded. It's a process–a process of intervention if not invention; we must venture for prevention and palliation, if not cure.

SUGGESTED READING

1. Altman AJ, Schwartz AD. Malignant disease of infancy, childhood and adolescent. WB Saunders Company, Philadelphia 1983;1-21.
2. Childhood cancer.www.kidshealth.com.
3. Darenreliler F, Livesey EA, Hindmarsh PC, et al. Growth and growth hormone secretion in children following treatment of brain tumors with radiotherapy. Acta Pediatr Scand. 1990;79:950-6.
4. Donaldson SS, Kaplan HS. Complication of treatment of Hodgkin's disease in children. Cancer Treat Rep. 1982;66:977-89.
5. Eifel PJ, Sampson CM, Tucker SL. With multiple radiation fractionation sensitivity of epiphyseal cartilage in weaning rat model. Int J Radiat Oncol Biol Phys. 1988;15:141-5.
6. Eifel PJ. Decrease bone growth arrest in weaning rats with multiple radiation fractions per day. Int J Radiat Oncol Biol Phys. 1988;15:141-5.
7. Green EM, Brecher ML, Yaker D, et al. Thyroid dysfunction in pediatric patients after neck irradiation for Hodgkin's disease. Med Pediatr Oncol. 1980;8:127-36.
8. Haas-Kogan DA, Fisch BM, Wara WM, et al. Intraoperative radiation therapy for high-risk pediatric neuroblastoma. Int J Radiat Oncol Biol Phys. 2000;47:985-92.
9. Hopewell JW. Radiation injury to the central nervous system. Med Pediatr Oncol Suppl. 1998;1:1-9.
10. ICRU Report 50. Prescribing, recording and reporting photon beam therapy. International Commission on Radiation Units and Measurements. 1993.
11. ICRU Report 62. Prescribing, recording and reporting photon beam therapy. (Supplement to ICRU Report 50). International Commission on Radiation Units and Measurements. 1999.
12. Muiherh RK, Ochs J, Fairclough D, et al. Intellectual and academic achievement status following CNS relapse: a retrospective analysis of 40 children for acute lymphocytic leukemia. Clin Oncol. 1987;5:933.
13. Perez CA, Tefft M, Nesbitt ME Jr, et al. Radiation therapy in the multimodal management of Ewing's sarcoma of bone: report of IESS. Natl Cancer Tnst Monogr. 1981;56:263-70.

14. Samaan NA, Viecto R, Schulz PN, et al. Hypothalamic, pituitary and thyroid dysfunction after radiotherapy to the head and neck. Int J Radiat Oncol Biol Phys. 1982;8:1857-67.

15. Shalet SM, Gibson B, Swindell R, Pearson D. Effect of spinal irradiation on growth. Arch Dis Child. 1987;62:461-4.

16. Thomas PRM, Perez CA, Neff JR, et al. The management of Ewing's sarcoma: role of radiotherapy in local tumor control. Cancer Treat Rep. 1984;68:703-10.

17. Thomas PRM, Tefft M, Compann PJ, et al. Results of two radiotherapy randomizations in the third National Wilms' Tumor Study (NWTS-3). Cancer. 1991;68:1703-7.

18. Tucker MA, et al. Bone sarcomas linked to radiotherapy and chemotherapy in children. Engl J Med. 1987;317:588-93.

19. Wheldon TE, Wilson L, Livingstone A, et al. Radiation studies on multicellular tumor spheroids derived from human neuroblastoma: absence of sparing effects of dose fractionation. Eur J Cancer Clin Oncol. 1986;22:563-6.

32 Pediatric Oncologic Emergencies

Dipankar Gupta

In the practice of pediatric oncology five primary etiologies are there which underlie most emergencies. This write-up gives a brief overview of the pathophysiology of the pediatric oncologic emergencies.

1. Infectious emergencies
2. Inflammatory emergencies
3. Hematologic emergencies
4. Metabolic emergencies
5. Mechanical emergencies.

INFECTIOUS EMERGENCIES

Immunosuppression is the primary underlying factor that predisposes patients with cancer to infectious complications. Patients are variably subjected to quantitative and qualitative decreases in granulocyte function (neutropenia), B cell function (hypogammaglobulinemia), T cell function, splenic function, and normal immunologic and integument barriers. In addition, alteration of typical body flora can result in the overgrowth of pathogenic organisms. Alone and combined, these factors increase the risk of serious systemic infection by bacterial, viral, fungal, and other opportunistic organisms (Table 32.1).

Bacterial Infections

Bacterial pathogens may induce focal or systemic infections, and the incidence of bacterial infections increases as the ANC decreases from 1000–500 to 100/mm. The most common etiologic agents are bacteria that colonize the host's skin and GI tract. Neutropenia is the primary risk factor for bacterial infections, and fever is the most common presenting symptom. In this context, **febrile neutropenia** commonly is defined as an ANC $< 0.5 \times 10^9$/L (< 500/mm^3), and fever may be defined as a temperature $> 38.0°C$ twice in 24 hours or a temperature $> 38.3–38.5°C$ once. The institution of empiric antibiotic therapy for a patient with neutropenia who is febrile decreases infection-related mortality rates, particularly that related to Gram-negative organisms.

Initial antibiotic therapy should consist of broad-spectrum monotherapy with cefepime, ceftazidime, or imipenem. Dual therapy consisting of an aminoglycoside in combination with an antipseudomonal beta-lactam is an equivalent alternative and should be considered, particularly when the patient's presentation suggests Gram-negative bacteremia or sepsis.

Initial empiric use of vancomycin in combination with single or dual therapy is appropriate in the setting of severe mucositis, quinolone prophylaxis, known colonization with resistant strains of *S. aureus* or *S. pneumoniae*, catheter-related infections, or hypotension-sepsis syndrome. Vancomycin should be discontinued after 48–72 hours if the clinical course or culture results warrant it. Antibiotics beyond empiric coverage may be needed to treat a confirmed or suspected focus of infection. Typhlitis or a suspected perirectal abscess should be managed with increased antibiotic coverage for anaerobic organisms. *C. difficile* enterocolitis requires treatment with metronidazole or vancomycin. Additional coverage should be based on organism sensitivities and clinical syndromes.

Table 32.1: Oncology-associated infections

Immunodeficiency	Etiology	Infection			
		Bacterial	Fungal	Parasite Protozoan	Viral
Neutropenia	Leukemia Chemotherapy Irradiation	Staphylococcus species Streptococcus species Enterococcus species Pseudomonas aeruginosa Aeromonas hydrophila Bacillus species Corynebacteria Enterobacteriaceae	Candida species Aspergillus species Fusarium species	NA	HSV
Decreased B cell—mediated immunity and decreased immunoglobulin levels	Leukemia Chemotherapy Corticosteroids	Streptococcus pneumoniae Haemophilus influenzae Neisseria meningitidis Salmonella species Escherichia coli P. aeruginosa	NA	P. carinii Giardia lamblia	Echovirus
Decreased T cell—mediated immunity	Leukemia Lymphoma Chemotherapy Corticosteroids	Listeria monocytogenes Legionella species Nocardia species Mycobacterium tuberculosis Atypical mycobacterium Salmonella species	Candida species Aspergillus species Cryptococcus neoformans Coccidioides immitis	P. carinii Cryptosporidium species Toxoplasma gondii Strongyloides stercoralis	Herpes viruses (HSV, CMV, varicella) Adenovirus Influenza Parainfluenza Measles Respiratory syncytial virus (RSV)
Splenic dysfunction	Splenectomy Hodgkin disease Irradiation	S. pneumoniae N. meningitidis H. influenza	NA	Babesia	NA
Interrupted barriers	Catheters Procedures Rashes Mucositis	Endogenous flora	Candida species Aspergillus species Fusarium species	NA	HSV Varicella
Loss of normal flora	Antibiotics	Overgrowth of Clostridium difficile	Overgrowth of Candida species	NA	NA

Fungal Infections

Fungi are broadly categorized by morphology as yeasts or filamentous molds. In children with cancer, infection by these and other opportunistic fungal pathogens has increased since the 1980s. The increase reflects the intensive immunosuppression that results from current antineoplastic treatment regimens. Candidal organisms are now the fourth most common bloodstream pathogen, and undiagnosed invasive fungal infections are identified increasingly at autopsy. This observation suggesting that fungal infections are underdiagnosed. Consistent with these findings is the result of a series of 61 pediatric autopsies in 1990. Mycotic infection, and not bacterial infection, was most common, as the clinician initially believed.

INFLAMMATORY EMERGENCIES

Pneumonitis, pancreatitis, hemorrhagic cystitis, and extravasation of vesicant chemotherapy products are clinically significant noninfectious inflammatory conditions that require emergency treatment in pediatric patients with malignancy.

Pneumonitis, pancreatitis, hemorrhagic/cystitis, and extravasation of vesicant chemotherapy products are clinically significant noninfectious inflammatory conditions that require emergency treatment in pediatric patients with malignancy. Typhlitis and *C. difficile* enterocolitis are considered infectious conditions and are addressed above.

Noninfectious pneumonitis is a complication of radiation therapy, chemotherapy, stem cell transplantation, and transfusion. Clinical presentations vary and range from no symptoms to respiratory failure. Chest radiographs may demonstrate an interstitial infiltrate or interstitial-alveolar pattern that may be unilateral or bilateral. Bronchoalveolar lavage is performed to exclude infectious etiologies and typically reveals a lymphocytic infiltrate. Pulmonary function tests demonstrate decreased compliance and decreased diffusion capacity. Corticosteroid therapy is the primary treatment. Specific chemotherapeutic agents are associated with acute lung injury. Bleomycin is the drug most commonly associated with pneumonitis and fibrosis. Other drugs frequently reported to cause pulmonary injury are carmustine, mitomycin, vinca alkaloids and methotrexate.

Pancreatitis

Pancreatitis is a complication of immunosuppressive therapy, and approximately 18% of all pediatric cases occur in the context of antineoplastic therapy. In particular, pancreatitis is associated with L-asparaginase chemotherapy and systemic steroid administration. Treatment is primarily supportive, with an emphasis on bowel rest, fluid resuscitation, and close monitoring of electrolytes, particularly for hypocalcemia and hyperglycemia.

Hemorrhagic Cystitis

Hemorrhagic cystitis is hematuria that results from an inflammation of the bladder. The condition is defined as painful urination with leukocytes and erythrocytes or clots in the urine. Cyclophosphamide and ifosfamide are the most common chemotherapeutic agents that cause hemorrhagic cystitis. An acrolein dye byproduct of their metabolism medicates this effect. The byproduct chemically irritates the bladder mucosa and the renal collecting system. Previous or concurrent pelvic irradiation is a risk factor for hemorrhagic cystitis, and a hemorrhagic cystitis is significantly and positively associated with infection by adenovirus and/or by the BK virus). Mesna combines with the metabolites of ifosfamide and cyclophosphamide to form nontoxic compounds in the urine. These preventive measures appear to reduce the incidence of cystitis to < 5%, and they likely account for a recent decrease in incidence of hemorrhagic cystitis.

Extravasation

Extravasation of chemotherapy products is reported to occur in 0.1–6.5% of chemotherapy infusions and may cause severe, irreversible, local injury. Chemotherapeutic agents may be classified as irritant, vesicant, or nonvesicant on the basis of their local toxicity to subcutaneous tissues. Irritant drugs cause pain at the injection site, and they may be associated with local inflammation. Vesicant drugs cause local tissue necrosis or induce blister formation. Table 32.2 lists drugs with the highest potential to cause local tissue damage after extravasation. Nonvesicant drugs produce acute reactions only occasionally.

HEMATOLOGICAL EMERGENCIES

Hematologic abnormalities that require emergency treatment result from abnormal hematopoiesis or

Table 32.2: Chemotherapeutic agents causing local tissue damage

Class		Drugs
Drugs with high potential for local tissue damage	Anthracycline or anthracycline analog	• Doxorubicin • Daunorubicin • Idarubicin • Mitomycin C
	Vinca alkaloid	• Vincristine • Vinblastine
	Epipodophyllotoxin	• Etoposide • Teniposide
	Heavy metal	• Cisplatin
Drugs with moderate potential for local tissue damage		• Dactinomycin • Fluorouracil • Mitoxantrone

coagulopathy. With respect to hematopoiesis, underproduction of specific cell lines is more common than overproduction. Underproduction is due to disease infiltration of the bone marrow, syndromes of bone marrow failure, or treatment-related myelotoxicity. Underproduction results in anemia, thrombocytopenia, neutropenia, or their combination. Overproduction of hematopoietic tissue is primarily observed as leukocytosis associated with acute leukemia. Coagulopathy manifests as hemorrhage, thrombosis, or both. Coagulopathy is a primary consequence of disease. It results from a primary toxicity due to treatment, or it is secondary to other known complications.

Bone Marrow Depression

Depression of normal bone marrow activity results in anemia, thrombocytopenia, and neutropenia. These signs are best treated with supportive care, regardless of their etiology. Supportive care often includes transfusion of individual blood components, which requires the following considerations in the context of the immunosuppressed patient with cancer.

• All blood, platelets, and granulocytes administered to immunosuppressed patients must be irradiated to prevent the lethal complication of graft versus host disease.

• Use of leukocyte-poor blood and platelets is recommended to minimize the risk of CMV contamination and to decrease both the risk of alloimmunization and the incidence of febrile transfusion reactions.

• Minimize the patient's exposure to blood products. Judicious use of blood products decreases infectious risks and is particularly important for patients with newly diagnosed aplastic anemia in whom engraftment of transplanted stem cells is inversely related to the number of exposures to previous donors.

Blood products may be obtained from the general blood supply or from directed donation. Directed-donor blood products appear to have an infectious risk equal to that of the general blood supply. Intrafamilial-directed donations should be discouraged in patients who may need stem cell transplantation to limit exposure to familial human lymphocyte antigens (HLAs).

Anemia

Pediatric patients who are not critically-ill usually tolerate anemia well and do not require transfusion unless their hematocrit is < 20–25% (Hb level 7–8), unless they have no evidence of recovery, or unless transfusion is necessary to improve symptoms. Transfusion of packed RBCs (PRBCs) may also be necessary to maintain optimal intravascular volume in a patient who is critically-ill or who has acute hemorrhage. The use of recombinant erythropoietin is limited by the weeks of therapy necessary to substantially increase hemoglobin (Hb) levels. Once severe anemia develops, patients usually require transfusion. Very often transfusion reaction may develop (Table 32.3).

Thrombocytopenia

In pediatric patients with cancer, thrombocytopenia results from underproduction or excessive consumption of platelets. Although thrombopoietin has strong positive effects on platelet production and though its use continues in clinical trials, the degree to which this cytokine affects platelet transfusion therapy remains unclear. Therefore, platelet transfusions remain the primary treatment for thrombocytopenia in pediatric patients with cancer. Platelet transfusions are used as prophylaxis

Table 32.3: Transfusion reactions

Reaction	Incidence	Etiology	Therapy
Fever	0.1–5 per 100	Commonly due to recipient antibodies to WBC or platelets in transfused blood product and subsequent release of pyrogens (IL-1, IL-6, TNF); rarely secondary to bacterial contamination of transfused blood product	Antipyretic for both acute management and pretreatment of subsequent transfusions
Rash, urticarial or allergic	0.5–4 per 100	Result of proteins in donor plasma that precipitates histamine release in the recipient. Immunologic memory may be exhibited on subsequent transfusions	Antihistamine for both acute management and pretreatment of subsequent transfusions
Transfusion-related acute lung injury (TRALI)	1 per 2000	Passive transfer of anti-HLA antibodies directed against recipient WBC. Less commonly, patient's anti-HLA antibody may be directed against donor WBC. Leukoagglutination and acute respiratory compromise may occur hours after transfusion	First, symptomatic respiratory support. Consider washed blood products on subsequent transfusion to remove antibody. HLA-specific blood products may be necessary
Anaphylaxis to first transfusion	1 per 800–1000	First transfusion: Recipient is IgA deficient and donor has IgA antibody present in the plasma	Stop transfusion. Emergency management of anaphylaxis, then test serum of both donor/blood and recipient for quantitative IgA level. Future blood products only from IgA-deficient donors. Recipient must be counseled regarding IgA deficiency
Anaphylaxis after first transfusion	Unknown	First transfusion: Recipient most likely had a mild, unrecognized allergic/urticarial response to a prior transfusion and current reaction results from amplified immune response	Stop transfusion. Emergency management of anaphylaxis using antihistamine, steroid, and epinephrine, as necessary
Hemolysis, acute	1/200,000	Intravascular: Recipient IgM antibody against transfused RBC antigen, usually ABO antigens. Less often results from exposure of a neoantigen. IgM antibody fixes complement and activates the coagulation cascade	Stop transfusion. Emergency management of hypotension, fever, chest pain and respiratory compromise. Expect renal failure and DIC. Approximately 40% of transfusion-related deaths result from acute hemolytic reactions
Hemolysis, delayed	1/800	Extravascular: Recipient IgG antibody against minor RBC antigen. Complement not usually fixed and hemolysis is extravascular with fever, malaise, weakness, anemia and indirect hyperbilirubinemia occurring days to weeks later	Symptomatic treatment
Graft versus host disease	Rare	Nonirradiated PRBC or platelets containing peripheral blood progenitor cells transfused to immunoincompetent recipient or homozygous donor to immunocompetent heterozygous recipient	Irradiate all blood products administered to immunocompromised hosts and directed donor products from relatives. GVHD is usually lethal

and as a treatment for bleeding. General considerations for the use of platelets in pediatric patients with malignancy include the following points:

- Avoid platelet transfusion in the absence of bleeding if thrombocytopenia is secondary to platelet consumption

- Consider empiric platelet transfusion in patients with platelet counts $< 10 \times 10^9$L ($< 10,000/mm^3$) if thrombocytopenia results from underproduction
- Consider empiric platelet transfusion in patients with platelet counts < 15–20×10^9L ($< 15,000$–$20,000/$

mm^3) if they have acute nonlymphocytic (myeloid) leukemia (ANLL) and if they are receiving induction chemotherapy, particularly if the platelet count is decreasing by 50% or more per day.

- Consider empiric platelet transfusion in patients with platelet counts $< 20 \times 10^9$L ($< 20,000$/mm^3) if the leukocyte count is $<100 \times 10^9$L ($> 100,000$/mm^3) in patients with ANLL or $< 300–400 \times 10^9$L ($> 300,000$-$400,000$/mm^3) in those with ALL.

Hyperleukocytosis

Hyperleukocytosis is the most common hematologic overproduction syndrome in pediatric patients with cancer that requires emergency treatment. Hyperleukocytosis is defined as a peripheral leukocyte count $> 100 \times 10^9$L ($> 100,000$/mm^3). Hyperleukocytosis is present at diagnosis in 6–15% of pediatric patients with ALL, 13–22% of patients with ANLL, and nearly all children with chronic myelogenous leukemia. Hyperleukocytosis is a poor prognostic indicator in the setting of ALL or ANLL because it is associated with metabolic and hemorrhagic complications. Respiratory complications are most prominent with elevated leukocyte counts in patients with ANLL. Hemorrhagic complications and death rates notably increase when peripheral leukocyte counts are $> 100 \times 10^9$L ($> 100,000$/mm^3) in the context of ANLL and $>300–400 \times 10^9$L ($> 300,000$-$400,000$/mm^3) in the context of ALL.

Coagulopathy

Pediatric patients with cancer are subject to have clinically significant abnormalities in procoagulation, inhibitors of coagulation, and fibrinolysis. The abnormalities result in hypocoagulable and hypercoagulable conditions that manifest as hemorrhage or thrombosis. Hemorrhage and thrombosis are considerable problems in the setting of hyperleukocytosis. Hemorrhage is also a notable complication during induction chemotherapy for class M 3, M 4, or M 5 AML, even with relatively low peripheral leukocyte counts.

Bleeding predominates in this setting secondary to the relative excess of fibrinolytic proteases compared with prothrombotic thromboplastic materials released from blast cells. Hemorrhage may also result from the consumption of coagulation factors in the setting of chronic activation of the procoagulation cascade, or it may result from underproduction of necessary coagulation factors in the setting of severe systemic illness and relative hepatic insufficiency.

Disseminated Intravascular Coagulation

Disseminated intravascular coagulation (DIC) is characterized by excessive activation of blood coagulation with the consumption of clotting factors. DIC causes hemorrhage, microangiopathic hemolytic anemia, and thrombosis of various degrees. DIC may contribute to hemorrhagic and thrombotic events. In children with cancer, DIC is most commonly associated with ANLL induction chemotherapy in which thromboplastic materials are released from leukemic blast cells. DIC also occurs in patients with sepsis or, less frequently, in those with widely disseminated solid tumors.

Primary therapy is supportive care and treatment of the inciting etiology. Patients with clinically significant hemorrhage or thrombosis associated with DIC may benefit from low-dose heparin therapy (7.5 U/kg/h). Thrombocytopenia is treated with platelet transfusion. Most specifically, fibrinogen is replaced by using cryoprecipitate. Hyperfibrinolysis, as evidenced by low antiplasmin levels, is treated with epsilon-aminocaproic acid if evidence of hematuria is lacking.

Thrombosis

Thrombosis is relatively uncommon oncologic emergency in children than in adults. In the pediatric population, symptomatic thrombosis may be associated with central venous catheters. However, thrombosis is most common in the setting of hyperleukocytosis and ALL treated with L-asparaginase in which severe thromboembolism, primarily of the cerebral venous sinus, is reported in 2.4–11.5% of patients. L-asparaginase therapy is associated with decreased plasminogen, antithrombin III and, to a lesser extent, protein C and protein S levels.

A coordinated *in vivo* increase in thrombin generation has been identified after L-asparaginase therapy. Thrombotic events are substantially most likely to occur in patients with at least 1 prothrombotic defect, such as factor V *G1691A* (Leiden) mutation, prothrombin *G 20210 A* mutation, or deficiency of protein C, protein S, or antithrombin III. Clinical presentations of patients with thrombosis of the sagittal sinus vary and range from asymptomatic to life threatening. Most patients present with headaches, seizure, focal motor deficits, cognitive deficits including aphasia, or a combination of signs. Treatment of patients with thrombosis associated with L-asparaginase therapy is primarily supportive, and good long-term recoveries were observed in most reported cases.

Metabolic Factors

Tumor Lysis Syndrome

This syndrome may be seen with any tumor that is undergoing rapid cell turnover as a result of high growth fraction or high cell death due to therapy. In general acute leukemia, high and intermediate grade lymphoma, and less commonly, solid tumors such as germ cell cancers undergoing therapy are the most commonly associated tumor types. Tumor lysis syndrome is characterized by the metabolic abnormalities of hyperuricemia, hyperkalemia, and hyperphosphatemia leading to hypocalcemia. Patients with underlying chronic renal insufficiency are more susceptible to developing tumor lysis syndrome because of their limited capacity to excrete the products of rapid tumor cell destruction.

Emergency Treatment of Patients with TLS

Table 32.4 summarizes emergency treatment of specific abnormalities found in patients with TLS. Intervention beyond the prophylactic measures outlined above is focused on maintaining normal end-organ function. The patient's specific response to serum abnormalities is best modulated by considering both the absolute serum level and the rate of change.

Hypercalcemia

Cause of Tumor Hypercalcemia

1. Associated tumors: Hypercalcemia is relatively common in patients with malignancy. The most common cause of hypercalcemia in hospitalized patients is malignancy. Hypercalcemia of malignancy can be associated with bone metastasis, or it may occur in the absence of any direct bone involvement by the tumor. Patients with hematologic malignancies accounted for approximately 15% of the cases. These patients usually have hypercalcemia in the presence of diffuse tumor involvement of bone, although in a small percentage there was no evidence of bone involvement.

2. Humoral mediators: In approximately 10% of the cases with malignancy, hypercalcemia develops in the absence of radiographic or scintigraphic evidence of bone involvement. In this group of patients, the pathogenesis of hypercalcemia appears to be secondary to humoral mediators, dominant of which is parathyroid hormone (PTH)-related protein (PTHrP), as well as other osteoclast activating factors (OAFs).

Symptoms, Signs and Laboratory Findings

Hypercalcemia often produces symptoms in patients with cancer and in fact may be the patients major problem. Polyuria and nocturia, resulting from the impaired ability of the kidneys to concentrate the urine occur early. Anorexia, nausea, constipation, muscle weakness, and fatigue are common. As the hypercalcemia progresses, severe dehydration, azotemia, mental obtundation, coma, and cardiovascular collapse may appear.

Treatment

Traditional treatment of pediatric patients with hypercalcemia and malignancies has relied on forced diuresis and calcitonin, corticosteroids, and mithramycin use. Table 32.5 summarizes indications, dosages, and features of these agents.

Bisphosphonates are useful for treatment of hypercalcemia. Bisphosphonates have a chemical structure similar to inorganic pyrophosphate, but they are resistant to hydrolysis in an acidic environment. Although their exact mechanism of action and spectrum of activity are incompletely understood, these compounds are potent inhibitors of both normal and pathologic osteoclast-mediated bone resorption.

Bisphosphonates that most closely resemble inorganic pyrophosphate (e.g. clodronate, etidronate, tiludronate) are metabolically incorporated into nonhydrolyzable

Table 32.4: Emergency management of tumor lysis syndrome

Problem	Severity	Intervention	Notes
Hyperkalemia	Mild to moderate: > 5.5 mEq/L or rapid rise	– ECG and cardiac monitoring – Remove potassium from all IV fluids – Administer sodium polystyrene resin (Kayexalate): 1–2 g/kg mixed with 3 mL sorbitol/g resin PO q6h – Give loop diuretic: Furosemide 0.5–2 mg/kg IV q6–24h	Sodium polystyrene induces allergic reaction in sensitive individuals
	Severe: > 6 mEq/L and rapid rise or ECG changes	– Insulin and dextrose: 0.1 U/kg regular insulin IV with 2 mL/kg 25% dextrose q30–60 min – Sodium bicarbonate: 1–2 mEq/kg IV infuse over 5–10 minutes – If ECG changes: Calcium gluconate 10%: 100 mg/kg/dose IV infuse over 3–5 minutes; may repeat in 10 min – Dialysis may be required	Calcium gluconate not compatible with sodium bicarbonate
Hyperphosphatemia	Moderate to severe	– Aluminum hydroxide: 50–150 mg/kg/d PO divided q4–6h – Normal saline IV bolus and mannitol 0.25-1 g/kg IV bolus – Consider dialysis if >10 mg/dL or poor renal function	Compensatory hypocalcemia may coexist
Elevated uric acid level	Mild to severe	– Recombinant urate oxidase (Rasburicase) 0.2 mg/kg IV q12–24h – Continue hyperhydration – Continue maintenance fluid, increasing to 2–3 fold more than normal maintenance dose – Continue allopurinol: 300 mg/m²/d – Alkalinize urine with sodium bicarbonate – Start dialysis if level >10 mg/dL or if renal failure occurs	Best management is prophylaxis; recombinant urate oxidase is a new, effective therapy for severe hyperuricemia and may obviate dialysis

analogs of adenosine triphosphate (ATP), which accumulate intracellularly and induce osteoclast apoptosis. Relatively potent nitrogen-containing bisphosphonates (e.g. pamidronate, alendronate, risedronate, zoledronate, ibandronate) appear to act as transitional-state analogs of isoprenoid diphosphates to inhibit the production of farnesyl diphosphate synthase and the mevalonate pathway. Inhibition of the mevalonate pathway prevents the necessary post-translational modification of small guanosine triphosphatases (GTPases) necessary for intracellular osteoclast signaling.

Hyponatremia

Severe hyponatremia, defined as a serum sodium level of < 125 mEq/l, is a complication in pediatric patients with malignancy. Severe hyponatremia can result from systemic illness, the syndrome of inappropriate secretion of antidiuretic hormone (SIADH), or iatrogenic factors acting individually or collectively. Symptoms are primarily neurologic, but early, mild hyponatremia causes no clinically significant symptoms. Anorexia, nausea, and malaise are the first overt findings. These progresses to headache, confusion, lethargy, seizure, coma, and

Table 32.5: Treatment of hypercalcemia

Drug or agent	Indication	Dosage	Onset of action	Advantage	Disadvantage
Normal saline	Hypovolemia, dehydration	2–3X maintenance	12–24 h	Simple	Hypervolemia
Furosemide	Hypervolemia or combination therapy with normal saline	0.5–2 mg/kg/dose IV	Immediate	Increased urinary excretion of calcium	Hypokalemia, hypomagnesemia
Corticosteroid	Hypercalcemia due to lymphoma	Prednisone 20–40 mg/m²/d PO	3–7 d	PO administration	Hyperglycemia, gastritis, osteopenia
Calcitonin	Acute control of hypercalcemia	2–8 U/kg SC/IM q6–12h	1–4 h	Rapid onset of activity; minimal toxicity	Nausea, hypersensitivity
Mithramycin	Severe hypercalcemia	10–50 mcg/kg IV Infused over 2–4 h	24–48 h	Highly effective; severe hematologic toxicity limits use	Significant toxicity; replaced by bisphosphonates

death. Although the CNS may tolerate a gradual change in serum sodium concentrations, rapid changes of 1–2 mEq/l/h lead to cerebral edema and neurologic dysfunction. Severe life-threatening symptoms almost uniformly occur when the serum sodium concentration is < 110 mEq/l or when the level decreases to 120 mEq/l within 24 hours.

Hyponatremia most often results from water retention combined with the administration of normal or excessive amounts of fluid. Hyponatremia associated with edematous states is most common in patients with cancer and may result from liver disease, veno-occlusive disease, infection, drug toxicity, or many other etiologies. Patients with hyponatremia are usually oliguric with urine sodium levels < 15 mEq/l. Excessive renal salt wasting may also cause hyponatremia and can result from drug-induced nephropathy, adrenal insufficiency, or use of thiazide diuretics. Patients with renal-induced hyponatremia are usually nonoliguric and have inappropriately high urine sodium levels. Abnormal release of ADH may also lead to hyponatremia, as in SIADH. The rate at which hyponatremia develops depends on the rate and volume of fluid administration. SIADH occurs in the context of CNS disturbances, pulmonary disease, use of specific drugs, and a variety of tumors.

Cyclophosphamide is the chemotherapeutic agent most commonly associated with impaired renal excretion of water. This complication is most often observed in patients receiving high dose regimens more commonly associated with stem cell transplant conditioning regimens (>30 mg/kg or >1 g/m²). Vincristine, vinblastine, melphalan, and thiotepa have had similar effects but effect less than those of cyclophosphamide. Hyponatremia is also a frequent iatrogenic consequence of underlying systemic illness. Overhydration with hypotonic solutions frequently results in mild or moderate hyponatremia. Failure to administer stress-dose levels of glucocorticoids to patients who are adrenally suppressed also results in hyponatremia.

Treatment is based on the patient's symptoms and underlying pathophysiology. These factors determine the optimal rate at which the serum sodium level should be corrected and the optimal volume of fluid to achieve the correction. In an asymptomatic patient, serum sodium concentrations should be corrected at a rate of 0.5 mEq/l/h during the first 24 hours of intervention or 12 mEq/l total. Rapid correction to 1–2 mEq/L/h is indicated only if a patient is symptomatic and only for the first 1–3 hours of therapy, with a goal to improve the serum sodium concentration to 12–15 mEq/l in the first 24 hours.

Hypoglycemia

Hypoglycemia is often defined as a serum glucose level of < 40 mg/dl. However, initial symptoms may occur at levels higher than this, particularly if the blood glucose level is decreased rapidly. Symptoms are often worst in the early morning. They may include weakness, dizziness, diaphoresis, and nausea. Symptoms may progress to diffuse neurologic deficits, seizure, coma, and death.

Hypoglycemia most commonly results from insulin-producing islet cell tumors that occur alone or as part of multiple endocrine neoplasia syndromes. Symptomatic hypoglycemia may also result from tumoral production of compounds with low molecular weight and non-suppressible insulin-like activity. Of these compounds, those best characterized are insulin-like growth factor (IGF)-1, IGF-2, somatomedin A, and somatomedin C. A graded response to hypoglycemia is appropriate. Mild hypoglycemia may be managed best by increasing the frequency of feedings or, if necessary, by administering IV infusions of dextrose-containing solutions. Relatively severe or symptomatic hypoglycemia may require corticosteroid and glucagon administration.

Adrenal Failure

Adrenal failure or adrenal insufficiency is rare in pediatric patients with cancer. The usual cause is adrenal suppression from the extended use of glucocorticoids at supraphysiologic dosages combined with an abrupt termination of therapy. Symptoms of adrenal insufficiency are exaggerated in the setting of physiologic stress and can include mild acidosis, hyponatremia, and hypokalemia. Severe circulatory collapse and shock are uncommon.

Lactic Acidosis

In pediatric patients with malignancy, lactic acidosis is rare and most frequently associated with hypo-perfusion and tissue hypoxia, as seen in patients with sepsis, low cardiac output, or extreme anemia. Lactic acidosis resulting from rapidly progressive hematologic malignancy or extensive liver involvement is best documented in adults with cancer. Treatment is appropriately directed at the underlying etiology of acidosis. A serum lactate level > 4 mEq/l is associated with a poor prognosis.

Mechanical Factors

Neurologic Emergencies

The principal neurologic mechanical emergencies that require acute medical treatment manifest as spinal cord compression, increased intracranial pressure (ICP) in association with cerebral herniation, and status epilepticus.

Spinal Cord Compression

Tumors: The most common tumors resulting in spinal cord compression are occurring with sarcoma, and lymphoma in children (Fig. 32.1). Purely intradural or epidural lesions are uncommon because more than three fourths of cases arise from either metastasis to a vertebral body or other bony parts of the vertebra or less commonly, direct extension from a paravertebral soft tissue mass.

Symptoms and signs: The most common early symptoms seen in patients with spinal cord compression are localized vertebral or radicular pain. These are not from the cord compression *per se* but rather from involvement of the vertebral structures and nerve roots at the level of the compression. Localized tenderness to pressure or percussion over the involved vertebrae is often found

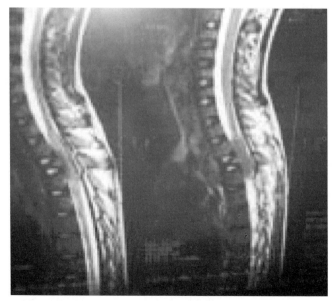

Fig. 32.1: MRI picture showing NHL with vertebral destruction and spinal compression

on physical examination. Because pain is seen initially in up to 90% of patients, localized back pain, radicular pain, or spinal tenderness in a patient with cancer should evoke the clinical suspicion of the physician and prompt further evaluation to determine whether the patient has potential or early cord compression.

Diagnosis: Magnetic resonance imaging (MRI) is the investigation of choice, although HRCT with myelography is an alternative. Plain radiographs and bone scans give evidence of metastases to vertebrae, but they are not diagnostic of spinal cord involvement. When there is evidence of bony involvement of the spine on a plain radiograph. An MRI for those patients who have subjective or objective evidence of weakness, radicular pain, paresthesia, or sphincter dysfunction because these patients are at the highest risk of spinal cord compression.

Treatment: Because of potentially precipitous deterioration when neurologic deficits have developed, treatment should be started immediately.

1. **Corticosteroids:** When a radiologic study identifies the level of cord compression or a neurologic deficit is detected on physical examination, dexamethasone should be started to reduce spinal cord edema. The recommended dose is 10 to 20 mg IV as a loading dose and then 4 to 6 mg PO or IV every 6 hours, to be continued through the initial weeks of radiation therapy.
2. **Radiotherapy:** Although the preferences of individual centers vary, it is generally recommended that immediate initiation of radiotherapy should be done once cord compression is diagnosed. Radiation therapy is most frequently given to a total dose of 40–45 Gy with daily dose fractions of 200 to 250 cGy. Alternatively, 400 cGy daily may be given initially for the first 3 days of therapy and then subsequently decreased to standard-dose levels for the completion of the radiation course. Short course therapies with higher dose fractions have also been used.

Cerebral Edema
Clinical Evaluation
Neurologic signs and symptoms: Intracranial metastases commonly manifest as a variety of neurologic symptoms and signs, including, headache, change in mentation, visual disturbances, cranial nerve deficits, focal motor or sensory abnormalities, difficulty with coordination, and seizures. In the more critical condition of brain stem herniation, there may be gradual to rapid loss of consciousness, neck stiffness, unilateral or bilateral pupillary abnormalities, ipsilateral hemiparesis, or respiratory dysfunction; the specific findings depend on whether there is uncal, central or tonsillar herniation.

Radiologic studies: MRI is the diagnostic modality of choice because it has greater sensitivity than CT in detecting the presence of metastatic lesions, evaluating the posterior fossa, and determining the extent of cerebral edema. CT is substituted for MRI in many institutions because of availability, ease of administration, shorter test time and less cost.

Treatment
Symptomatic therapy: Once the presence of cerebral edema is established, dexamethasone should be started. The rationale for the use of steroids centers on the etiology of cerebral edema. It appears that the invasion of malignant cells releases leukotrienes and other soluble mediators responsible for vasodilation increased capillary permeability, and subsequent edema. Dexamethasone inhibits the conversion of arachidonic acid to leukotrienes, thereby decreasing vascular permeability. Patients with severe cerebral edema leading to a life-threatening rise in intracranial pressure or brain stem herniation should also receive mannitol (in a 20 to 25% solution) infused IV over approximately 30 minutes. This may be repeated every 6 hours if needed although serum electrolytes and urine output must be monitored closely.

Cardiovascular Emergencies
In pediatric patients, mechanical emergencies of the cardiovascular system are uncommon, but they may result from compromise in cardiac function or vascular flow. Although anthracycline chemotherapy may depress myocardial contractility and result in long-term medical complications, it is an unusual acute emergency. The primary acute emergency is tamponade resulting from malignant or reactive pericardial effusion. Although vascular compression from a tumor mass frequently occurs, it rarely precipitates a medical emergency. The primary

exception to this is superior vena cava (SVC) syndrome, which is often observed in association with a large mediastinal mass.

Cardiac Tamponade

Cardiac tamponade is defined as the inability of the ventricle to maintain cardiac output because of extrinsic pressure or an intrinsic mass. Although pericardial and pleural effusions are frequently observed, tamponade physiology is a rare complication of pediatric malignancy. Clinical findings of impending tamponade are similar to those of heart failure and include chest pain, cough, dyspnea, hiccups, nonspecific abdominal pain, and pulsus paradoxus >10 mm Hg. Chest radiographs may reveal the classic water-bag cardiac silhouette. ECG may demonstrate low-voltage QRS complexes and flattened or inverted T waves. Echocardiography is the best single study, and it demonstrates pericardial effusion and atrial or ventricular collapse with hemodynamic compromise. Percutaneous catheter drainage is the treatment of choice and may be performed under echocardiographic or fluoroscopic guidance. Pericardial fluid may contain malignant cells and should be evaluated accordingly. Resolution of the effusion is expected when the underlying malignancy is treated.

Superior Vena Cava Syndrome (SVCS)

The superior vena cava is responsible for the venous drainage of the head, neck, and arms. Its location places it near lymph nodes that are commonly involved by malignant cells from primary lung tumors and from lymphomas. Lymph node distention or the presence of a mediastinal tumor mass may compress the adjacent superior vena cava, leading to superior vena cava syndrome (SVCS) (Figs 32.2 and 32.3). Similarly, the presence of a thrombus due to a hypercoagulable state secondary to underlying malignancy or a thrombus developing around an indwelling central venous catheter may also lead to the development of this syndrome.

Symptoms and signs: Patients who develop SVCS commonly complain of dyspnea, orthopnea, paroxysmal nocturnal dyspnea, and facial, neck and upper-extremity swelling. Associated symptoms may include cough, hoarseness, and chest or neck pain. Headache and mental status changes may also be seen.

Treatment: Initially patients with SVCS may be treated with oxygen for dyspnea, furosemide 20 to 40 mg IV to reduce edema, and dexamethasone IV in divided doses. The benefit of dexamethasone is not clear. In patients with lymphoma, there is probably a lympholytic effect with resultant decrease in tumor mass; in patients with

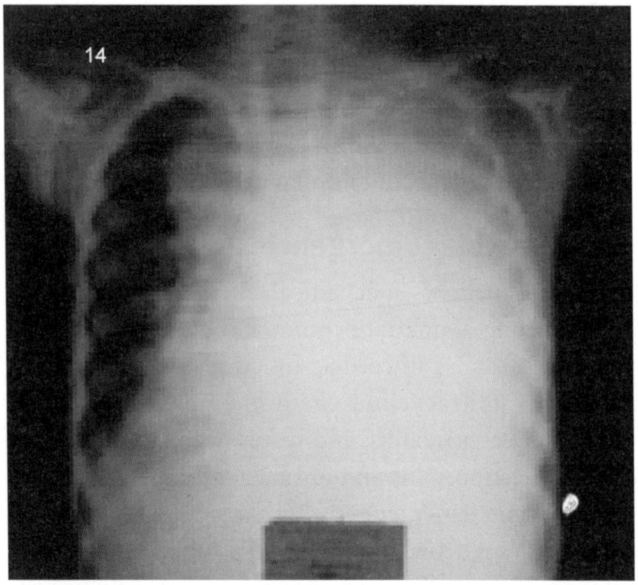

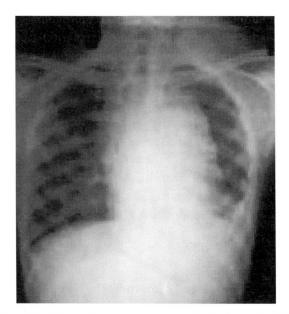

Fig. 32.2: X-ray chest showing mediastinal mass following non-Hodgkin lymphoma

Fig. 32.3: SVC syndrome caused by mediastinal mass in NHL

most other tumors, the effect is probably limited to decreasing any local inflammatory reaction from the tumor and from subsequent initial radiotherapy.

Anaphylaxis

Causes: Anaphylaxis, although infrequent, is one of the most catastrophic potential side effects of biologic and chemotherapy. Anaphylaxis is a hyperimmune reaction mediated by the release of immunoglobulin E. This emergency situation may arise in oncology patients who are exposed to serum products, bacterial products such as L-asparaginase, certain cytotoxic agents, antibiotics such as penicillin, iodine-based contrast material, latex and monoclonal antibodies. However, virtually any drug can lead to a hyperimmune response resulting in anaphylaxis.

Clinical manifestations: Patients may display anxiety, dyspnea, and presyncopal symptoms. Urticaria, generalized itching, and evidence of bronchospasm and upper–airway angioedema may occur. Peripheral vasodilation may manifest as facial flushing or pallor, can result in significant hypotension, and may lead to syncope.

Management: Prompt recognition and treatment can be invaluable in blunting an adverse response and may prevent a reaction from becoming life threatening. Patients must be assessed rapidly to ensure that an open airway is present and maintained. Supplemental oxygen should be given for respiratory symptoms. Endotracheal intubation may be necessary. If severe laryngeal edema rather than bronchospasm is the cause of respiratory distress, tracheostomy or cricothyrotomy is necessary.

Respiratory Failure

Respiratory failure in patients with cancer may have many potential causes:
1. Bacterial or other pneumonias, especially in patients who are neutropenic due to therapy.
2. Overwhelming parenchymal pulmonary metastases (Fig. 32.4).
3. Radiation injury.
4. Lung damage from chemotherapy agents such as bleomycin, mitomycin, high dose cyclophosphamide, or methotrexate.

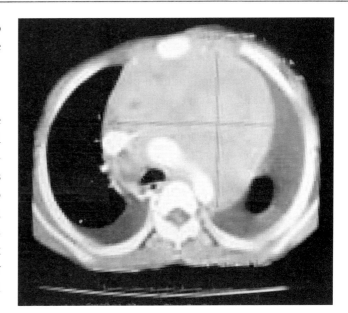

Fig. 32.4: CT scan of chest showing mediastinal mass with diffuse lung involvement in NHL

5. Pulmonary edema secondary to cardiac damage from cytotoxic agents such as doxorubicin, or capillary leak syndrome from biologic agents such as IL-2.
6. Sepsis and other causes of the systemic inflammatory response syndrome.
7. Interstitial pulmonary spread of cancer.
8. Retinoic acid syndrome from tretinoin (all trans-retinoic acid) therapy of acute promyelocytic leukemia.
9. Pulmonary emboli, either multiple small or single large.

Gastrointestinal Emergencies

GI obstruction, pseudo-obstruction, and ileus are seen in children with cancer. Although uncommon, GI obstruction in children is most commonly due to intussusception in which a neoplasm in the bowel wall creates a lead point to initiate the process. Burkitt lymphoma in the terminal ileum frequently comes to medical attention in this manner. In addition, intussusception is reported in patients with adenomyoma of the Meckel diverticulum, hamartoma of the ileum, acute lymphoblastic leukemia, leiomyosarcoma, or after resection of Wilms' tumor. GI obstruction has also been reported after a volvulus resulting from a mesenteric lymphangioma. Obstruction of the large colon primarily occurs in the context of large pelvic tumors and as a complication of constipation-obstipation induced by chemotherapy, e.g. vincristine, narcotic analgesia, or both. Typhlitis, sepsis, or other severe illness may precipitate a temporary ileus. Abdominal ultrasonography or fluoroscopy performed with air-or water-soluble contrast material is the recommended diagnostic procedure. Fluoroscopic procedures can also be therapeutic. Surgery may be necessary for reduction, tissue diagnosis, or both. Reduction of the intussusception and treatment of the primary pathology are the principal approaches used in patients with GI emergencies. In general, large tumor masses that cause GI obstruction because of external compression are best

treated with chemotherapy, surgery, radiation therapy, or their combination. Treatment-related complications respond to interim GI decompression and supportive medical treatment.

SUGGESTED READING

1. Davis MP, et al. Modern management of cancer-related intestinal obstruction. Curr Oncol Rep. 2000;2:343.
2. Dropcho EJ. Remote neurologic manifestations of cancer. Neurol Clin. 2002;20:85.
3. Vaitkus PT, et al. Treatment of malignant pericardial effusion. JAMA. 1994;272:59.
4. Vim BT, et al. Rasburicase for the treatment and prevention of hyperuricemia. Ann Pharmacother. 2003;37: 1047.

Intensive Care Issues in Pediatric Oncology Patients

Agni Sekhar Saha

THE INTERFACE BETWEEN PEDIATRIC ONCOLOGY AND PEDIATRIC INTENSIVE CARE MEDICINE

Pediatric oncology patients often get critically ill, both at presentation and during therapy, resulting admission to the pediatric intensive care unit (PICU). However, unlike the overall prognosis of pediatric oncology patients which has improved remarkably over the last 50 years outcome of patients who end up being admitted to the PICU had been poor. Most studies quoting a mortality of 40 to 50% as opposed to the general PICU mortality of < 10%. The figures became significantly worse once the patients were ventilated and even more so if they had shock requiring ionotropes. Fatality was almost universal if 3 or more organ systems needed support. This even led some to question whether it is appropriate to institute intensive care to these patients. However, over the last ten years, studies are consistently being published reporting better outcome data for this patient population. Some of these studies have even reported a significant correlation between outcome and the time period of admission. So, there is now hard evidence that oncology patients do benefit from PICU service. However, the bad prognostic factors like, need for ventilation, shock needing ionotropes, multiple organ dysfunction syndrome, higher disease severity score, more or less remained the same. Prognosis of patients needing 3 or more organ system support is still universally bleak. This has led to the present thinking that oncology patients should be transferred to PICU early in order to get the benefit of

better outcome. There is probably one exception to this general improvement, i.e. patients with bone marrow transplant (BMT), who continue to pose the greatest of challenges to the intensivist and is often considered the 'Holy grail' of pediatric intensive care medicine.

OVERVIEW

Critically ill children with malignancy are in most ways similar to the general PICU population, vulnerable to different organ system failures and needing similar support. However, they are also significantly different in a number of ways. We would now briefly consider these differences, their consequences. There are also certain complications which are typically or exclusively seen in pediatric oncology patients. These complications and their managements would also be briefly reviewed.

a. General condition: These children are adversely affected both by the primary disease and the prolonged therapy. This effect is often global involving multiple systems which reduce their 'physiological reserve'. As a result they can deteriorate very quickly. These patients are 'fragile' and need to be 'handled with care'.

   Implication: Early identification of problems, close monitoring and proactive institution of intervention is the key to success.

b. Immunosuppression and sepsis: They are often immunosuppressed both as a result of the malignancy and the therapy.

   Implications: The importance of strict handwashing simply cannot be overemphasized. All hygiene measures should be scrupulously maintained. Asepsis for all procedures is desirable. All access to central lines must be aseptic. Ideally immunecompromised patients should be treated in isolated cabins with positive pressure so that air flow is from inside out. Barrier nursing is also another consideration.

c. The usual features of sepsis may be masked or subtle. So be vigilant.

Think of cytomegalovirus (CMV), fungi (Both *Candida and Aspergillus*), *Pneumocystis carinii*, etc. Consider Septran and Fluconazole prophylaxis.

d. Prolonged hospital stay makes them prone to nosocomial infections.

Implications: Cover pseudomonas and methycillin resistant *Staphylococcus aureus* (MRSA).

Consider the profile of organisms prevalent in the institute and their sensitivities.

e. Often they have already received multiple or prolonged courses of broadspectrum antibiotics.
Implication: Consider fungi.

f. They often have indwelling vascular catheters like multiple lumen central lines or surgical lines like Portacath or Broviac lines making them prone to catheter related infections.

Implications – In addition to venipuncture sample, always send a sample from the catheter. If it is a multilumen catheter then send separate samples from each lumen and remember to label them so that the lumens could be identified from the samples.

Cover coagulase negative staphylococcus and also consider Candida.

If any catheter or lumen is suspected or confirmed as the source of infection, administer antibiotics through that catheter or lumen and give an 'Antibiotic lock'. If a catheter or lumen is culture positive, always send repeat cultures to ensure clearance of infection. Catheter infections are notoriously difficult to treat and often needs removal of the catheter. Although this is frustrating, never hesitate to take this step and avoid the temptation to wire in a central line through the same tunnel! If possible, do not reinsert another 'clean' line until the infection is cleared.

g. They often have extensive mucositis which acts as the port of entry for the infection.

Implication: Cover *Streptococcus viridans*.

h. Many patients start with a compromised cardiac function due to chemotherapy (anthracyclines, cyclophosphamde, 5-FU) or chest radiation.

Implication: Look for a cardiac component and get an echocardiography early. Echo also would exclude cardiac tamponade which is relatively common, difficult to diagnose and can present as shock (see later).

i. These patients fair worse in the presence of organ dysfunction, especially multiple organ dysfunction, than the general population.

Implications: Do everything possible to prevent organ failure and start organ system support early. This is especially important for renal replacement therapy (RRT). RRT not only support the renal function but also makes room for further administration of volumes and also prevent lysis of membranes and lung injury that are often associated with renal failure in these patients.

COMPLICATIONS REQUIRING ADMISSION IN PICU

Febrile Neutropenia

Neutropenia is seen commonly. Indeed, all neutropenic patients certainly do not require PICU admission. At the same time, patients who are ill enough to get admitted to the PICU and neutropenic as well have worse outcome. If a child is needing organ support and having neutrophil counts < 200/cmm or < 500/cmm which is decreasing, G-CSF should be considered, which reduces length of stay and duration of neutropenia (adult study). However, no study has yet demonstrated significant survival benefit, possibly due to the size of the trials. If fungal infection is proved or suspected, then GM-CSF is indicated, although evidence is even more scarce.

Shock

Although the outcome was once thought to be poor, now there are many studies quoting survival of around 70% in non-BMT subjects. Hence, it is definitely worthwhile treating this aggressively. The baseline blood pressure (BP) of patients receiving chemotherapy is often lower than normal. This effect is more pronounced for diastolic than systolic pressure.

Implications: If possible, always check the baseline BP from previous patient records. Be suspicious if the low BP is mainly diastolic and not associated with tachycardia and poor perfusion. As always, give at least a couple of fluid boluses and check the response before moving onto ionotropes.

These patients often have already received steroids in recent past for a number of reasons.

Implication: Consider steroids early. The standard practice of considering steroids only after the shock is proven to be resistant to adequate volume and ionotrope therapy is probably not appropriate in this patient population.

Pulmonary

They often present with respiratory failure. There may be pre-existing pulmonary fibrosis due to therapy or chest radiation. They are also prone to pneumonia and ARDS. All these scenarios are characterized by 'stiff lung' having a low compliance.

Implication

While ventilating, use an open lung, low volume lung protective strategy. Use high PEEP, often 8-10 cm of H_2O and tidal volume of 6-8 mL/kg.

High Frequency Oscillatory Ventilation (HFOV)

The same theme is true here as well. HFOV did not offer any advantage when used only as a rescue therapy after 'adequate' trial of conventional ventilation and people started questioning its role. However, evidence is now gathering which suggests early (within the first 6 hours of mechanical ventilation) institution of HFOV may improve outcome. High mean airway pressure, open lung strategy (which is now employed almost universally in all groups of patients anyway) is to be used.

Massive Hemoptysis

Although not very common but is a dramatic event with considerable mortality. Invasive pulmonary aspergilosis (often in the recovery phase from prolonged neutropenia) is the commonest cause. Other infective etiologies are *Pseudomonas, Staphylococcus aureus, Klebsiella*, etc. Non-infective causes include tumor extension, diffuse alveolar hemorrhage, etc. Risk is asphyxia with clots within the airway. Patients often need intubation which can be difficult. The glottis is often not visualized. If so, aim towards the point from where active bleeding is coming! Once in, take extra care in fixing the endotracheal tube (ET). Use and maintain high PEEP (>10 cm H_2O) until bleeding is controlled for at least 24 hours. Tracheal toileting should be judicious. If done sparingly then there is every risk of ET blockage with clots needing re-intubation. On the other hand, every time the ET is suctioned, the PEEP is lost which increases the chance of recurrence of bleeding. Transfuse packed red cells and platelets as indicated and correct clotting abnormalities.

If aspergilosis is confirmed or suspected, consider combination anti-fungal therapy with high dose liposomal amphotericin B (6 mg/kg), caspofungin and voriconazole. Bronchoscopy with endoluminal therapy or bronchial arteriography followed by transcatheter embolization by trained personnel are options for poor risk non-surgical patients with continuing bleeding. Segmental or lobar resection is a much better option having higher survival and lower recurrence rates.

Superior Mediastinal Mass/SVC Syndrome/ Anterior Mediastinal Mass

Causes are numerous. It is an emergency if it is affecting the airways and causing obstructive respiratory symptoms. An urgent CT scan is needed to understand the anatomy. The dilemma is whether to start radiotherapy or steroids, both of which can effectively reduce the mass but also have the potential of subsequent interference with tissue diagnosis or to go for a biopsy which usually needs general anesthesia that can be tricky. The decision is a multidisciplinary one involving the oncologist, anesthetist, surgeon and the intensivist. Pitfalls, if any child with a central neck line develops SVC syndrome, always rule out thrombosis first before considering other diagnoses.

These patients are treacherous for airway management. Their airway may obstruct with slight provocation like change in posture, loss of tone due to anesthetics, etc. and

Intubation can be difficult! If airway control is absolutely necessary, gas induction is preferred. General anesthesia should not be given, if the cross-section of trachea on CT scan, and the peak expiratory flow rate are less than 50% of expected values irrespective of whether the patient is symptomatic or not.

Cardiac

These patients often have subnormal cardiac function secondary to chemotherapy or radiotherapy. A baseline echocardiography to assess functional reserve is always warranted.

Cardiac Tamponade

Usual causes are local or metastatic spread of tumor or lymphatic obstruction. Bleeding diathesis often contributes.

If suspected, echocardiography must be obtained which is both sensitive and specific and also gives a functional assessment. Chest X-ray is not sensitive and ECG is not specific. These patients tolerate hypovolemia badly. Make sure patient is adequately 'filled'. Give generous fluid bolus. Diuretics are contraindicated. Pericardiocentesis under fluoroscopic and ECG control should be done as soon as possible. Some patients might end up needing surgical pericardiotomy.

Gastrointestinal (GI) System

These patients are prone to GI complications like obstruction, perforation, peritonitis, abdominal compartment syndrome, hemorrhage, etc. and the management is similar as in any other group of patients. Because of the immunosuppression and frequent administration of steroids, the features of abdominal complications like pain, muscle guard, etc. can be subtle and difficult to recognize. They can also have the so-called 'silent' perforation.

Typhlitis

This is also called neutropenic enterocolitis. The exact pathophysiology is uncertain but is thought to be related to inflammation and mucositis secondary to chemotherapy which is complicated by bacterial translocation. Cecum is the most commonly affected part. Typical clinical triad of fever, abdominal pain and diarrhea is not present in many cases. Sepsis and perforation are the major complications. Investigation of choice is CT scan and a bowel wall thickness of > 4 mm confirms the diagnosis. Ultrasound is an alternative tool which could be performed on bedside even in very ill patients thereby obviating the need to transfer the patient to the radiology department. Management is supportive with bowel rest until bowel sounds are heard, nasogastric suction, broad-spectrum antibiotics and parenteral nutrition. Surgery is a difficult choice because of the often poor general condition and should be considered only in perforated cases.

Acute Appendicitis

Although the incidence is the same as in general pediatric population, the diagnosis is difficult due to both the subtler signs and the similarity of presentation between typhlitis and appendicitis. Studies have shown that in as many as 37.5% of cases in this patient group, the diagnosis may be delayed. Series has been reported where 5 out of 7 patients had incorrect preoperative diagnosis. This forms the other strong reason to get a CT scan (or ultrasound scan) in any patient with suspected typhlitis. Management is appendicectomy. Prognosis is worse than that in the general population, possibly due to both the general condition of these patients, immunosuppresion and the delayed diagnosis.

Central Nervous System (CNS)

CNS again may be affected both by the primary disease or metastases or the therapy.

Seizure

These patients are at increased risk of seizures compared to the general pediatric population and seizure accounts for about 60% of CNS indications for PICU admission in this group of patients. The management is as for other patients. Carbamazepine and valproate causes myelosuppression and should be avoided.

Raised intracranial pressure (ICP): There may be many causes. Management is directed both at initial stabilization, active control of ICP as well as specific treatment of the cause. Management of raised ICP is as usual. Infra-tentorial tumors often present with raised ICP secondary to obstructive hydrocephalous which constitutes an emergency indication for surgical decompression. Intracranial tumor or metastasis is possibly the only current indication for dexamethasone in raised ICP.

Metabolic

Dyselectrolytemias especially that of sodium are often seen because of both renal and CNS pathologies. Acidosis is also seen frequently. Management is standard.

Tumor Lysis Syndrome

This complication occurs secondary to very rapid lysis of large tumor tissue mass, usually after cytoreductive chemotherapy but can also occur after steroids or radiotherapy. Commonly seen in acute fluid cancers, i.e. acute leukemias (except AML) and lymphomas as well as bulky solid tumors that are very sensitive to chemotherapy, i.e. neuroblastoma, meduloblastoma, etc. Highest risk in patients with B-cell ALL and Burkitt's lymphoma with lactate dehydrogenase of > 500 U/L. Characterized by triad of raised uric acid, potassium and phosphate levels with secondary hypocalcemia due to high phosphate levels. Symptoms are secondary to the metabolic abnormalities, i.e. malaise, weakness, vomiting and features of hypocalcemia like tetany, carpopedal spasm, seizures, etc. Two primary concerns are acute renal failure due to deposition of calcium phosphate and uric acid crystals in renal tubules and arrhythmia due to hyperkalemia. Both are worsened by acidosis.

Management

In high-risk cases it is often prudent to start therapy prophylactically before initiation of chemotherapy. This decision would come from the oncologist involved.

Allopurinol

Reduces production of uric acid but has no role in lowering existing hyperuricemia. Therefore, it should be started 24–48 hours before starting chemotherapy.

Rasburicase

Reduces hyperuricemia by converting uric acid to allantoin. Rasburicase is contraindicated in patients with glucose-6-phosphate dehydrogenase deficiency which should be checked. There is some evidence that rasburicase is more effective than allopurinol in this setting.

Fluids

This is the cornerstone of therapy. Usual recommendation is to keep patient on 0.25% saline with 5% dextrose with 50-100 mmol $NaHCO_3$/L at 2-4 times maintenance to keep urine output > 100 mL/m^2/h, urinary pH at 7–7.5 and urine specific gravity < 1.010. Hydration must be started early, i.e. early morning on the day of starting therapy. Aggressive alkalinization should be avoided as this further decreases the level of ionized calcium.

Diuretics

Usually avoided as the chance of both urate and phosphate crystal deposition in the renal tubules is increased especially in hypovolemic patients. Osmotic diuretics and furosemide may have some role in the volume overloaded patient with low urine output (< 60 mL/m^2/h).

Electrolyte Disturbances

Intake of potassium and phosphate should be restricted. Hyperkalemia is treated as usual. Oral phosphate binders (calcium carbonate, aluminium hydroxide, etc.) are used. Calcium supplements may worsen or cause deposition of calcium phosphate crystals as the solubility product factor (Ca X PO$_4$ = 60) is reached. Therefore, hypocalcemia is treated only if symptomatic.

Renal Replacement Therapy

Goals of therapy are either treatment of acute renal failure (associated with either resistant hyperkalemia or acidosis or symptomatic fluid overload), reduction of phosphate and/or uric acid level to prevent further renal damage or to create more 'space' to enable administration of further 'volume' as part of the therapy in an oliguric patient. Continuous veno-venous hemifiltration (CVVH) is the most commonly applied method although either hemodialysis or peritoneal dialysis can also be employed. In some centers in selected patients CVVH is started prophylactically to prevent any renal damage although there is no evidence to support this approach.

Retinoic Acid Syndrome

This is a complication seen in acute pro-myelocytic leukemia patients days to weeks after starting all-trans-retinoic acid (ATRA) therapy. It can be seen in up to 25% of patients and mortality as high as 13% has been reported. Features are of water retention associated with renal failure. Weight gain, respiratory distress, plural and pericardial effusion, hypotension and fever has been reported. Chext X-ray reveals pulmonary edema with infiltrates with or without plural and/or pericardial effusion. Therapy is dexamethasone 0.5 – 1 mg/kg/12 H. Atra may be stopped temporarily until features subside.

ETHICAL CONSIDERATIONS

This can be the most difficult aspect of the management. As stated earlier, mortality is much higher in critically-ill oncology patients. Once intensive care and life-supporting measures have been initiated, it is the intensivists primary responsibility to continually assess the whole picture and ensure that continuation of intensive care is appropriate, ethical, and serves the child's best interests. Often withdrawal of invasive care is to be considered. Although the intensivist usually leads, the decision has to be a team decision of which the parents (and the child if appropriate) must be important members along with other specialists and nursing staffs. Western studies have consistently shown that most parents would prefer to play an active part in the decision making rather than not and an empathetic, open and honest approach from the clinical team is appreciated by the parents. This also helps grieving and subsequent coping. Although social and cultural values are different, there is as yet no evidence to suggest that it might be any different in India or the sub-continent.

It is extremely important for the lead to remain clear about the basis for such decisions and communicate this clearly to the team. 'Futility' provides a much more acceptable, clear and robust ethical ground for withdrawal than 'Quality of life' considerations. However, 'Quality of life' decisions are not entirely avoidable. Always try to resist mixing 'Futility' and 'Quality of life' principles to support the decision about a single patient. Usually this represents uncertainty and confusion of the leader rather than the reality. If in doubt, seek the parents' opinion and err in favor of continuation rather than withdrawal.

SUGGESTED READING

1. Cesaro S, Toffolutti T, Messina C, et al. Safety and efficacy of caspofungin and liposomal amphotericin B, followed by voriconazole in young patients affected by refractory invasive mycosis. Eur J Haematol. 2004;73:50-5.

2. Clark OA, Lyman G, Castro AA, et al. Colony-stimulating factors for chemotherapy-induced febrile neutropenia. Cochrane Database Syst Rev. 2003;CD003039.

3. Edward C Wong, Anne L Angiolillo. Oncologic emergencies. In: Slonim AD, Pollack MM (Eds). Pediatric Critical Care Medicine, 1st Edition. Lippincott Williams & Wilkins 2006;585-96.

4. Fiser RT, West NK, Bush AJ, et al. Outcome of severe sepsis in pediatric oncology patients. Pediatr Crit Care Med. 2005;6:531-6.

5. Goldman SC, Holcenberg JS, Finklestein JZ, et al. A randomized comparison between rasburicase and allopurinol in children with lymphoma or leukemia at high risk for tumor lysis. Blood. 2001;97:2998-3003.

6. Hagen SA, Craig DM, Martin PL, et al. Mechanically ventilated pediatric stem cell transplant recipients: Effect of cord blood transplant and organ dysfunction on outcome. Pediatr Crit Care Med. 2003;4:206-13.

7. Hobson MJ, Carney DE, Molik KA, Vik T, Scherer LR 3rd, Rouse TM, et al. Appendicitis in childhood hematologic malignancies: analysis and comparison with typhlitis. J Pediatr Surg. 2005;40:214-9; discussion 219-20.

8. Meyer S, Gottschling S, Biran T, Georg T, Ehlayil K, Graf N, et al. Assessing the risk of mortality in paediatric cancer patients admitted to the paediatric intensive care unit: a novel risk score? Eur J Pediatr. 2005;164:563-7. Epub. 2005 May 24.

9. Rheingold SR, Lange BJ. Oncologic emergencies. In: Pizzo PA, Poplack DG (Eds). Principles and practice of pediatric oncology, 4th Edition. Philadelphia, PA: Lippincott Williams & Wilkins 2004;1177-1203.

10. Ricketts RR. Clinical management of anterior mediastinal tumors in children. Semin Pediatr Surg. 2001;10: 161-8.

11. Rodrigo Mejia, Jose A Cortes, Deborah L Brown, Gerardo Quezada, Michael E Rytting, Carroll J

King, Alan I Fields. Oncologic emergencies and complications. In: Nichols DG (Ed). Roger's Textbook of Pediatric Intensive Care, 4th Edition. Lippincott Williams & Wilkins 2008:1710-24.

12. Sivan Y, Schwartz PH, Schonfeld T, Cohen IJ, Newth CJ. Outcome of oncology patients in the pediatric intensive care unit. Intensive Care Med. 1991;17(1):11-5.

13. Tamburro RF, Barfield RC, Shaffer ML, Rajasekaran S, Woodard P, Morrison RR, Howard SC, Fiser RT, Schmidt JE, Sillos EM. Changes in outcomes (1996-2004) for pediatric oncology and hematopoietic stem cell transplant patients requiring invasive mechanical ventilation. Pediatr Crit Care Med. 2008;9:270-7.

14. van Gestel JP, Bollen CW, van der Tweel I, Boelens JJ, van Vught AJ. Intensive care unit mortality trends in children after hematopoietic stem cell transplantation: a meta-regression analysis. Crit Care Med. 2008;36: 2898-904.

34 Hematopoietic Stem Cell Transplant

Arpita Bhattacharya

INTRODUCTION

Hematopoietic stem cell transplant (HSCT) is now widely used to treat both malignant and nonmalignant conditions. These special cells are characterized by their ability to self-replicate and undergo terminal differentiation into erythroid, myeloid, lymphoid and megakaryocytic lineage.

History

Research in the field of stem cells was pioneered by E Donnall Thomas in the 1950's to 1970's. His team showed that infused bone marrow cells can migrate to and repopulate the host's bone marrow and produce viable functioning components of all lineages. This work later won him a Nobel Prize.

The first successful transplant was performed by Robert A Good.

Subsequent research in this field is directed at developing effective yet less toxic conditioning regimens, decreasing transplant related mortality and morbidity, improving survival, and improving understanding of the immune mechanisms associated both with adverse effects as well as the beneficial antitumor effects of the graft.

Types of HSCT

Autologous Transplantation

The patient's own stem cells are used as a rescue therapy after high-dose myeloablative therapy. This is generally used in chemosensitive hematopoietic and solid tumors to eliminate all malignant cells by administering high-dose chemotherapy and subsequent rescue of the host's bone marrow with previously harvested autologous stem cells. Immunosuppression is not required after autologous transplantation.

Allogeneic Transplantation

This refers to the use of stem cells from a human leucocyte antigen (HLA)—matched related or unrelated donor. This is used for a variety of malignant and non-malignant disorders to replace a defective host marrow or immune system with the normal donor marrow and immune system. The key to successful allogeneic transplantation is finding an HLA-matched donor, because it decreases the risk of graft rejection and graft versus host disease (GVHD).

The 3 HLA loci critical for matching are: HLA-A, HLA-B, and HLA-DR. HLA-C, HLA-DP and HLA-DQ were recently added to this list. A completely matched sibling donor is considered ideal. For unrelated donors, a completely matched or a single mismatch is considered acceptable for most transplantation protocols. Syngeneic transplantation is a form of allogeneic transplantation in which the donor is an identical twin sibling of the patient. Graft rejection is less of an issue for such transplants when compared to other allogeneic transplants.

CBT (Cord Blood Transplant)

Hematopoietic stem cells can be collected from the umbilical cord and placenta. The use of CBT has rapidly increased because of several favorable factors: Ease of collection, expanded and prompt availability, no risk to the donors, decreased risk of adverse effects (e.g. GVHD, transmission of infections), increased tolerance to HLA-mismatch, and no risk of donor loss at the time of transplantation.

Sources of Stem Cells

The traditional source of hematopoietic stem cells for use in autologous and allogeneic transplantations was bone marrow. Use of peripheral blood (PBSC) as a source of these cells later replaced bone marrow for all autologous and most allogeneic transplantations.

Stem cells may be harvested from the bone marrow, peripheral blood and umbilical cord blood.

Collecting Stem Cells

Clinically relevant sources for autografting are BM and PBSC, and for allografting, BM, PBSC and CB.

Table 34.1: Cellular characteristics of various sources of stem cells

	Source of stem cells		
	Bone marrow	Peripheral blood	Cord blood
Stem cell content	Adequate	Good	Low
Progenitor cell content	Adequate	High	Low*
T cell content	Low	High	Low, functionally immature
Risk of tumor cell contamination	High	Low	Not applicable

*Studies have shown that the cord-blood progenitor cells have greater proliferative potential than that of peripheral blood and marrow progenitor cells.

Bone Marrow

BM aspirations can be done regardless of age, and very young infants have successfully been used as donors. Young donors have a distinct advantage with a better yield of stem cells and reduced risk of graft vs host disease (GVHD).

Unrelated donors can volunteer between ages 18–55. Full medical history, clinical examination and laboratory investigations are required before accepting a person as a donor.

Marrow is generally harvested from the posterior iliac crests under general anesthesia. After collection into a closed system, the cell suspension is passed through filters of different kinds to remove aggregates, fat particles and bone fragments. The preparation is then dispatched to the laboratory for processing and cryopreservation.

For allogeneic donation, the maximum volume collected should not exceed 20 ml/kg. The minimum number of nucleated cells recommended for engraftment is 2×10^8/kg of the recipient.

Autologous marrow collections should contain a leucocyte number of at least 3×10^8/kg.

Marrow is infused into the recipient via an IV line over less than one hour.

Peripheral Blood Stem Cells (PBSC)

PBSC is mobilized prior to harvesting using cytotoxic chemotherapy, hematopoietic growth factors or a combination of both. Collection of PBSC is usually accepted in adult related transplants, for second transplants and for mismatched transplants where T-cell depletion is indicated. The speed of engraftment is faster, and incidence of acute GVHD is somewhat lower than in BM grafts. However, incidence of chronic GVHD is higher.

Table 34.2: Clinical characteristics with various sources of stem cells

	Different sources of stem cells		
	Peripheral Blood (PBSC)	Bone Marrow (BM)	Cord Blood (CBSC)
HLA matching	Close matching required	Close matching required	Less restrictive than others
Engraftment	Fastest	Faster than cord blood but slower than peripheral blood	Slowest
Risk of acute GVHD	Same as in bone marrow	Same as in peripheral blood	Lowest
Risk of chronic GVHD	Highest	Lower than peripheral blood	Lowest

The optimum time for harvesting PBSC after mobilization is when the leukocyte count is $5 \times 10^9/l$. Mononuclear cell apheresis is the standard procedure for collecting circulating PBSC. Central venous access is usually required for the donor. The donor is connected to a cell separator, and up to 16 liters of blood may be processed daily. Leukapheresis may be carried out over several days.

A minimum CD 34+ cell dose of $2 \times 10^6/kg$ will provide stable hamatopoietic recovery in most recipients. Higher thresholds of $3.5-5 \times 10^6/kg$ will increase the probability of rapid reconstitution and are usually optimum targets.

Cord Blood Hematopoietic Stem Cells

The first cord blood transplant was performed in 1988 on a patient with Fanconi anemia, from his HLA identical sibling. The patient was alive and apparently cured of his condition 10 years later. Since the first case, the number of CB collections and transplants are increasing rapidly, especially among HLA matched siblings. Successful grafts have been obtained from siblings differing for 1, 2 or 3 HLA antigens. The establishment of cord blood banks have enabled unrelated HLA matched or partially matched transplants.

CB banking for autologous or allogeneic HSCT has several advantages: Easy access, indefinite storage, speed of donor search, viral safety, and a source of stem cells for expansion and gene therapy.

Collection can be performed immediately after delivery in the labor room. The volume obtained is 40–150 ml.

Indications for HSCT

More than 30,000 autologous and 15,000 allogeneic transplantation procedures are performed every year worldwide. The list of diseases for which HSCT is being used is rapidly increasing. More than half of the autologous transplantations are performed for multiple myeloma and non-Hodgkin lymphoma, and a vast majority of allogeneic transplants are performed for hematologic and lymphoid cancers.

Table 34.3 summarizes the common indications for HSCT. Cord-blood transplants are being used for many of the allogeneic transplant indications whenever a suitable HLA-matched donor is unavailable or whenever time for identifying, typing, and harvesting a transplant from an unrelated donor is limited.

Conditioning Regimens

The three principal objectives of HSCT conditioning regimens are:
- **Space making:** It is believed that immature progenitor cells occupy niches within the bone marrow in order to obtain the necessary support for proliferation and differentiation. Conditioning frees these spaces for the donor cells to settle in.
- **Immunosuppression:** This is necessary to prevent rejection of the graft by the host. This is obviously not needed in autologous transplants.
- **Disease eradication:** The conditioning regimen eliminates residual disease as in hematological malignancies. In diseases with hyperplastic marrow, e.g. thalassaemia, this is also a very essential factor.

Table 34.3: Common indications for HSCT

Autologous transplantation		Allogeneic transplantation	
Malignant disorders	*Nonmalignant disorders*	*Malignant disorders*	*Nonmalignant disorders*
• Neuroblastoma • Non-Hodgkin lymphoma • Hodgkin disease • Acute myeloid leukemia (AML) • Medulloblastoma • Germ cell tumors	• Autoimmune disorders • Amyloidosis	• AML • Non-Hodgkin lymphoma • Hodgkin disease • Acute lymphoblastic eukemia (ALL) • Chronic myeloid leukemia (CML) • Myelodysplastic syndromes	• Aplastic anemia • Fanconi anemia • Severe combined immunodeficiency • Thalassemia major • Diamond-Blackfan anemia • Sickle cell anemia • Wiskott-Aldrich syndrome • Osteopetrosis • Inborn errors of metabolism • Autoimmune disorders

Conditioning regimens can be classified as myeloablative, nonmyeloablative, and reduced intensity.

Myeloablative regimens: These are designed to kill all residual cancer cells in autologous or allogeneic transplantation and to cause immunosuppression for engraftment in allogeneic transplantation. Total-body irradiation (TBI) and cyclophosphamide or busulfan and cyclophosphamide are the commonly used myeloablative therapies. These regimens are especially used in aggressive malignancies, such as leukemias.

Nonmyeloablative regimens: Use doses of chemotherapy drugs and radiation substantially lower than those of myeloablative regimens. These regimens are immunosuppressive but not myeloablative and rely on a graft-versus-tumor effect to kill tumor cells with donor T-lymphocytes. Because of their decreased acute and chronic toxicity, these regimens can be used in patients aged 55 years or older and in patients with notable comorbidities.

Such regimens are usually beneficial for slow-growing tumors, such as those of chronic myelogenous leukemia, and are also beneficial for a variety of nonmalignant disorders, such as thalassemia and autoimmune disorders.

Reduced-intensity regimens: These are between myeloablative and nonmyeloablative regimens and involve drugs such as fludarabine, melphalan, antithymocyte globulin, and busulfan. Such regimens also reduce acute and chronic toxicity compared with myeloablative regimens. The incidence of GVHD is comparable to that of myeloablative regimens, though its onset is delayed with this.

Outcome

Over the years, transplantation-related mortality and morbidity rates have considerably decreased because of improved conditioning regimens, HLA typing, supportive care, and prevention and treatment of serious infections. However, overall and event-free survival rates are based on the individual's disease pathology and on the stage of disease. Table 34.4 lists the survival rates of different diseases after HSCT.

Patients undergoing HLA-matched sibling allogeneic transplantation have the best 5-year survival rate of all treated patients.

Table 34.4: Malignancy-wise five-year survival data

Disease	Stage	Survival rate, %		
		Autologous transplantation	Allogeneic transplantation	
			Sibling donor	Unrelated donor
ALL	CR 1	NA	65	45
	CR 2	NA	55	35
AML	CR 1	60	65	30
	CR 2	40	45	50
	No remission	20	NA	25
CML	Chronic phase < 1 y	NA	70	55
	Chronic phase > 1 y	NA	60	50
Hodgkin disease	CR 1	80	NA	NA
	CR 2	70	NA	NA
	No remission	45	NA	NA
Diffuse large-cell lymphoma	CR1	65	25	30
	CR 2	50	25	NA
	No remission	45	20	NA
Neuroblastoma		40	NA	NA

Note.—CR = complete response; NA = not applicable.
*Based on Kaplan-Meier curves of data from the Center for International Blood and Marrow Transplant Research (CIBMTR) and the National Marrow Donor Program (NMDP) data.

Complications

HSCT related complications can be classified as early and late effects.

Early Effects

These are characterized by endothelial damage, which may be a direct effect of the conditioning regimen or may be caused indirectly through the production of cytokines (IL-1, TNF-α).

Mucositis

Mucositis is one of the most common adverse effects of transplantation. It can involve the entire gastrointestinal tract, leading to painful mouth sores, diarrhea, nausea, and abdominal pain. It is usually managed symptomatically with narcotics and topical anesthetics.

Graft Versus Host Disease

Acute GVHD is a common complication of allogeneic transplantation and occurs within first 100 days of the procedure. It is an immune response of donor T lymphocytes against host cells. It is the result of a multistep cascade that include:

1. Tissue damage due to conditioning regimen causing activated host cells to secrete inflammatory cytokines (IL-1, TNF-α).
2. Donor T cell activation.
3. Effector phase (cytokine storm): Dynamic interactions between cells with amplification and dysregulation of complex cytokine networks.

Onset of acute GVHD is marked by the appearance of rash, which may painfully denude, followed by liver dysfunction, diarrhea, fever and weight-loss.

Prevention of GVHD can be achieved by:
- Choice of best donor to avoid HLA incompatibility and gender mismatch.
- T cell depletion of graft.
- Reducing intensity of conditioning regimen.

Post-transplant immunosuppressive treatment includes cyclosporine A (CsA) alone or in combination with methotrexate, tacrolimus and mycophenolate mofetil (MMF).

Current research is focusing on improving our understanding of the pathophysiologic pathways of GVHD to design targeted therapies and genetic modifications of donor T-cells to prevent and treat GVHD.

The severity of GVHD is inversely related to the risk of relapse because GVHD and graft versus leukemia (GVL) effect are interrelated. Therefore, strategies reducing GVHD may increase relapse rates. New strategies are being developed to separate these two effects to decrease the incidence and severity of GVHD without increasing the risk of relapse.

Veno-occlusive Disease

Veno-occlusive disease (VOD), also known as sinusoidal obstruction syndrome, is a potentially fatal syndrome of tender hepatomegaly, direct hyperbilirubinemia, ascites, and weight gain that generally occurs within three weeks of transplant. VOD is caused by damage to the sinusoidal endothelium and nonthrombotic sinusoidal obstruction. TBI and drugs, such as oral busulfan and cyclophosphamide, predispose to this syndrome. Pre-existing liver disease and certain genetic mutations that alter drug metabolism may increase the risk of VOD. No standard effective therapy is currently available. Defibrotide is a novel agent that elicits responses in severe VOD; it is under investigation in a phase III trial.

Transplantation-related Lung Injury

Transplantation-related lung injury (TRLI) is an acute inflammatory response that leads to severe lung injury. TRLI is seen in allogeneic transplants. The risk factors include higher dose of total body irradiation (TBI), older age, HLA disparity and GVHD. Early treatment with corticosteroids and etanercept, an anti-tumor-necrosis factor (TNF) agent, can reduce the extent of this injury. Mortality is high (50–70%).

Transplantation-related Infections

Life-threatening bacterial, fungal, and viral infections (e.g. those due to *Aspergillus* or Cytomegalovirus) are common in patients undergoing HSCT. Causes include prolonged neutropenia, use of steroids, and immunodeficiency associated with GVHD. Bacterial sepsis occurs early in the course of transplantation whereas viral infections such as those caused by cytomegalovirus usually occur after engraftment. Fungal infections such as those caused by *aspergillus* may occur anytime after 7–10 days of onset of neutropenia until engraftment. Early recognition and treatment are vital. Following engraftment, the ongoing risk of infection relates to the degree of immunosuppression.

Late Effects

Chronic GVHD

Chronic GVHD is most common in patients who develop acute GVHD, but it can develop in its absence. Chronic GVHD is characterized by an immune phenomenon that clinically resembles lupus, scleroderma, or Sjögren syndrome. The common target organs are skin (80%), liver (75%), oral mucosa (70%), and eyes (50%). The immune system is also involved resulting in greater susceptibility to infection and higher morbidity and mortality.

Immunosuppression with corticosteroids, CsA, tacrolimus, and MMF are the mainstays of treatment. Hydroxychloroquine, an antimalarial drug, is effective in several autoimmune disorders, including chronic GVHD.

Ocular Effects

Posterior subcapsular cataract formation is common in HSCT recipients. TBI is the predisposing risk factor. Keratoconjunctivitis sicca, or dry eyes, is part of the chronic GVHD syndrome. Other adverse effects include retinopathy, infectious retinitis, and hemorrhage. Treatment includes the use of topical lubricants and steroids.

Endocrine Effects

In children, growth and development are impaired, and they may require growth-hormone supplements. Puberty is delayed. Hypothyroidism is also common in these patients. Patients need to be counseled prior to HSCT regarding the inevitability of infertility and need to be offered the option of sperm or egg banking.

Pulmonary Effects

Pulmonary effects include restrictive and chronic obstructive lung disease. Conditioning regimens, infections and GVHD are important risk factors. Bronchiolitis obliterans is a specific form of obstructive lung disease seen in HSCT recipients.

Musculoskeletal Effects

Osteoporosis and avascular necrosis are common adverse effects in HSCT recipients.

Neurocognitive and Neuropsychological Effects

Cranial irradiation and neurotoxic chemotherapy with methotrexate are known to be associated with leukoencephalopathy, cerebral atrophy, microangiopathy and demyelination.

A low intelligence quotient (IQ), sleep disorders, fatigue, memory problems, and developmental delays have all been reported in HSCT recipients. These issues must be addressed appropriately to improve the person's overall quality of life.

Immune Effects

Host immunity is suppressed for months to years after HSCT. This effect is more pronounced in allogeneic transplantation than in autologous transplantations. Factors responsible for depressed immunity include severe myelosuppression due to the myeloablative conditioning of the host, acute GVHD that further suppresses host immunity, and the use of immunosuppressants to prevent or treat GVHD.

In allogeneic transplant recipients, complete immune reconstitution takes a few years and depends on the ability of naïve prethymic donor T cells to mature in the host's thymus and to become host tolerant and antigen specific. This process is most efficient in children and young adults because they have an active thymus. Older patients may never completely recover their immunity because their thymic tissue might not be fully functional.

These immune effects in HSCT patients should be kept in mind, as these patients are prone to serious infections long after the initial HSCT procedure. It also raises the issue of revaccinating these patients after HSCT. No formal guidelines for revaccinating HSCT patients are established, though the current literature suggests that most vaccine-acquired immunity wanes after HSCT. Most killed vaccines are considered safe, but use of live virus vaccines is generally contraindicated. Appropriate timing for revaccinating is 12–18 months after the HSCT, though this period may need to be individualized on the basis of the patient's immune function. Vaccinations earlier than this do not result in an appropriate immune response.

SUGGESTED READING

1. Apperly JF, Gluckman E, Gratwohl A, Craddock C. Blood and Marrow Transplantation (Eds). 2000.
2. Copelan EA. Hematopoietic stem-cell transplantation. N Engl J Med. 2006;354:1813-26.

3. Cutler C, Antin JH. Peripheral blood stem cells for allogeneic transplantation: a review. Stem Cells. 2001;19:108-17.

4. Iwasaki T. Recent advances in the treatment of graft-versus-host disease. Clin Med Res. 2004;2:243-52.

5. Koh LP. Unrelated umbilical cord blood transplantation in children and adults. Ann Acad Med Singapore. 2004;33:559-69.

6. Matthay KK, Villablanca JG, Seeger RC, et al. Treatment of high-risk neuroblastoma with intensive chemotherapy, radiotherapy, autologous bone marrow transplantation, and 13-cis- retinoic acid. Children's Cancer Group. N Engl J Med. 1999;341:1165-73.

7. Siena S, Schiavo R, Pedrazzoli P, Carlo-Stella C. Therapeutic relevance of CD34 cell dose in blood cell transplantation for cancer therapy. J Clin Oncol. 2000;18:1360-77.

8. Singhal S, Mehta J. Reimmunization after blood or marrow stem cell transplantation. Bone Marrow Transplant. 1999;23:637-46.

9. Socie G. Current issues in allogeneic stem cell transplantation. Hematology. 2005;10 Suppl 1:63.

10. Socie G, Salooja N, Cohen A, et al. Nonmalignant late effects after allogeneic stem cell transplantation. Blood. 2003;101:3373-85.

35 Growth Factors and Biologicals in Pediatric Oncology

Madhumita Nandi

Biologicals are a group of proteins or glycoproteins which are produced naturally in the body but have also been synthesized and used for treatment of various infectious, malignant and immunological diseases. This group of natural proteins, sometimes broadly named cytokines, are a group of soluble proteins that are released by a cell to send messages which are delivered to the same cell (autocrine), an adjacent cell (paracrine), or a distant cell (endocrine). The cytokine binds to a specific receptor and causes a change in function or in development (differentiation) of the target cell. Cytokines are involved in reproduction, growth and development, normal homeostatic regulation, response to injury and repair, blood clotting, and host resistance (immunity and tolerance). Unlike cells of the endocrine system, many different types of cells can produce the same cytokine, and a single cytokine may act on a wide variety of target cells. The response of a target cell may be altered by the context in which it receives a cytokine signal. The context includes other cytokines in the milieu, and extracellular matrix. Thus has developed the concept of cytokines as alphabet letters that combine to spell words which make-up a molecular language.

Cytokines may be divided into six groups: Interleukins, colony-stimulating factors, interferons, tumor necrosis factor, growth factors, and chemokines.

BIOLOGICALS IN CANCER SUPPORTIVE CARE

Several hemopoietic growth factors have been purified, cloned, and produced in bacteria. These molecules are able to modulate selectively the activity of mature blood cells as well as stimulating the production of specific lineages of blood cells. Each of the growth factors has a unique spectrum of biological activities. These growth factors enhance the recovery and function of circulating blood cells after cancer therapy or bone marrow transplantation. Some of the hemopoietic growth factors which are in clinical use at present are erythropoietin, granulocyte colony stimulating factor (G-CSF), Granulocyte-monocyte colony stimulating factor (GM-CSF), monocyte-colony stimulating factor (M-CSF), and thrombopoietin.

Erythropoietin (EPO)

History

Hematologist Dr John Adamson and nephrologist Dr Joseph W Eschbach looked at various forms of renal failure and the role of the natural hormone EPO in the formation of red blood cells. Studying sheep and other animals in the 1970s, the two scientists helped establish that EPO stimulates the production of red cells in bone marrow and could lead to a treatment for anemia in humans.

EPO is a glycoprotein hormone that stimulates the production of red blood cells in bone marrow. It is produced mainly by the kidneys and is released in response to decreased levels of oxygen in body tissue. Erythropoietin is also referred to by the names epogen, procrit, epoetin alfa, and EPO. Recently a genetically engineered form of the hormone, called recombinant erythropoietin (rEPO), has been made. It is a drug approved by the Food and Drug Administration (FDA) in 1989 to treat low red blood cell counts caused by cancer chemotherapy treatment and kidney failure.

Erythropoietin stimulates the erythropoietic progenitor cells in bone marrow. Patients need an adequate supply of iron in the body for erythropoietin to work best. If a patient's iron is low, the patient may need oral iron supplementation. The increase in red blood cell levels should be seen in two to six weeks after beginning therapy in cancer-related anemia patients.

Dosage

Erythropoietin is a clear, colorless liquid which is administered by intravenous or subcutaneous routes. Erythropoietin starting dose is 50–100 units per kilogram of body weight three times a week. This would be adjusted based patient response. It can be given at a maximum dose of 300 units per kg.

Side Effects

The common side effects are iron deficiency anemia and raised blood pressure. So adequate iron stores should be ensured during EPO therapy. In addition to taking oral iron replacement, patients should increase their intake of iron in their diet. Also, blood pressure monitoring is essential.

A common side effect due to erythropoietin administration is pain or burning at the site of the injection. This can be decreased by making sure that the erythropoietin is at room temperature before giving the infection. Other side effects of patients who receive erythropoietin include diarrhea and local swelling. Less common side effects in cancer patients include fever, nausea and vomiting, fatigue, shortness of breath, and weakness.

Thrombopoietin (TPO)
History

Thrombopoietin was cloned by five independent groups in 1994. Before its identification, its function has been hypothesized for as much as 30 years as being linked to the cell surface receptor *c-Mpl*, and in older publications *thrombopoietin* is described as *c-Mpl ligand* (the agent that binds to the c-Mpl molecule). Thrombopoietin is one of the Class I hematopoietic cytokines.

Thrombopoietin (TPO) is a glycoprotein hormone produced mainly by the liver and the kidney that regulates the production of platelets by the bone marrow. It stimulates the production and differentiation of megakaryocytes, the bone marrow cells that fragment into large numbers of platelets.

Thrombopoietin is an experimental drug that may increase the number of platelets in the bloodstream. Thrombocytopenia is a common side effect from many common chemotherapy agents, such as carboplatin. By reducing the severity of platelet-related side effects, thrombopoietin could allow the antitumor medication to be used at higher doses and/or for longer periods of time.

Genetics

The thrombopoietin gene is located on the long arm of chromosome 3 (q26.3-27). Abnormalities in this gene occur in some hereditary forms of thrombocytosis (high platelet count) and in some cases of leukemia. Thrombopoietin shares its first 153 amino acids with erythropoietin.

Therapeutic Use

Despite numerous trials, thrombopoietin is not used therapeutically. Theoretical uses include the procurement of platelets for donation and recovery of platelet counts after myelosuppressive chemotherapy. A modified recombinant form, termed "megakaryocyte growth and differentiation factor" (MGDF), caused a paradoxical reaction, delaying the development of therapeutic thrombopoietin. A quadrivalent peptide analogue is undergoing development, as well as several small molecule agents. A non-peptide ligand of *c-Mpl*, which acts as a thrombopoietin analogue, is under investigation.

Colony-stimulating Factors

Colony-stimulating factors (CSFs) are secreted glycoproteins, which bind to receptor proteins on the surfaces of hemopoietic stem cells and thereby activate intracellular signaling pathways which can cause the cells to proliferate and differentiate into a specific kind of blood cell.

The name "colony-stimulating factors" comes from the method by which they were discovered. Hemopoietic stem cells were cultured on a so-called semi-solid matrix, which prevents cells from moving around, so that if a single cell starts proliferating, all of the cells derived from it will remain clustered around the spot in the matrix where the first cell was originally located. These are referred to as "colonies." It was, therefore, possible to add various substances to cultures of hemopoietic stem cells and then examine which kinds of colonies (if any) were "stimulated" by them.

The substance which was found to stimulate formation of colonies of macrophages, for instance, was called macrophage colony-stimulating factor, and so on.

Colony-stimulating factors include:

- *CSF1*—macrophage colony-stimulating factor
- *CSF2*—Granulocyte macrophage colony-stimulating factors (also called GM-CSF and sargramostim)
- *CSF3*—Granulocyte colony-stimulating factors (also called G—CSF and filgrastim)
- Synthetic—Promega poietin
- Interleukin—3(Multi-colony stimulating factor)

Granulocyte-macrophage colony-stimulating factor, often abbreviated to **GM-CSF**, is a protein secreted by macrophages, T cells, mast cells, endothelial cells and fibroblasts.

GM-CSF is a cytokine that functions as a white blood cell growth factor. GM-CSF stimulates stem cells to produce granulocytes (neutrophils, eosinophils, and basophils) and monocytes. Monocytes exit the circulation and migrate into tissue, whereupon they mature into macrophages. It is, thus, part of the immune/inflammatory cascade, by which activation of a small number of macrophages can rapidly lead to an increase in their numbers, a process crucial for fighting infection.

GM-CSF is also known as molgramostim or, when the protein is expressed in yeast cells, sargramostim (Leukine®).

GM-CSF is used as a medication to stimulate the production of white blood cells following chemotherapy. It has also recently been evaluated in clinical trials for its potential as a vaccine adjuvant in HIV-infected patients. The preliminary results have been promising but GM-CSF is not presently FDA-approved for this purpose.

Leukine is the trade name of sargramostim manufactured by Berlex Laboratories, a subsidiary of Schering AG. Its use was approved by US Food and Drug Administration for acceleration of white blood cell recovery following autologous bone marrow transplantation

in patients with non-Hodgkin's lymphoma, acute lymphocytic leukemia, or Hodgkin's disease in March 1991. In November 1996, the FDA also approved sargramostim for treatment of fungal infections and replenishment of white blood cells following chemotherapy.

Granulocyte colony-stimulating factor (**G-CSF** or **GCSF**) is a hormone. It is a glycoprotein, growth factor or cytokine produced by a number of different tissues to stimulate the bone marrow to produce granulocytes and stem cells. G-CSF then stimulates the bone marrow to pulse them out of the marrow into the blood. It also stimulates the survival, proliferation, differentiation, and function of neutrophil precursors and mature neutrophils.

G-CSF is also known as **Colony-stimulating factor 3** (**CSF 3**).

G-CSF is produced by endothelium, macrophages, and a number of other immune cells. The natural human glycoprotein exists in two forms, a 174- and 180-amino-acid-long protein of molecular weight 19,600 grams per mole. The more-abundant and more-active 174-amino acid form has been used in the development of pharmaceutical products by recombinant DNA (rDNA) technology.

Mouse granulocyte colony-stimulating factor (G-CSF) was first recognized and purified in Australia in 1983, and the human form was cloned by groups from Japan and the United States in 1986.

The G-CSF-receptor is present on precursor cells in the bone marrow, and, in response to stimulation by G-CSF, initiates proliferation and differentiation into mature granulocytes.

The gene for G-CSF is located on chromosome 17, locus q11.2–q12. The GCSF gene has 4 introns, and that 2 different polypeptides are synthesized from the same gene by differential splicing of mRNA. The 2 polypeptides differ by the presence or absence of 3 amino acids. Expression studies indicate that both have authentic G-CSF activity.

G-CSF stimulates the production of white blood cells. In oncology and hematology, a recombinant form of G-CSF is used with certain cancer patients to accelerate recovery from neutropenia after chemotherapy, allowing higher-intensity treatment regimens. Chemotherapy can cause myelosuppression and unacceptably low levels of white blood cells, making patients prone to infections and sepsis. However, in a Washington University

School of Medicine study using mice, G-CSF is shown to lessen the density of bone tissue even while it increases the WBC count, if this is found to occur in human cases it would necessitate increased consumption of calcium and vitamins A and D. G-CSF is also used to increase the number of hematopoietic stem cells in the blood before collection by leukapheresis for use in hematopoietic stem cell transplantation.

Itescu planned in 2004 to use G-CSF to treat heart degeneration by injecting it into the blood-stream, plus SDF (stromal cell-derived factor) directly to the heart. The recombinant human G-CSF synthesized in an *E. coli* expression system is called filgrastim. The structure of filgrastim differs slightly from the structure of the natural glycoprotein. Most published studies have used filgrastim. Filgrastim (Neupogen®) and PEG-filgrastim (Neulasta®) are two commercially-available forms of rhG-CSF (recombinant human G-CSF). The PEG (poly-ethylene glycol) form has a much longer half-life, reducing the necessity of daily injections.

Another form of recombinant human G-CSF called lenograstim is synthesized in Chinese Hamster Ovary cells (CHO cells). As this is a mammalian cell expression system, lenograstim is indistinguishable from the 174-amino acid natural human G-CSF. No clinical or therapeutic consequences of the differences between filgrastim and lenograstim have yet been identified, but there are no formal comparative studies.

BIOLOGICALS FOR THERAPEUTICS

A. Interleukin

These are a class of naturally occurring proteins important in regulation of lymphocyte function. Several known types are recognized as crucial constituents of the body's immune system. Antigens and microbes stimulate production of interleukins, which induce production of various types of lymphocytes in a complex series of reactions that ensure a plentiful supply of T cells that fight specific infectious agents.

Interleukins are a group of cytokines (secreted signaling molecules) that were first seen to be expressed by white blood cells (leukocytes, hence the *-leukin* as a means of communication *inter-*). The name is something of a relic though (the term was coined by Dr Paetkau, University of Victoria); it has since been found that interleukins are produced by a wide variety of bodily cells. The function of the immune system depends in a large part on *interleukins*, and rare deficiencies of a number of them have been described, all featuring autoimmune diseases or immune deficiency.

At least 18 types of this important class, with varying origin and function, exist. Production of interleukins is now known not to be confined to lymphocytes or macrophages.

B. Monoclonal Antibodies

Antibodies or immunoglobulins are a crucial component of the immune system, circulating in the blood and lymphatic system, and binding to foreign antigens expressed on cells. Once bound, the foreign cells are marked for destruction by macrophages and complement. In the context of cancer immunotherapy, monoclonal antibodies have brought to light a wide array of human tumor antigens. In addition to targeting cancer cells, antibodies can be designed to act on other cell types and molecules necessary for tumor growth.

The approval of monoclonal antibodies (MAbs/ MOAB) as antibody-targeted therapy in the management of patients with hematologic malignancies has led to new treatment options for this group of patients. Three classes of therapeutic MAbs showing promise in human clinical trials for treatment of hematologic malignancies include unconjugated MAbs, drug conjugates in which the antibody preferentially delivers a potent cytotoxic drug to the tumor, and radioactive immunotherapy in which the antibody delivers a sterilizing dose of radiation to the tumor. A better appreciation of how MAbs are metabolized in the body and localized to tumors is resulting in the development of new antibody constructs with improved biodistribution profiles.

Types of monoclonal antibody that have been developed are as follows:

1. *Chimeric:* Chimeric antibodies are 65–90% human and consist of the constant or effector domain of the human antibody molecule combined with the murine variable regions (which bring about antigen recognition) by transgenic fusion of the immunoglobulin gene.

2. *Partially humanized:* Partially humanized antibodies are about 95% human and consist of the

A list of interleukins

Name	Source	Function
IL-1	Macrophages	Small amounts induce acute phase reaction, large amounts induce fever stimulates
IL-2	TH1-cells	growth and differentiation of T cell response. Can be used in immunotherapy to treat cancer or suppressed for transplant patients
IL-3	T cells	Stimulates bone marrow stem cells
IL-4	TH 2-cells, just activated naive [[CD 4+ cell]], [[memory CD 4+ cells]]	Involved in proliferation of B cells and the development of T cells and mast cells. Important role in allergic response (IgE)
IL-5	TH 2-cells	Role in differentiation of B cells, eosinophil production, and IgA production
IL-6	Macrophages, TH 2-cells	Induces acute phase reaction
IL-7	Stromal cells of the red marrow and thymus	Involved in B, T, and NK cell survival, development, and homeostasis
IL-8	Macrophages, epithelial cells, endothelial cells	Neutrophil chemotaxis
IL-9	T-cells, specifically by CD 4+ helper cells	Stimulates mast cells
IL-10	Monocytes, TH 2-cells, mast cells	Inhibits Th1 cytokine production
IL-11	Bone marrow stroma	Acute phase protein production
IL-12	Macrophages	NK cell stimulation, Th1 cells induction. May suppress food allergies
IL-13	TH 2-cells	Stimulates growth and differentiation of B-cells (IgE), inhibits TH1-cells and the production of macrophage inflammatory cytokines
IL-14	T cells and certain malignant B cells	Controls the growth and proliferation of B cells
IL-15	Mononuclear phagocytes (and some other cells) following infection by virus(es).	Induces production of Natural Killer Cells
IL-16	A variety of cells (including lymphocytes and some epithelial cells)	Chemoattracts immune cells expressing the cell surface molecule CD 4
IL-17	–	Induces production of inflammatory cytokines
IL-18	Macrophages	Induces production of Interferon-gamma (IFNγ)
IL-19		–
IL-20	–	Regulates proliferation and differentiation of keratinocytes
IL-21	–	Induces proliferation in natural killer cells (NK) and cytotoxic T cells
IL-22	–	Activates STAT 1 and STAT 3 and increases production of acute phase proteins such as serum amyloid A, Alpha 1-antichymotrypsin and haptoglobin in hepatoma cell lines
IL-23	–	Increases angiogenesis but reduces CD 8 T-cell infiltration
IL-24	–	Plays important roles in tumor suppression, wound healing and psoriasis by influencing cell survival
IL-25	–	Induces the production IL-4, IL-5 and IL-13, which stimulate eosinophil expansion
IL-26	–	Enhances secretion of IL-10 and IL-8 and cell surface expression of CD 54 on epithelial cells
IL-27	–	Regulates the activity of B lymphocyte and T lymphocytes
IL-28	–	Plays a role in immune defense against viruses
IL-29	–	Plays a role in host defenses against microbes
IL-30	–	Forms one chain of IL-27
IL-31	–	May play a role in inflammation of the skin
IL-32	–	Induces monocytes and macrophages to secrete TNF-α, IL-8 and CXCL 2

complementarity determining regions of the murine antibody (which determine antibody specificity) and a limited number of structural aminoacids grafted onto a CDR-depleted human antibody backbone by recombinant technology.

3. *Deimmunized:* Deimmunized antibodies have the immunogenic epitopes in the murine variable domains replaced with benign aminoacid sequences, resulting in a deimmunized variable domain. The deimmunized variable domains are linked genetically to human antibody constant domains.

4. *Primatized:* Primatized antibodies have a chimeric antibody structure of human and monkey that is close to an exact copy of a human antibody.

5. *Fully humanized:* Fully human antibodies have been developed by use of genetically engineered transgenic mice and advances in the generation of synthetic human antibody libraries.

At present, therapeutic monoclonal antibodies are being used in hematological and solid malignancies including non-Hodgkin's lymphoma, breast cancer and colorectal cancer. MOABs may be used in cancer treatment in a number of ways:

1. MOABs that react with specific types of cancer may enhance a patient's immune response to the cancer.

2. MOABs can be programmed to act against cell growth factors, thus interfering with the growth of cancer cells.

3. MOABs may be linked to anticancer drugs, radioisotopes (radioactive substances), other BRMs or other toxins. When the antibodies latch onto cancer cells, they deliver these poisons directly to the tumor, helping to destroy it.

Some of the biological agents used in oncologic therapeutics are Anti-TNF agents like infliximab and anti-CD-20 agents like rituximab.

Infliximab

It is a chimeric IgG1 antibody of human Fc fragment and murine Fab directed against TNF. It is an antibody that binds to TNF and inactivates them. It is given as IV infusion 0, 2, 6 weeks and then every 8 weeks. It is mainly used in Refractory JIA, lymphoma, etc.

Data of using infliximab is still limited. It can have some serious side effects like; a) Infections, b) Flare-up of tuberculosis, c) Lupus like diseases, d) Lymphomas, etc.

Anti-CD20 Agents

Rituximab is a chimeric monoclonal antibody directed against CD 20 antigen. CD 20 is a B lymphocyte marker. Its mechanism of action includes antibody mediated cytotoxicity, complement dependant cytotoxicity, B cell proliferation inhibition, apoptosis induction, etc. It is used mainly in CD 20+ non-Hodgkin lymphoma and also under trial in various autoimmune and immunological diseases. Overall, it has good efficacy and limited toxicity mainly related to infusion related events; though it's cost is a prohibitory factor.

C. Cancer Vaccines

Cancer vaccines are another form of biological therapy currently under study. Vaccines for infectious diseases, such as measles, mumps, and tetanus, are injected into a person before the disease develops. These vaccines are effective because they expose the body's immune cells to weakened forms of antigens that are present on the surface of the infectious agent. This exposure causes the immune system to increase production of plasma cells that make antibodies specific to the infectious agent. The immune system also increases production of T cells that recognize the infectious agent. These activated immune cells remember the exposure, so that the next time the agent enters the body, the immune system is already prepared to respond and stop the infection.

Researchers are developing vaccines that may encourage the patient's immune system to recognize cancer cells. Cancer vaccines are designed to treat existing cancers (therapeutic vaccines) or to prevent the development of cancer (prophylactic vaccines). Therapeutic vaccines are injected in a person after cancer is diagnosed. These vaccines may stop the growth of existing tumors, prevent cancer from recurring, or eliminate cancer cells not killed by prior treatments. Cancer vaccines given when the tumor is small, may be able to eradicate the cancer. On the other hand, prophylactic vaccines are given to healthy individuals before cancer develops.

These vaccines are designed to stimulate the immune system to attack viruses that can cause cancer. By targeting these cancer-causing viruses, doctors hope to prevent the development of certain cancers.

Early cancer vaccine clinical trials involved mainly patients with melanoma. Therapeutic vaccines are also being studied in the treatment of many other types of cancer, including lymphoma, leukemia, and cancers of the brain, breast, lung, kidney, ovary, prostate, pancreas, colon, and rectum. Researchers are also studying prophylactic vaccines to prevent cancers of the cervix and liver. Moreover, scientists are investigating ways that cancer vaccines can be used in combination with other BRMs.

D. Gene Therapy

Gene therapy is an experimental treatment that involves introducing genetic material into a person's cells to fight disease. Researchers are studying gene therapy methods that can improve a patient's immune response to cancer. For example, a gene may be inserted into an immune cell to enhance its ability to recognize and attack cancer cells. In another approach, scientists inject cancer cells with genes that cause the cancer cells to produce cytokines and stimulate the immune system. A number of clinical trials are currently studying gene therapy and its potential application to the biological treatment of cancer.

E. Other Non-specific Immunomodulating Agents

Non-specific immunomodulating agents are substances that stimulate or indirectly augment the immune system.

Often, these agents target key immune system cells and cause secondary responses, such as increased production of cytokines and immunoglobulins. Two non-specific immunomodulating agents used in cancer treatment are bacillus calmette-guerin (BCG) and levamisole.

SUGGESTED READING

1. Gallin J, Snyderman R (Eds). Inflammation: basic principles and clinical correlates. 3rd edition, Philadelphia, Lippincott William and Wilkins, 1999.
2. http://www.cancer.gov/cancertropics/factsheet/therapy/gene.
3. Janeway CA, et al. (Eds). Immunobiology. The immune system in Health and Disease, 4th edition, New York, Garland, 1999.
4. Kaushansky K. Lineage-specific hematopoietic growth factors. N Engl J Med 2006;354:2034-45. PMID 16687716.
5. Kuter DJ, Goodnough LT, Romo J, DiPersio J, Peterson R, Tomita D, Sheridan W, McCullough J. Thrombopoietin therapy increases platelet yields in healthy platelet donors. Blood 2001;98:1339-45. Fulltext. PMID: 11520780.
6. Mendelian Inheritance in Man (OMIM) 600044.
7. Morstyn G, Burgess AW. Hemopoietic growth factors: a review. Cancer Res. 1988 Oct 15;48(20):5624-37.
8. Nakamura T, Miyakawa Y, Miyamura A, Yamane A, Suzuki H, Ito M, Ohnishi Y, Ishiwata N, Ikeda Y, Tsuruzoe N. A novel non-peptidyl human c-Mpl activator stimulates human megakaryopoiesis and thrombopoiesis. Blood. 2006;107:4300-7. PMID 16484588.
9. Roitt I, et al. (Eds.) Immunology. 5th edition, London, Mosby, 2002.
10. Science Vol. 311 No. 5769, pp. 1875-76, 31 March 2006 DOI: 10.1126/science.1126030.

36 Nutritional Support in Pediatric Cancer Patient

Anirban Chatterjee

Pediatric cancers are very different from adults. The most common cancers are leukemia and lymphoma, brain tumor, soft-tissue sarcoma, neuroblastoma, Wilms' tumor, and bone cancer. The prognosis of pediatric cancers has gradually improved in the last 20 years. The responsibility of nutritional support in the medical management of pediatric cancer go along similar speed with this progress. Most pediatric cancers are acute onset. So weight loss may not be found at early-diagnosed tumors, it most frequently present during treatment and cancer progression. Children are greatly affected by malnutrition due to decreased calorie stores. Extra calories are also required for growth and development. The literature reveals that up to 46% of pediatric cancer patients can suffer malnutrition. Poor nutritional conditions have an impact on different clinical outcomes, including treatment failure, quality of life and cost of care. Malnutrition causes further reduction in immune functions which result in delayed wound healing and altered drug metabolism. Consequently, it can be a causative factor to mortality and poor prognosis.

The cancer is well-known for its cancer cachexia. However, this is different from wasting (Table 36.1). Cachexia is a progressive muscle wasting due to increased protein or calorie requirements. Cytokines released by the tumor are the major cause to lose both fat and lean body mass, i.e. skeletal muscle. Cachexia causes decrease in response to treatment and death.

ETIOLOGY

Malnutrition and obesity are due to imbalance between energy of intake and expenditure

Table 36.1: Difference between cachexia and wasting

Factors	Cachexia	Wasting
Decreased body cell mass (BCM)	Present	Present
Weight loss	Absent or small compare to BCM	Present
Increase resting energy expenditure	Frequently	Not essentially
Reduction of functional status	Present	Present
Increased cytokine production	Present	Absent
Increased mortality	Present	Absent
Treatment	Anticytokine, Anabolic hormone	Increased intake

- Energy intake = Total energy expenditure (TEE)
  - TEE = REE + E (activity) + E (growth) + E (loses) + SDA
- REE = Resting energy expenditure
- E (activity) = Energy needs for activity
- E (growth) = Energy needs for normal growth
- E (loses) = Energy needs for obligatory losses in urine and stool
- SDA= Specific dynamic action of food (the energy needs for digestion and absorption)

Weight loss found when any of the elements of TEE are higher than requirement and not coordinated by increase in energy intake.

PATHOPHYSIOLOGY

The pathogenesis of cancer malnutrition is not well-understood.

Changes in Energy Expenditure

Quickly multiplying cells increase the basal metabolic rate from 20 to 90%. It is not probably so important for the cause of MN. In adult study, suggest that 33% is hypo-metabolic, 25% is hypermetabolic, and 40% is normal. TEE reduces due to reduced physical activity.

Reduced Food Intake

Anorexia is an early and most important factor, but it is more multifaceted than simple chronic starvation. Cause of anorexia in children cancer is varied widely, for instance appetite-depressing factors produced by the tumor cells themselves or by the immune cells of the host, chemotherapy, radiotherapy, surgery, recurrent infections, nausea, uncontrolled pain, changes in smell and taste perception, intestinal motility disorders, early satiety, low physical activity, and psychological factors. Low protein-calorie intake related to anorexia may be aggravated by loss of nutrients by vomiting and malabsorption.

Alteration of Micronutrient Metabolism

Carbohydrate → (insulin resistance) due to increased glucose intolerance, increased neoglucogenesis, etc.
Lipid → Increase FFA turnover, Increase FFA oxidation, increase glycerol turn over, increase lypolysis, lipogenesis
Protein → Hypoalbuminemia, acute phase protein high, increase protein breakdown related to falling levels of insulin-like growth factors and IGF binding protein.

Cytokines like TNFα, IL 6, IL 1 and interferon γ are also increased. TNFα is responsible for cancer cachexia,

increased FFA turnover, increased glycerol turnover, increased whole body protein turnover. TNFα and IL6 decreases lipoprotein lipase action and facilitate lipolysis (Table 36.2).

CLINICAL ASSESSMENT

History

Nutritional history must include symptom of cancer, its therapy and effect on nutrient intake, absorption. History includes growth data, past cancer treatment and effects on nutritional status. Development history includes particularly feeding capabilities and swallowing skill.

Physical examination—among them arm anthropometrics are most essentials.

Investigation

Measurement of Body Composition

Lean body mass is metabolically active component of body. It is lost in cancer cachexia. Bioelectrical impedance is an expensive and increasingly available method of assessing body composition. At present, Dual Energy X-ray Absorptiometry (DEXA) is becoming increasingly more available. DEXA can measure directly lean body mass, fat mass and bone mass.

Laboratory Evaluation

Biochemical parameters used for nutritional assessment include visceral protein levels. There is increase of positive acute phase protein (C reactive protein, ferritin, ceruloplasmin) and decrease of negative acute phase protein (albumin, prealbumin, transferrin, retinol binding protein) in catabolic conditions and infections. Albumin is the most abundant, least expensive, and easiest to measure. Therefore, albumin is the most commonly used biochemical marker to measure protein status. Hypoalbuminemia is not specific for diagnosis of malnutrition as it may be due to reduced synthesis, increased loss and increased third place loss. Prealbumin circulates in plasma in 1:1 ratio with retinol binding protein. It has short half-life; that is two days and more sensitive to assess nutritional status.

Table 36.2: Different cancer related factors and their effects

Cause	Effect
TNFα	Anorexia
Chemotherapy	Anorexia + gastrointestinal side effect
High dose chemotherapy, continuous infusion, Total body irradiation	Mucosal damage, esosphagitis, enteritis, malabsorption, diarrhea
Psychological-depression	Reduced intake

Stomatitis, xerostomia, dental problems and dysphagia may also contribute to a low protein-calorie intake.

NUTRITIONAL INTERVENTION TECHNIQUE

The method of nutritional support depends on clinical situation and nutritional requirement. Nutritional supports are oral feeding, enteral nutrition or parenteral nutrition. Several prospective randomized controlled trials were not able to demonstrate the clinical usefulness of supplying nutritional support in malnutrition in adult cancer patients in respect to morbidity, mortality and duration of hospitalization. A weight loss approximately 5–10% is tolerable during chemotherapy. Without supporting aggressive nutritional management to prevent it, it should be recovered between two segments. *Short-term nutritional support* (5–10 days) is commonly used in pediatric cancer patients with temporary impairment of oral nutritional intake. Its principal aim is to cover water and electrolyte needs and to provide some protein-calorie intake with the hope of a protein-sparing effect. Such a short-term nutritional support is less common in adult cancer patients because their rate of dehydration and weight loss is much less rapid. *Long-term nutritional support* (several weeks) is indicated when a low oral intake is expected for a long time according to the type of cancer and the therapeutic protocol.

Oral Feeding

Adequate calorie must be supplemented for proper weight gain. Change of texture of food, adjustment of electrolyte and mineral content may be required. Sanitary food practices, washing raw food before preparation adequate hand-washing can prevent food-borne infection in the immunocompromised children. Food sharing and street foods are to be avoided.

Enteral Nutrition

When a nutritional support is required to preserve weight, tubefeeding via the gut must be the method of choice. Enteral nutrition is the minimal invasive and the most physiological system. It retains the anatomic and immunologic function of gastrointestinal mucosa. It also hinders bacterial toxins, which are liberated in pediatric cancer due to several factors. It also has many advantages in terms of feasibility, cost, and quality of life. Enteral nutrition can provide nutritional support in cancer children with adequate gastrointestinal function and suboptimal oral intake. Nasogastric tubes are most frequently used, but are badly tolerated for more than 6–8 weeks. It has been shown to be a safe and effective method of reversing malnutrition in children with cancer. Initial resistance decreases when the family learns the simplicity of feeding via a tube. Home-care organizations enable families to administer enteral nutrition at home, a good way to increase the independence of the child. A weight gain of more than 10% was observed in patient after three months. Quality of life increased subjectively, and hospitalizations for dehydration were reduced.

Parenteral Nutrition

Parenteral nutrition is indicated when the child's nutritional status cannot be maintained by the enteral route (Table 36.3). This may occur for instance with tumors producing gastrointestinal tract obstruction or in cases of protracted nausea and vomiting. Reversal of energy deficit, improved weight gain and an increase in serum albumin by parenteral nutrition have been reported. A usual indication for parenteral nutrition in oncology is bone marrow transplantation, which requires intensive treatments causing relevant gastrointestinal toxic effects. Morbidity and mortality rates are decreased by parenteral nutrition in this indication. However, its use should be strictly limited in other types of cancer, because a significant increase in infections and mechanical complications has been reported. Central venous access must be obtained. Peripheral line can provide < 900 mOsm/L, 10% dextrose, 1.5% to 2% amino acid.

Specific Nutrients

As stressed above, early nutritional support is encouraged, not only when severe malnutrition is present. The

Table 36.3: Parenteral nutrition

Nutrient	Start with	Rate of increase	Final setting
Dextrose	3–4 mg/kg/hr	2–3 mg/kg/hr	8–18 mg/kg/hr
Amino acid	1 gm/kg/day	0.5–1 gm/kg/day	1.5–3 gm/kg/day
Lipid	1 gm/kg/day	0.5–1 gm/kg/day	1–3 gm/kg/day

Home-care organizations are useful in enabling a stable pediatric cancer patient with severe and long-term involvement of the gastrointestinal system to receive parenteral nutrition at home.

failure of conventional nutritional support to improve clinical outcome in severely malnourished cancer patients, which has been reported principally in adults under parenteral nutrition, might be related to the fact that standard nutrients do not address or reverse metabolic abnormalities that result in cancer cachexia. The use of specific nutrients is currently under considerations are L-glutamine, L-arginine, and ω-3 polyunsaturated fatty acids, which are known to modulate the immunologic system, are the best studied. L-glutamine is a nonessential amino acid synthesized by skeletal muscle. It is necessary for normal cellular proliferation, in particular for enterocytes and lymphocytes. Its role in maintaining gut mucosal integrity and function is essential. Better nitrogen balance, reduced incidence of clinical infection, lower rates of microbial colonization and shortened hospital stays have been reported. In another recent trial, oral and parenteral L-glutamine seemed to be of limited early benefit for patients having allogeneic or autologous stem cell transplantation for hematologic or solid malignancies. L-Glutamine may also protect the intestinal mucosa from radiation therapy in an animal model. It may also prevent chemotherapy-induced stomatitis. L-arginine is a nonessential amino acid in humans. L-arginine may play a role in the nutritional treatment of cancer patients in different ways, either by enhancing natural killer cell cytotoxicity, or by stimulating protein synthesis in tumors and increasing the response to chemotherapy, or by activating nitric oxide synthesis. ω3 polyunsaturated fatty acids and dietary ω3 polyunsaturated fatty acids from fish oil might restore immunodeficiency and prolong survival in severely-ill patients with generalized malignancy. It has also been suggested that a fish oil-enriched diet could reduce tumor-induced cachexia in an animal model.

Pharmacotherapeutics: Pharmacological therapies of cancer anorexia and cachexia are still not satisfactory. It includes appetite-stimulating medicine like corticosteroids, progestational substance, anabolic steroids, melatonine, insulin, growth hormone, insulin-like growth factor, and anticytokine drugs, such as thalidomide, pentoxifylline.

SUGGESTED READING

1. Albrecht JT, Canada TW. Cachexia and anorexia in malignancy. Hematol Oncol Clin North Am. 1996;10:791-800.

2. American College of Physicians. Parenteral nutrition in patients receiving cancer chemotherapy. Ann Intern Med. 1989;110:734-6.

3. Andrassy RJ, Chwals WJ. Nutritional support of the pediatric oncology patient. Nutrition. 1998;14:124-9.

4. Aquino VM, Smyrl CB, Hagg R, McHard KM, Predstridge L, Sandler ES. Enteral nutritional support by gastrostomy tube in children with cancer. J Pediatr. 1995;127:58-62.

5. Body JJ. Metabolic sequelae of cancers (excluding bone marrow transplantation). Curr Opin Clin Nutr Metab Care. 1999;2:339-44.

6. Den Broeder E, Lippens RJJ, van't Hof MA, et al. Effects of nasogastric tubefeeding on the nutritional status of children with cancer. Eur J Clin Nutr. 1998;52:494-500.

7. Gough DB, Heys SD, Eremin O. Cancer cachexia: pathophysiological mechanisms. Eur J Surg Oncol. 1996;22:192-6.

8. Mathew P, Bowman L, Williams R, Jones D, Rao B, Schropp K, et al. Complications and effectiveness of gastrostomy feedings in pediatric cancer patients. J Pediatr Hematol Oncol. 1996;18:81-5.

9. McGeer AJ, Detsky AS, O'Rourke K. Parenteral nutrition in cancer patients undergoing chemotherapy: a meta-analysis. Nutrition 1990;6:233-40.

10. Mercadante S. Parenteral versus enteral nutrition in cancer patients: indications and practice. Support Care Cancer. 1998;6:85-93.

11. Pietsch J, Ford C. Children with cancer: measurements of nutritional status at diagnosis. Nutrition in clinical practice. 2000;185-88.

12. Reilly J, Ventham J, Newell J, Aitchison T, Wallace W, Gibson B. Risk factors for excess weight gain in children treated for acute lymphoblastic leukaemia. In J of Obes. 2000;24:1537-41.

13. Taminiau JAJM, Lingbeek L, Israëls T, de Kraker J. Nutritional support for children with cancer. Ballière's Clin Paediatr. 1997;5:291-304.

14. Tisdale MJ. Cancer cachexia: metabolic alterations and clinical manifestations. Nutrition. 1997;13:1-7.

37 Palliative Care in Pediatric Oncology

Madhumita Nandi

Despite remarkable improvements in survival rates, a good percentage of children suffering from cancer still die. And they die a painful, agonizing and distressing death. Palliative care is the effort to reduce this pain, distress and agony as far as possible while taking care of their psychological, social and spiritual concerns also. Optimal care of children with advanced cancer includes early integration of this palliative care with continuing efforts to treat the underlying illness and continuing with optimal palliation when curable treatment is no longer possible.

Though this aspect of cancer care is receiving due importance in western setting, it is still grossly lacking in Indian scenario. The terminal symptoms and sufferings are never adequately relieved while a child is dying, availability of symptom-control specialists are lacking though there are good number of pediatric oncology specialists in general, and we often don't even acknowledge the dying in our quest for cure.

In general, the various obstacles for optimal palliative care are:
1. Lack of specific pediatric palliative care specialists.
2. Lack of availability of appropriate tools to use for symptoms and quality-of-life assessments in children.
3. Financial barriers for adequate palliation.
4. Most importantly, the emotional turmoil experienced while caring for a dying child may sometimes be very difficult to cope up with for some physicians and care-givers. So they often tend to 'give up' rather than address this aspect optimally.

The important tenets of palliative care are:
1. Communication and decision making.
2. Cancer directed therapy—to continue or not.
3. Symptom assessment and control.
4. Quality of life at end of life and imminent death.
5. Bereavement.

COMMUNICATION AND DECISION MAKING

Optimal palliation requires open and ongoing communication amongst all medical team members, the child and the family. Earlier recognition by the physician or the parent that there is no realistic chance for cure is associated with better palliative care. Open ended questions directed at the possibility of the child's death might go a long way in easing the suffering at the end of life.

Sometimes, communicating directly with the child may be needed. While doing so, the communicator must have the knowledge of developmental understanding of death of the child. The Table 37.1 gives an overview of the children's concept of death.

One important aspect of communication is making an appropriate decision for resuscitation for children with advanced cancer. But, as this is an emotionally trying topic, most caregivers avoid discussing this until

Table 37.1: Table showing concept about death in children

Birth to 2 years	Death is perceived as separation or abandonment No cognitive understanding of death
2 to 6 years	Death is reversible or temporary Death is often seen as punishment Magical thinking that wishes can come true
6 to 11 years	Gradual awareness of irreversibility and finality Concrete reasoning with ability to see cause and effect relationship
Above 11 years	Death is reversible, universal and inevitable Abstract and philosophical reasoning

collapse seems imminent. But, parents may be to handle this decision making better when they are not in the midst of an acute crisis. The physician should give realistic information while allowing the parents to take the decision.

While communicating, it is also important to decide about the location of end-of-life care, whether it should at home or hospital. Family preferences should be given due importance. For hospital care, the hospitals need to develop palliative care units and for home care, a proper home-care team should be in place.

CANCER-DIRECTED THERAPY

There may sometimes be efforts to continue treatment for the underlying cancer even when there is no prospect for cure. This may be prompted by a desire to extend the child's life as far as possible, or to palliate symptoms related to progressive disease. This effort should be delicately balanced with the possible impact on the quality of life. Rather than complete dichotomizing the approach to care as purely 'curative' or 'palliative', attention should be focused on controlling the cancer as long as reasonably possible.

Sometimes, the terminally-ill cancer afflicted children may be the subjects of phase I trials to determine the toxicities and maximum tolerated dose of an investigational therapeutic agent. Effective communication with the parents is essential while undertaking such trials, so that they are not carried away by false hopes of therapeutic benefit.

Large dose radiation over shorter period of time is sometimes administered to relieve symptoms like for pain relief, bone or pulmonary metastasis, control of bleeding, relief of large airway obstructions, spinal cord compression and superior vena caval obstruction. Here late arising complications are not of major concern and complete tumor elimination is also not necessary.

SYMPTOM ASSESSMENT AND CONTROL

Terminally-ill cancer afflicted children have a number of symptoms, which may give rise to significant suffering and these should be tackled with high priority. Any symptom causing significant distress and agony warrants

immediate evaluation and intervention. There should be a holistic approach to symptom relief and both physical and psychological factors should be taken into account. The commonly experienced symptoms, which might cause significant agony to these children and their families include fatigue, pain, anemia and bleeding, depression and anxiety, CNS symptoms like seizures and spinal cord compression, fever, infections, significant nausea, vomiting and diarrhea leading to increasing cachexia and respiratory discomfort.

Fatigue

This is one of the most common symptoms. The etiology is multi-faceted and includes anemia, infections, malnutrition, sleep disturbances and psychological factors. Thus, the treatment of fatigue requires identification of the underlying cause and treatment of the same if possible.

Pain

More than 80% of children with terminal cancer experience pain. Physicians should use a developmentally appropriate scale to evaluate the degree of pain in these children. The basic approach should be World Health Organization (WHO) Analgesic Ladder Programme. It involves a step-wise approach to pain-relief, starting from the weak analgesics (paracetamol and NSAIDs) to the stronger ones (morphine, fentanyl).

Paracetamol is the drug of choice for mild pain. Pain due to bony metastasis may need NSAIDs for relief, but reduced platelet numbers may preclude it's use. Newer NSAIDs like rofecoxib, a selective COX II inhibitor may be safer in children with advanced cancer but further research is needed to recommend its definitive role.

Oxycodone, hydrocodone and codeine are reserved for moderate pain. Morphine is advocated for severe and chronic cancer related pain.

It is important to monitor the patient closely for drug related side-effects as pain management is initiated. Sedation may be a side effect of opioid therapy. Dextroamphetamine and methylphenidate have been used to relieve excessive somnolence. Flushing, itching, rash, nausea and constipation are other side-effects of opioid therapy. Rash and itching may be effectively treated by antihistaminics like hydroxize and phenothiazine. Constipation may have to be treated by laxatives. Respiratory depression is a rarely encountered side effect of opioid therapy. Opioid dose may have to be lowered if this occurs.

Neuropathic pain, which occurs due to compression or infiltration of neural tissue by tumor may need tricyclic antidepressants and anticonvulsants for pain relief. Gabapentin, a newer anticonvulsant, is being used increasingly for neuropathic pain. Refractory neuropathic pain may need epidural and intrathecal catheters and neurolytic nerve blocks. Pain due to bony destruction, visceral distention and cerebral edema may need corticosteroids for relief.

Other therapeutic modalities, which have been tried for pain relief include guided imagery, hypnosis, meditation, massage, acupuncture and acupressure.

Depression and Anxiety

Psychostimulants, selective serotonin reuptake inhibitors and tricyclic antidepressants are used for treatment of depression in terminally-ill cancer afflicted children. Lorazepam has been used as an antianxiety agent in these settings. But, benzodiazepines are best only for short-term or intermittent use because prolonged use may give rise to psychomotor impairment.

Central Nervous System Symptoms

Seizures, features of raised intracranial pressure and spinal cord compression are common CNS complication of terminally-ill patients. Anticonvulsants are used for seizures. Raised intracranial pressure may be problematic in children dying of brain tumor. If maximum radiation doses have already been administered, the only option remains is to increase the dose of dexamethasone. But, this again may be limited by the appearance of side-effects of steroids such as hypertension, weight gain and cushingoid appearance, etc.

Spinal cord compression may result from epidural metastasis. Corticosteroids help decrease the edema and pain. Radiotherapy may be used for radiosensitive tumors. Otherwise, surgical debulking may be necessary.

Anemia and Bleeding

Symptoms like anemia and thrombocytopenia often occur in hematological malignancies or solid tumors metastatic to bone marrow. Periodic transfusion of red cells and platelets may be required.

Fever and Infections

While deciding whether to start antibiotics and go for a diagnostic work up in a terminally-ill cancer child, factors such as how responsive the infection may be to antibiotics, the possible side effects of antibiotics and how uncomfortable the child will be if those are not administered should be taken into account. Paracetamol alone on in combination with ibuprofen may be given for fever.

Nutrition and Hydration

The cancer anorexia-cachexia syndrome is often difficult to manage in terminal children and is also emotionally charging. The cause of cachexia is often multifactorial. Gastrostomy tubes and intravenous rehydration may have to be used when appropriate.

Nausea and vomiting may be a problem because of tumor invasion, opioid therapy, and raised intracranial pressure. Raised ICP may be treated with dexamethasone. 5-HT3 antagonists may be effective antiemetics. Lorazepam may have to be considered for refractory symptoms.

Constipation may be a distressing problem. Causes may be immobility, poor fluid intake, drugs like opioids. Laxatives have to be used in addition to providing attention to appropriate hydration.

Dyspnea

Respiratory distress may result in substantial suffering. Treatment of the underlying cause like antibiotics for pneumonia, diuretics for cardiomyopathy, pleural effusion drainage, chest tube placement and instillation of sclerosant drugs may alleviate this symptom to some extent. Supplemental oxygen may be helpful even when there is no hypoxia.

WHEN DEATH IS IMMINENT

The child experiences weakness, loss of interest in food, drowsiness and delirium in the face of imminent death. Only the essential medications should be continued. The need for terminal sedation may arise because terminal restlessness and agitation. Opioid dose may have to be increased or a second agent such as benzodiazepine or barbiturate may have to be added.

BEREAVEMENT

The death of a child is so shockingly abnormal that the bereavement period may extend much longer than other anticipated deaths. Bereaved parents and siblings need support and follow-up for a long time. All that is needed is a kind word and a caring attitude.

Last, but not the least, caregivers of dying children including physicians also need support. Repeated experiences of loss of life may be very stressful to bear.

SUGGESTED READING

1. Dreyer ZE, Blatt J, Bleyer A. Late effects of childhood cancer and its treatment. In: Principles and Practice of Pediatric Oncology. Editors-Pizzi PA, Poplack DG. Fourth Edition. Lippincott, Williams and Wilkins Philadelphia. 2002;1431-61.
2. Hobbie W, Ruccione K, Harvey J, Moore IM. Care of survivors. In: Nursing Care of Children and Adolescents with Cancer, Baggott CR, Kelly KP, Fochtman D, Foley GV (Eds), 3rd Edn. WB Saunders; Philadelphia 2002;426-65.
3. Marina N. Long-term survivors of childhood cancer: the medical consequences of cure. P Clin N Am. 1997;44:1021-42.
4. Wolfe J, Friebert S, Hilden J. Caring for children with advanced cancer integrating palliative care. Pediatr Clin N Am. 2002;49:1043-62.

Psychological Issues in Pediatric Oncology

Rakesh Mondal, Nibedita Chatterjee

As the management of pediatric oncology has revolutionized in last decades there are some interesting issues are coming up regarding the psychosocial aspect.

The issues can be broadly seen as impact of disease and medication on mental health. Some childhood cancers even mimic the symptoms of psychiatric disorders.

CHILDHOOD CANCERS RELATED TO PSYCHOLOGICAL ISSUES

Perhaps the greatest difference between patients in the adolescent and other age groups is in supportive care, particularly psychosocial care. Adolescents and young adults have special needs that are unique, broader in scope, and often more intense. Cancer therapy causes practical problems in social arenas. The dependence of adolescent and young adult patients on peer-group approval poses greater challenges when confronted with a diagnosis of cancer. Self-image, a critical determinant during this phase of life, is compromised by many of the adverse effects of therapy, such as alopecia, weight gain or loss, mucositis, dermatitis (acne, mouth sores), bleeding, infection and contagiousness, susceptibility to infection and need for isolation. Impaired sexuality, e.g. intimacy, impotency, risk of tetratogenicity, and mutilating surgery also poses problems. Other challenges include the loss of time from school, work, and community and the financial hardships that occur at an age when economic independence from family is an objective. A wide range of financial challenges occurs in this age group. There are the usual limitations in affording life, much more

once confounded by the costs of cancer treatment. There may be guilt if not attending to these responsibilities or stress and fatigue if trying to keep up a semblance of normal activity. Partner relationships are tested by the strain of the cancer diagnosis and its therapy. Whether a partner stays in the relationship is challenged by fear of relapse or infertility and may be influenced unduly in either direction by guilt or sympathy. Those contemplating having children may fear passing on a genetic predisposition to cancer. Medical professionals are often poorly equipped to deal with the psychosocial challenges within the age group and are often pressured by the need in these patients to increase compliance, reduce stress, and improve the quality of life.

Overall, the vast majority of cases of cancer diagnosed before the age of 30 years appear to be spontaneous and unrelated to either carcinogens in the environment or family cancer syndromes. This contrasts with known etiologies and contributing factors in older adults in whom many cancers have been strongly linked to environmental causes. Rare exceptions include clear cell adenocarcinoma of the vagina or uterine cervix and breast cancer caused by prenatal diethylstilbestrol, second malignant neoplasms in patients treated with chemotherapy and/or radiotherapy for a prior cancer, melanoma induced by ultraviolet light, cervical carcinoma resulting from human papillomavirus, Kaposi sarcoma and non-Hodgkin lymphoma arising in persons infected with human immunodeficiency virus, and Hodgkin and Burkitt's lymphomas resulting from Epstein-Barr virus. Given that the duration of exposure to potential environmental carcinogens is directly proportional to age, it is not surprising that tobacco, sunlight, or diet-related cancers are less likely to occur in older adolescents and young adults than in older persons. Skin cancer, lymphoma, sarcoma, thyroid cancer, and hepatic cancers may also occur at higher frequency during this period of life in persons with inherited conditions. In total, however, cancers attributable to environmental or inherited factors account for a small proportion of the cancers that occur during adolescence.

Nonetheless, adolescents should be made aware of environmental carcinogens, including tobacco, ultraviolet rays from the sun and tanning lamps, recreational drugs, alcohol, and sexually transmitted diseases, since exposure to these agents starts or intensifies during this age, and lifestyles are often established during adolescence. Cancer control efforts to reduce exposure to these carcinogens are unlikely to affect rates of cancers in young adults, but should decrease their rates as older adults.

Adolescent Care Facilities

Adolescent patients are seen by specialists, including house physicians, gynecologists, emergency physicians, gastroenterologists, dermatologists, neurologists, and other specialists. When the referral of an adolescent patient is made to an oncologist, it may be to a medical, radiation, surgical, gynecologic, or other oncologic specialist. The majority of 15- to 19-year-olds diagnosed with cancer are treated at adult facilities. In the end, the health care facility decision should be based in large part on which setting will provide the patient with the best outcome. If these are equivalent, social or supportive factors should next weigh into the decision.

Young adults with malignant melanoma, colorectal carcinoma, breast cancer, or epithelial ovarian cancer should be better served by medical oncologists, gynecologic oncologists, and surgical oncologists familiar with the cancers of adults. That most adult oncology centers have access to few services dedicated to older adolescent patients limits the comprehensiveness of care of the age group in the adult oncology setting.

Determining which facility is most appropriate certainly will vary from cancer-to-cancer and from case-to-case. Patients at any age who have a "pediatric"

tumor, such as rhabdomyosarcoma, Ewing sarcoma, and osteosarcoma, will probably benefit from the expertise of a pediatric oncologist. Individuals between the ages of 16 and 24 years may have varying levels of maturity and independence, and the choice of physician and setting for their care should be individually determined. They may be less aggressive with chemotherapy dosing than the pediatric oncologist whose patients, like young adults, can tolerate higher doses. Pediatric oncologists have also pioneered risk-adapted therapies to preserve fertility and reduce adverse effects on body image. On the other hand, services to facilitate gamete preservation are more limited in pediatric than in adult centers.

Ideally, centers and oncologists devoted to the care of this group of patients could be available to provide age-specific nursing care, recreation therapy, and peer companionship. There should be a discipline of adolescent oncology with its own training programs, science, research, clinical trials, and managed care institutions.

Communicating the Diagnosis

It follows certain principles as stated below:
1. Establish a protocol for communication.
2. Communicate immediately at diagnosis and follow-up later.
3. Communicate in a private and comfortable space.
4. Communicate with both parents, and other family members if desired.
5. Hold a separate session with the child.
6. Solicit questions from parents and child.
7. Communicate in ways that are sensitive to cultural differences.
8. Share information about the diagnosis and the plan for cure.
9. Share information on lifestyle and psychosocial issues.
10. Encourage the entire family to talk together.

MENTAL HEALTH PROBLEM AND CHILDHOOD CANCERS

People with mental disorders, especially clinical depression and bipolar disorder, have a high risk of developing certain cancers at younger ages, including brain and lung cancer.

Smoking and alcohol abuse are obvious reason in this pattern, both linked with clinical depression and lung cancer in studies. However, people with mental disorders were more likely to develop cancer at a younger age and had more brain and respiratory tumors. As expected, adolesent with mood disorders had higher odds of developing tobacco-related cancers, e.g. cancers of the mouth, throat, lung, etc. People with mental disorders have high rates of smoking and alcohol abuse, both of which increase the risk of tobacco-related cancers. Mood disorders were the most common mental disorder linked to cancer. A significant percent of women and men had anxiety disorders prior to their cancer diagnosis. Women who had a long history of chronic clinical depression have a higher risk of dying from breast cancer, which might be due to lack of compliance with treatment.

CHILDHOOD CANCERS MIMICKING THE PSYCHIATRIC DISORDERS

Fatigue is often found with lymphoma could be mistaken for depression. Leukemia and lymphoma and pancreatic cancer in some studies shown to have clinical depression as the primary symptom in recent years. When a patient has a sudden mood change, residents should be trained to look for organic causes of depression, like brain tumors at the earliest. Some mental health diseases are caused by the cancer. Mood disorders like clinical depression have been recognized as an early symptom of brain tumors. The increased pressure in the brain caused by the tumor can cause a variety of symptoms, such as seizures or mental disturbances including depression. These patients should have brain imaging and other tests. The current question that makes oncologist wonder if the cancer itself is causing depression with alteration in immune system.

Psychosocial Support

The Internet technology that has seen an explosion of usage, may be a way for patients with cancer to obtain information and support through websites as well as online communication platforms. Many of these adolescents are also accessing the internet for health care information. Websites; by logging on to the World Wide Web, patients with cancer can access a wealth of information about cancer from sources, such as national cancer organizations, voluntary associations, and personal websites created by individuals with cancer. Websites are being increasingly used as sources of health information and support. Cancer-related websites revealed that most users of the site believed that information from the internet helped them to cope better with cancer. The internet may be a particularly appropriate mode of intervention for adolescents with cancer. It can provide information to young people who feel frustrated by restricted access to health care resources or who feel anxious about asking sensitive health questions. Online support groups can be a valuable source of information and social support. Bulletin boards, newsgroups, and chatrooms are now being used by people with cancer to find each other online and offer advice and peer support. These are online platforms where users can post, read and respond to text messages on particular topics. Facebook, chatrooms are online communication systems that allow users to exchange text messages. An online computer network; can provide information and support, websites can be surfed for information, and online support groups and bulletin boards. Facebook can provide contact with peers. These are all disparate sources of support reported significantly lower degrees of pain intensity, pain aversiveness, and anxiety. Support is available to childhood cancer survivors and their families who have anxiety and depression after treatment. These are just a few of the many resources available:

a. American Cancer Society (www.cancer.org); This site provides web-based support network, other programs and services, and stories of hope for cancer survivors and their families.

b. Candlelighters Childhood Cancer Foundation (www.candlelighters.org); This site offers education, support, service, and advocacy for childhood cancer survivors, their families and the professionals who care for them.

c. Cure Search (www.curesearch.org); This site provides parents and families with information related to specific cancer type, treatment stage and age group as well as tips on navigating the health care system, getting and giving support, and maintaining a healthy lifestyle.

d. Patient Centered Guides (www.patientcenters.com/survivors); This site provides a list of follow-up clinics for childhood cancer survivors and articles related to psychosocial aspects of survivorship.

e. The Anxiety Disorders Association of America (www.adaa.org): This site provides information that can help people with anxiety disorder find treatment and develop self-help skills.

SUGGESTED READING

1. Barr RD. On cancer control and the adolescent. Med Pediatr Oncol. 1999;32:404-10.
2. Biermann JS, Golladay GJ, Greenfield ML, Baker LH. Evaluation of cancer information on the internet. Cancer. 1999;86:381-90.
3. Chen X, Siu LL. Impact of the media and the internet on oncology: survey of cancer patients and oncologists in Canada. Journal of Clinical Oncology. 2001;19: 4291-7.
4. Cotterill S. Pediatric oncology and the Internet. Pediatric Hematology and Oncology. 2001;18:393-5.
5. Eysenbach G, et el. Empirical studies assessing the quality of health information for consumers on the world wide web: a systematic review. Journal of the American Medical Association. 2002;287:2691-2700.
6. Giuseppe Masera, SIOP Working Committee on Psychosocial Issues in Pediatric Oncology: Guidelines for Communication of the Diagnosis; Medical and Pediatric Oncology. 1997;28:382-5.
7. Kupst MJ, Bingen K. Stress and coping in the pediatric cancer experience. In: RT Brown (Ed.) Pediatric Hematology/Oncology: A Biopsychosocial Approach. New York: Oxford University Press 2006.
8. NCCN. NCCN Clinical Practice Guidelines in Oncology: Distress Management, 2006. http://www.nccn.org/professionals/physician_gls/PDF/distress.pdf.
9. Pao M, Ballard E, Rosenstein D, Wiener L, Wayne A. psychotropic medication use in pediatric oncology patients. Archives of Pediatrics and Adolescent Medicine. 2006;160:818-22.
10. Sharp J. The internet: Changing the way cancer survivors receive support. Cancer Practice. 2000;8:145-7.
11. Tamaroff MH, Festa RS, Adesman AR, Walco GA. Therapeutic adherence to oral medication regimens by adolescents with cancer. II. Clinical and psychologic correlates. J Pediatr. 1992;120:813-7.
12. Wiener L, Hersh SP Kazak A. Psychiatric and psychosocial support for child and family. In: Principles and Practice of Pediatric Oncology. (5th Edition) Pizzo, PA and Poplack, DG (Eds). Lippincott, Philadelphia, 2006.

39 Nursing Practices in Pediatric Oncology

Madhumita Nandi, Dipti Bhattacharya

Optimal nursing care for children and adolescents with cancer is as important as the actual treatment of cancer. The expertise in oncology nursing practice should be such that it has the vision to deliver the highest quality of care to children and adolescents diagnosed with cancer. The pediatric oncology nurse's role should be focused on the dying child and bereaved family. A pediatric oncology nurse should have a broad knowledge base of childhood cancer, its treatment, side effects including late effects.

Advances in treatment, improved supportive therapies and the use of clinical trials have led to dramatic increase in survival rates for children diagnosed with malignancies. Eighty percent of children diagnosed with cancer are surviving these previously fatal diseases and re-entering society "cured" of their primary cancer. These children, after they are 'cured', look forward to a bright, fruitful and productive future which is expected to be 'disease free'.

But, their future life may not be always 'event-free' as they are always at risk for the development of physical and psychosocial late effects due to specific chemotherapeutic, surgical and radiation treatments. The risk of late effects is varied and the intensity and type is dependent on several factors including individual patient characteristics, the diagnosis or disease process, and the type treatment received. Some of these late effects include alterations in growth and development, fertility problems, cognitive impairment, organ system damage, psychological problems including quality of life issues, employment, and marriage.

Since the majority of survivors do not seek long-term cancer–related or treatment-related follow-up care, risk factor identification and early detection of health care problems may be compromised. Additionally, early detection of problems and subsequent treatment may be compromised by survivor's lack of knowledge regarding risk and the need for follow-up care. Due to knowledge deficits and the lack of cancer-related or treatment-related health care follow-up, the impact of treatment on the development of future healthcare problems cannot be fully evaluated.

Pediatric oncology nursing is developing as the professional stream for promoting optimal nursing care for children suffering from cancer and the survivors from this disease. The focus of care for these patients, from the nurses' perspective must involve education, early detection and intervention for deleterious physical or psychosocial effects of therapy, and modified health behaviors to promote wellness. The goal of care is to promote the development of young adults who are capable of leading fulfilling and productive lives physically, psychologically and socio-economically. These professionals play an integral role in the care of this growing population of pediatric cancer survivors and in educating the community at large regarding their specific needs.

Pediatric oncology nursing care must encompass the evolving area of long-term toxicities including the physical and psychosocial needs of the pediatric cancer patient matures. They should be able to explore the issues concerning care of pediatric cancer survivors and make several recommendations to improve survivor health care and quality of life.

Pediatric oncology nursing is yet to gain momentum as a separate specialty in India. In 1978, the Association of Pediatric Oncology Nurses (APON) developed *standards of nursing practice* for pediatric oncology nurses. These standards were later revised in 1987 to reflect both nursing process and outcome standards, including statements. To address continuing changes in pediatric cancer care, the nursing document has been periodically updated.

The *Pediatric Oncology Nursing Scope and Standards of Practice* (2007) is a revision of the Scope *and Standards of Pediatric Oncology Nursing Practice* (2000). It incorporates key aspects of previously published standards from organizations such as the American Nurses Association, the Society of Pediatric Nursing, and the Oncology Nursing Society. Currently the *Scope and Standards* reflects the ongoing changes in nursing practice, describes, and defines the role of the professional pediatric oncology registered nurse and the pediatric oncology advanced practice registered nurse.

APHON (Association of Pediatric Hematology/Oncology Nurses) is the leading professional organization, with more than 2,500 members, for registered nurses caring for children, adolescents, and young adults with cancer and blood disorders and their families in west. Its mission is to provide and promote expert practice in pediatric hematology/oncology nursing to its members and the public at large.

The following is the skilled development of Association of Pediatric Hematology/Oncology Nurses:

1. Pediatric oncology nurses acquire knowledge about late effects of cancer therapy to provide expertise in heath care maintenance, early identification of recurrence or second malignancy, and timely identification/treatment of physical and psychosocial sequel.
2. Pediatric oncology nurses facilitate the development of optimal adaptation to long-term survival for the survivor and family. This can be accomplished by assisting survivors or families in acquiring

developmentally appropriate knowledge of the cancer diagnosis, the cancer treatment and implications of the treatment on future health outcomes.

3. Pediatric oncology nurses should review, utilize, participate in or disseminate research relevant to the cancer survivor population.
4. Pediatric oncology nurses act as advocates for cancer survivors by fostering public education about survivorship issues and promoting awareness of survivor health care needs.
5. Whenever possible, pediatric oncology nurses should participate in efforts to decrease barriers to cancer survivor care and should encourage survivors to seek appropriate cancer-related follow-up care.
6. Programs need to be developed which focus on the medical and psychosocial care of the pediatric cancer survivor. These programs should include a multidisciplinary team with expertise to address survivor needs. Ideally, the team should consist of the survivor and family, a pediatric oncology nurse, a pediatric oncologist, social worker, subspecialists or consultants, and access to adult health care providers when health care issues are outside the expertise of the pediatric multidisciplinary team. Adult health care providers should become integral participants in the care of the adult cancer survivor.

The APHON further envisages the following duties and responsibilities of a Pediatric Nurse Practitioner.

CLINICAL

- Works in conjunction with the medical staff and nursing to facilitate patient management through the health care system, thus exercises independent judgment in the assessment, diagnosing and initiation of delegated medical processes or procedures.
- Performs and documents comprehensive health histories and physical assessments on assigned pediatric patients and episodic evaluation on others, to include initiation of resuscitation or other appropriate emergency therapy as needed.
- Formulates diagnoses and identifies problems and health risk profiles of selected pediatric patients and

documents and communicates this information to other members of the health care team.

- Performs orders and interprets diagnostic studies, such as X-rays and laboratory tests, in consultation with pediatric consultant.
- Performs procedures within scope of practice.
- Orders medications, treatments and therapies in accordance with oncologist.
- Requests consultation and initiates referrals to other health care providers.
- Evaluates and analyzes patient responses to the disease process or therapeutic or diagnostic interventions.
- Provides information and support to patients and families regarding disease process and treatment plan, thus facilitating communication between patients, families and health care team.
- Educates patient and families regarding planned diagnostic procedures, medications, treatments and post-hospital care.
- Writes discharge orders and coordinates plans for follow-up care.
- Evaluates and consults with selected patients and families in outpatient setting at the time of follow-up appointments regarding post-hospitalized course of care.

QUALITY IMPROVEMENT INITIATIVES

- Examines systems and processes in pediatric oncology populations and recommends, develops, implements and evaluates strategies for improvement.
- Facilitates communication between medical and nursing teams.
- Promotes timely and compassionate communication between families and health care team.
- Participates in multidisciplinary discharge rounds.
- Participating in medical and nursing research projects. Identifying areas related to nursing practice that requires classification or advancement through the research process.

LEADERSHIP

- Serves on selected committees of nursing, medical and administrative personnel.
- Serves as a member of "Acute Care Clinical Leadership Team".
- Actively participates in the clinical experience of undergraduate and graduate nurses.
- Actively participates in the clinical experience of medical students, interns and residents.

EDUCATION

- Participates in activities that contribute to the education of other health care professionals.
- Serves as preceptor for undergraduate, graduate and advanced practice nurses.
- Develops and presents educational programs to the medical and nursing personnel.
- Participates in the design and development of teaching materials for patients and families.

PROFESSIONAL DEVELOPMENT

- Updates practice through continuing education by attending pediatric conferences, rounds, reports, lectures, journal clubs, conferences, etc.
- Serves as clinical resource in the care of pediatric oncology patients to nursing, medical and allied health care practitioners.
- Seeks professional growth opportunities that enhance professional practice through both formal and informal activities.
- Contributes to the community by being active in selected local or state volunteer activity.

FUTURE IMPLICATIONS

Pediatric oncology nurses are in a position to continually affect health related outcomes in the growing population of pediatric cancer survivors. By acquiring knowledge about late toxicities of cancer therapy, pediatric oncology nurses will become key health care providers and educators for the survivor population. They should work in tandem with other health care providers for childhood center.

SUGGESTED READING

1. Eshelman D, Childhood Cancer Survivor Care APON Position Paper. Association of Pediatric Oncology Nurses, 2003.
2. Jacobs LA (Ed). Statement on the scope and standards of advanced practice nursing in oncology. 3rd edition Pittsburgh, PA: Oncology Nursing, 2003.
3. Nelson MB, Forte K, Freiburg D, Hooke MC, Kelly KP, O'Neill JB. Pediatric Oncology Nursing: Scope and Standards of Practice, 2007.
4. Oncology Nursing Society. Oncology nursing society position paper on quality cancer care. Oncology Nursing Forum, 1997;24:951-3.
5. Sanders J, Glader B, Cairo M, Finklestein J, Forman E, Green DM, et al. Section on hematology/oncology executive committee: Guidelines for the pediatric cancer center and role of such centers in diagnosis and treatment. Pediatrics. 1997;99:139-41.
6. http///www.aphon.org

40 Managing Pediatric Cancer Patients with Limited Resources

Sanat Ghosh

INTRODUCTION

Treatment of malignancy in developed countries is highly specialized. The essential features of such specialized centers are the availability of improved diagnosis, use of modern uniform protocol-based therapy, ample supply of medicines, ready access to intensive care, written evidence-based supportive care guidelines, improved identification and treatment of co-morbid conditions (malnutrition, infections).

In developing countries only a few such centers are available, as centers with such features are difficult to establish in poor socio-economic conditions. Thus, 60% of world's cancer patients have little or no access to specialized treatment centers and their survival rates are predictably inferior to those in centers with advance health care system.

Clearly, there remains a significant gap between an 80% cure rate of acute lymphoblastic leukemia in resource rich countries and 35% cure rate in many resource poor countries. The inequality in cancer treatment between developing and developed countries possesses the great challenge that has only began to be addressed.

Perhaps, the most compelling reason against investing in better cancer treatment for children in poor countries is that millions of deaths can be prevented by combating infectious diseases with relatively inexpensive strategies. Indeed, the World Health Organization and many international charities have committed to use their resources in reducing the mortalities from infectious diseases by two-thirds during the next decade. Naturally, non-communicable diseases and chronic childhood diseases are not among the priorities of these organizations. The profile of childhood morbidity and mortality is rapidly changing in resource poor countries with control of infectious diseases. As a result, the rate of death from cancers is becoming the leading cause of childhood mortality. In children, aged 1–14 years cancer is the leading cause of disease-related childhood death in the United States but the third leading cause in Brazil and forth in El Salvador. Although giving priorities in using resources to fight infections clearly has the potential to save most of the children in developing countries, we have always reason to argue for wider access to effective cancer treatment. This argument is not only based on humanitarian considerations, but it also addresses the rapidly changing profile of causes of illness and death among the children in countries with limited resources.

Because of high incidence and curability, acute lymphoblastic leukemia is the logical initial target for pediatric cancer programs. In the present article also, emphasis will be given on acute lymphoblastic leukemia among childhood malignancies for the same reason.

CAUSES OF TREATMENT FAILURE IN RESOURCE POOR COUNTRIES

To understand the causes of treatment failure of childhood cancers in resource poor countries, the reports of some series of cases treated in resource poor conditions are evaluated.

On retrospective evaluation of 168 patients of acute lymphoblastic leukemia, treated in Honduras, abandonment of treatment (n=38) and treatment related toxic effects (n=35) were found to be the common cause of treatment failure. It was realized that prolonged travel time to the treatment facility was the main cause of abandonment of treatment. Outcome could be substantially improved by interventions that help to prevent abandonment of therapy, e.g. funding for transport, satellite clinics and support groups and by prompt treatment of therapy-related complications.

Relapse, abandonment of therapy, delayed diagnosis, co-morbid conditions, death from toxicity due to sub-optimal supportive care were found to be the main cause of treatment failure and establishment of a dedicated pediatric oncology program in El Salvador with strategies to reduce some of these problems was associated with increase in ALL survival from 5 to 48%.

In the 1970's, survival rates after treatment of ALL in children in India were poor even in specialized cancer centers. The introduction of a standard treatment protocol (MCP 841) and improvement of supportive care in the three major cancer centers in India Cancer Institute, Chennai, Tata Memorial Hospital, Mumbai, All India Institute of Medical Sciences, Delhi, led to an increase in the event-free survival rate from less than 20% to (45–60)% at four years. When patient characteristics from all three Indian centers were compared to the published series from western nations, more extensive disease at presentation was found in Indian patients which might be due to delayed diagnosis. The worse outcome of treatment in Indian patients was due to higher rate of toxic death likely to have arisen from a combination of more extensive disease at diagnosis, co-morbid conditions, e.g. inter-current infections, difference in the level of hygiene, poor access to acute care and limited supportive care facilities in Indian hospitals.

It is also reviewed that in India, although there are several oncology institutions and regional cancer centers, very few patients have access to specialized treatment. The reasons for this are low socio-economic status, long distance from the treatment center, the financial burden of chemotherapy, lack of supportive treatment and simultaneous support to the family backbone.

Outcome of 375 children with ALL diagnosed between 1980 to 2002 at a pediatric hospital in the resource poor city of Recife, Brazil was evaluated. During the early period (1980–1989) patients were treated at a public general hospital with no pediatric oncology unit, protocol-based therapy, consistent supply of medicines, specially trained nurses, 24 hours physician coverage and little access to intensive care. During the middle period (1994–1997), the children were treated with definite protocol but were cared for in the general wards by nurses who had no specialized oncology training. During the recent period (1997–2002), patients were treated with a definite protocol in a dedicated pediatric oncology unit staffed continuously by pediatric oncologists and oncology trained nurses and had rapid access to intensive care. The five years event-free survival estimate was 32% for the early period, 47% for the middle period and 63% for the recent period. The hazard ratio for treatment failure was high for high-risk versus standard-risk ALL. The later emphasized the need for improved diagnosis for risk categorization of ALL patients.

In summary, treatment failure for childhood cancers in poorly developed pediatric centers and in early part of the recently developed pediatric oncology centers in resource-poor countries are caused by relapsed disease, abandonment of therapy and death from infections and hemorrhage. The high rate of relapse resulted from the absence of improved diagnosis, standardized protocol-based therapy, unreliable supply of medicines and delayed diagnosis resulting in extensive disease at diagnosis. Abandonment of therapy is caused by long distance of the treating center, cost related to travel and long stay of the patient and the family members at the treating centers, cost of therapy, absence of support to the family backbone while staying at the treating center long distance away. Death from toxicity was caused by lack of oncology trained nurses, 24 hours on-site pediatric oncologist, ready access to intensive care, written evidence-based supportive care guidelines, improved identification and treatment of co-morbid conditions, adequate and regular supply of medicines and blood products.

REQUIREMENTS TO IMPROVE THE OUTCOME

Based on the causes of treatment failure, leaders in international pediatric oncology have summarized key elements of successful treatment of cancer in resource poor countries, which are as follows:

Identification of Local Needs

Effective treatment of childhood cancers requires specialized treatment center which is a dedicated multi-disciplinary hospital with ready access to intensive care facility, improved supportive care, 24 hours on-site oncologist and oncology trained nurses. For poor socio-economic conditions number of such centers is scanty. Thus, most of the pediatric cancer patients of resource poor countries do not have access to specialized treatment facility. This leads to high rate of abandonment of treatment. If anything is to be done to bring the benefits of the modern cancer treatment to more children, it is to expand the access to treatment centers. This can be achieved by increasing the number of specialized cancer treatment centers and establishing satellite centers and satellite clinics under each specialized treatment center.

Mobilization of the Community

Mobilization of the community is required to support the family. Community mobilization may result in establishment of childhood cancer support groups in the form of non-profit, non-government foundation to support the needs of the children with cancer by raising fund in the private sector to assist families with lodging, transportation and the cost of treatment not covered by the hospitals. They would identify the correctable defects in the health care system and lobby for the required changes.

Partnership with Established Center

This strategy emphasizes a partnership (twinning) between institutions in developed countries and those in underdeveloped countries to have long-term success. Twinning fosters interactions between public hospitals in developing countries and established cancer treatment centers in developed countries with the goal of improving survival rates of childhood cancer patients. Such alliance has generated sufficient momentum to allow some hospitals in Central and South America to begin sharing their expertise with other oncologists in the developing regions. Examples of such twinning approach are existing in Central and South America, north-east Africa and south-east Asia for as long as ten years.

Development of Multi-disciplinary Health Care System with Improvement of Supportive Care

Treatment of childhood cancers has improved to a great extent with establishment of specialized cancer treatment center. The essential features of such centers are improved diagnosis, ample supply of medicines and blood products, access to intensive care facility, improved supportive care, 24 hours on-site pediatric oncologists and oncology trained nurses. They would function as specialized pediatric cancer treatment centers and provide necessary support to the satellite centers or clinics. Such centers along with their satellite centers and clinics would function as a backbone to the childhood cancer treatment program.

Use of Standardized Definite Treatment Protocol

Use of a uniform standardized protocol for treatment of childhood cancer is a very essential and primary requirement to improve survival.

Clinical Research

Finally clinical research is essential to identify the cause of treatment failure and adopt treatment protocols to local conditions as demonstrated in Honduras, Chile and Maxico.

The high cure rates of childhood malignancy in Europe and United States are achieved during last 40 years. It is proved that proven treatment regimens can be adopted for use in a resource poor condition in much less time. In Recife, the five years event-free survival increased from 32 to 63% in a decade despite little change in region's economy and rate of infant mortality (85 per 1000 live births in 1991 versus 74 in 2000).

CONCLUSION

Treatment of childhood cancers in a dedicated pediatric oncology unit using a comprehensive multi-disciplinary team approach, protocol based therapy, wide access to treatment facility, locally funded family support system is associated with improved outcome even in areas with limited economic resources.

SUGGESTED READING

1. Cambell M, Salgado C, et al. Improved outcome for ALL in children of a developing country: results of the Chi Lean National Trial PINDA 87. Med Pediatr Oncol. 1999;33:88-94.
2. Howard SC, Pedrosa M, Lins M, et al. Establishment of a pediatric oncology program and outcomes of acute lymphoblastic leukemia in a resource poor area. JAMA. 2004;291:2471-5.
3. Magrath I, Shanta V, Advani S, et al. Treatment of acute lymphoblastic leukemia in countries with limited resources, lessons from use of a single protocol in India over a twenty-year period. Eur J of Can. 2005;41:1570-83.
4. Menon J, Mathews L, Purushothaman KK. Treating leukemia in a resource-poor setting. Indian Pediatrics. 2008;45:410-2.
5. Metzger M, Howard S, Fu L, et al. Outcome of childhood acute lymphoblastic leukemia in resource poor countries. The Lancet. 362(9385):706-8.
6. Pedrosa F, Bonilla M, Liu et al. Effect of malnutrition at the time of diagnosis in the survival of children treated for cancer in El Salvador and Northern Brazil. J Pediatr Hematol Oncol. 2000;22:502-5.
7. Pui Ch, Cheng C, Leung W, et al. Extended follow-up of long-term survivors of childhood acute lymphoblastic leukemia. N Engl J Med 2003;349:640-9 [Erratum, N Engl J Med. 2003;349:1299].
8. Pui CH, Ribeiro RC. International collaboration on childhood leukemia. Int J Hematol. 2003;78:383-9.
9. Raul C, Ribeino, Ching-Hon Pui. Saving the children-improving childhood cancer treatment in developing countries. N Eng J Med. 2005;352;21:2158-60.
10. Rivera-luna R, et al. B-lineage ALL of childhood: an institutional experience. Arch Med Res. 1997;28:233-9.
11. Unicef. State of the world's children 2004. Available at http:/www.unicef.org/sowe04/index.html.
12. Wilimas JA, Ribeiro RC. Pediatric hemotology oncology outreach for developing countries. Hematol Oncol Clin North Am. 2001;41:136-40.
13. World Health Organization. Statistical information. available at http:/www.who.int/whosis/menu.cfm.

Training and Research in Pediatric Oncology

Rakesh Mondal, Ashish Mukherjee, Sumantra Sarkar

Training and research in pediatric oncology are tried to explain in question-answer format below.

WHAT DOES A PEDIATRIC ONCOLOGIST DO?

A pediatric oncologist is a physician, who has completed a minimum of 6 years of training after medical school. The training begins with a 3-year residency in pediatrics. During this time, residents gain some exposure to pediatric hematology-oncology as part of required and elective inpatient and outpatient rotations. Some residency programs also offer opportunities to engage in a short-term clinical or laboratory research project. Many who enter the field develop their initial interest as pediatric residents experiencing the challenges and joys of caring for children with complex disorders such as cancer. Another related specialty is medical oncology. The duration of training for this specialty is similar; however, medical oncologists care for adult patients. Their residency is in internal medicine rather than pediatrics, and their fellowship training emphasizes disorders common in adults. Pediatric oncology deals primarily with acute lymphoblastic leukemia, and embryonal tumors. Adult specialists, on the other hand, focus more on oncology (especially solid tumors). Other specialties that overlap with pediatric oncology are radiology and pathology, with a focus on cancer diagnosis or transfusion medicine; laboratory hematology; and cytogenetics. Although these specialists are engaged in teaching and research, they have little or no direct patient contact, unlike pediatric

hematologists-oncologists. The link between pediatric oncology has a historical basis. Children with acute leukemia, the most serious of the relatively common oncologic disorders, are usually referred to and cared for by hematologists. As chemotherapy and other treatment approaches were developed during the 1950s and 1960s, these hematology specialists, who were familiar with cancer chemotherapy, began to also care for and study children with solid tumors. Today pediatric oncology specialists are involved with a wide range of tumors, from hemangiomas and other benign vascular malformations to malignant brain neoplasms.

IS PEDIATRIC ONCOLOGY DEPRESSING?

Cancer remains the leading cause of death from disease in children younger than 15 years old. Most of us have been touched by loved ones who have succumbed to cancer. Dealing with death and dying scenarios can be depressing, but the field of pediatric oncology is certainly not. Survival rates for most childhood cancers have increased; almost all children are now treated with curative intent and in most cases treatments are successful. Cure rates for all childhood cancers are approximately 75%, and most centers have "off therapy" programs to follow these children. Death rates for other diseases that pediatric oncologists have declined dramatically, so many children with hematologic disorders are expected to have a nearly normal lifespan. Pediatric oncology specialists now practice as part of multidisciplinary teams, with many providing care and comfort to dying children and their families. Many find it rewarding to care for patients with complex diseases and to provide long-term care for patients during treatment and after therapy. The emerging field of palliative care provides extensive support and resources for dying patients, families, physicians and the treatment team.

WHAT IS THE LIFESTYLE OF A PEDIATRIC ONCOLOGY SPECIALIST?

Personal time and family life are important for every person. Despite the hard work, most pediatric oncology specialists are able to design their career so that their professional life is well balanced with leisure and family time. However, virtually all work more than 40 hours a week, so those considering a pediatric oncology career should be prepared to work hard during training and thereafter.

WHAT ABOUT REMUNERATION?

Pediatric hematology-oncology specialists generally earn salaries similar to those of other pediatric subspecialists. Salaries in private practice are often somewhat higher than in the academic arena, although less so than in previous years. However, most employment opportunities for pediatric oncology specialists offer a comfortable lifestyle.

WHAT ARE THE CAREER CHOICES FOR A PEDIATRIC ONCOLOGY SPECIALIST?

Though widely varied, the most common pathway after completing a fellowship is a position as an instructor or assistant professor of pediatrics in an academic pediatric oncology division. Primary duties, which vary from day-to-day and are often unpredictable (one reason it is so interesting), are diagnosing and caring for children with blood diseases and cancer; teaching medical students, residents, fellows, and other healthcare professionals; and conducting clinical research through case studies and clinical trials. Most teaching activities are performed one-on-one in the clinic or at the bedside, rather than as didactic lectures in the classroom. Most pediatric

oncology specialists are part of a team of physicians, advanced practice nurses, social workers and other healthcare professionals in an academic group practice. A small but important subset of pediatric oncology specialists, after completing their standard fellowship training, devote extra years to laboratory experience, which sometimes follows or includes obtaining a doctoral degree. This research is usually performed in basic science laboratories. These individuals usually spend the majority of their time conducting laboratory research in a basic or translational research area of pediatric oncology. A smaller but important percentage of their time is devoted to the clinical duties outlined above. Determining the causes of these diseases and discovering improved treatments rest in better understanding of the fundamental biology of cancer and the blood, hence it is logical that some individuals in the specialty engage in laboratory research. Other researchers focus on clinical investigation. These individuals often receive extended training in epidemiology, biostatistics and protocol designing, and some obtain a master's degree in public health. They conduct studies for better understanding of the cause and nature of disease and to develop improved treatment strategies through randomized clinical trials or health services research. This is an exciting pathway for many young pediatric oncology specialists. A few other specialists are engaged in administrative activities as division chiefs, department chairs and deans. Still others pursue the private practice of pediatric oncology or are employed by pharmaceutical firms.

In addition, opportunities exist for the pediatric oncology specialist to travel and participate in exciting scientific meetings, to network and become friends with colleagues from around the world, and to design and participate in summer camping experiences and other support activities for patients and their families.

IS IT POSSIBLE TO FURTHER SUBSPECIALIZE IN SOME ASPECTS OF ONCOLOGY AFTER RECEIVING THE GENERAL TRAINING?

Many pediatric oncology specialists care for patients with diverse diseases. However others, especially those on larger medical school faculties or for whom research constitutes a significant portion of their duties, focus on the field in which they develop special expertise. Many individuals emphasize clinical oncology, and some narrow their expertise specifically to solid tumors or to a specific type of tumor (e.g. neuroblastoma, bone tumors). Others deal primarily with acute leukemia, neuro-oncology (brain tumors), cancer pharmacology, or development of experimental agents. An emerging field is bone marrow (stem cell) transplantation. Some pediatric oncology specialists devote most or all of their time to diagnosing and caring for the transplant patient and conducting clinical, translational or laboratory research in transplantation.

Following are some specialized fields of training, which may be taken by the aspirant oncologist to be expert in those fields:

General Pediatric Hematology-Oncology

It provides the trainees with instruction and experience in the pathophysiology of pediatric hematologic and oncologic disorders, as well as in the clinical diagnosis and management of these disorders. Upon completion of the training program, fellows will be competent in the clinical practice of pediatric hematology-oncology and will be prepared to conduct meaningful clinical, translational or laboratory-based research. The residents should receive training in ethics, biostatistics, administration and teaching.

Leukemia/Lymphoma Training

This training helps and teaches how to diagnose leukemia and lymphoma in children and adolescents, determine the appropriate treatment plan and enroll patients on clinical protocols.

Solid Tumor Training

Through this training, one can learn the essential clinical, radiographic and biologic characteristics associated with various solid tumors seen in children and adolescent and their management.

Bone Marrow Transplant Training

This provides an introduction to the principles of autologous and allogeneic hematopoietic stem cell transplantation and the general evaluation and management of patients with disorders treated by hematopoietic stem cell transplantation.

Neuro-oncology Training

This training helps to learn the essential clinical, radiographic and biologic characteristics associated with various brain tumors seen in infants, children and adolescent and their management.

Follow-up Clinic

This is for learning the outpatient management of newly diagnosed and continuing patients with hematologic and oncologic disorders.

Hemato-pathology Rotation

Familiarize the residents with the basic microscopic features of normal peripheral blood, bone marrow and lymphoid organs in pediatric patients. Provide the basic knowledge necessary to recognize the microscopic features of the main pediatric malignant hematopoietic tumors of bone marrow and lymph nodes.

Radiation Oncology

Residents in oncology are encouraged to spend time in radiation oncology to improve their understanding of the role of radiation therapy in the treatment of children. A one week rotation has been organized during which time the resident is expected to experience, through observation or participation: (a) A radiation oncology consultation; (b) Informed consent discussion; (c) Simulation procedure; (d) Treatment planning, and; (e) Treatment delivery.

Other Key Areas of Research

Molecular Oncology Program include oncogenes and tumor suppressors, cell cycle regulators, chimeric transcription factors, and molecules governing stress responses, apoptosis, and checkpoint control. The program encourages the application of emerging laboratory findings in a practical clinical setting. The Transplantation & Gene Therapy Program is focused mainly on diseases that may be treated by manipulation of hematopoietic stem cells and their progeny by effective transfer of genes.

Trainees participate in the research activities of the institution through patient care activities, by enrolling patients on protocols by their eligibility for protocol enrollment, following protocol guidelines and carefully documenting protocol events. Preparation for important institutional presentations often requires reviews of patient materials and these reviews occasionally lead to publishable results. Research mentors may be selected from any ongoing clinical or laboratory-based research program.

SUGGESTED READING

1. Agarwal BR, Marwaha RK, Kurkuse PA. Indian National Training Project Practice Pediatric Oncology (INTPPO): 2nd National teachers meeting, Consensus report. Med Pediatr Oncol. 2002;39:251.

2. Arora B, Banavali SD. Pediatric oncology in India: Past, present and future. Indian J Med Pediatr Oncol. 2009;30:121-3.

3. Dix D, Gulati S, Robinson P, et al. Demands and rewards associated with working in pediatric oncology and a qualitative study of Canadian healthcare providers. J Pediatr Hematol Oncol. 2012;34:430-5.

42 Cancer Vaccines

Pragya Pant, Goutam Mukherjee, Toshibananda Bag

Vaccines have been considered as one of the most significant inventions of the past century. They are among the safest and most cost-effective agents for disease prevention. In the past few decades, focus has shifted towards the search for vaccines against non-infectious diseases like malignancies.

Cancer vaccines are medicines that belong to a class of substances known as 'biological response modifiers'. Biological response modifiers work by stimulating or restoring the immune system's ability to fight infections and disease. Cancer vaccines are designed to boost the body's natural ability to protect itself, through the immune system, from dangers posed by damaged or abnormal cells such as cancer cells.

WHAT ARE CANCER VACCINES?

The term cancer vaccine refers to a vaccine that either prevents infections with viruses which predispose to malignancies, treats already existent malignancy, or prevents the development of cancer in certain high-risk individuals.

There are two broad types of cancer vaccines:

- Preventive (or prophylactic) vaccines, which are intended to prevent cancer from developing in healthy people. Preventive vaccines, which are commercially available for cervical cancer and liver cancer, block infection with the causative agents of human papillomavirus and hepatitis B virus, respectively. So, they are not cancer vaccines in the true sense.
- Treatment (or therapeutic) vaccines, which are intended to treat an existing cancer by strengthening the body's natural defenses against the cancer. Cancer vaccines are thought of as active immunotherapies because they "boost" the body's own immune system response to cancer cells, which is generally low. They should be specific because they should only affect the cancer cells. These vaccines do not just boost the immune system in general; they cause the immune system to attack cells with one or more specific antigens. Because the immune system has special cells for memory, it's hoped that the drugs will help keep cancer from coming back.

A true cancer vaccine has cancer cells, parts of cells, or pure antigens. It may be combined with other substances or cells called adjuvants that help boost the immune response even further.

Using vaccines in the treatment of cancer is relatively new, and chiefly experimental. Therapeutic vaccines for breast, lung, colon, skin, renal, prostate and other cancers are now being investigated in clinical trials.

HOW DO CANCER PREVENTIVE VACCINES WORK?

Persistent infection by several microbial agents is responsible for at least 15 to 25% of cancer globally, including most cancers of the liver, stomach and cervix. The percentage is lower in developed than developing countries.

Cancer preventive vaccines target infectious agents that cause or contribute to the development of cancer.

These vaccines do not target cancer cells; they target the viruses that can cause these cancers. They are similar to traditional vaccines, which help prevent infectious diseases, such as measles or polio, by protecting the body against infection. Both cancer preventive vaccines and traditional vaccines are based on antigens that are carried by infectious agents and that are relatively easy for the immune system to recognize as foreign.

WHAT CANCER PREVENTIVE VACCINES ARE AVAILABLE IN THE MARKET?

The Food and Drug Administration (FDA) has approved two vaccines, Gardasil® and Cervarix®, that protect against infection by the two types of HPV—types 16 and 18—that cause approximately 70 percent of all cases of cervical cancer worldwide. At least 17 other types of HPV are responsible for the remaining 30 percent of cervical cancer cases. HPV types 16 and/or 18 also cause some vaginal, vulvar, anal, penile and oropharyngeal cancers.

In addition, gardasil protects against infection by two additional HPV types, 6 and 11, which are responsible for about 90 percent of all cases of genital warts in males and females but do not cause cervical cancer.

Gardasil, manufactured by Merck and Company, is based on HPV antigens that are proteins. These proteins are used in the laboratory to make four different types of "virus-like particles," or VLPs, that correspond to HPV types 6, 11, 16 and 18. The four types of VLPs are then combined to make the vaccine. Because gardasil targets four HPV types, it is called a quadrivalent vaccine (11). In contrast with traditional vaccines, which are often composed of weakened whole microbes, VLPs are not infectious. However, the VLPs in gardasil are still able to stimulate the production of antibodies against HPV types 6, 11, 16 and 18.

Cervarix, manufactured by GlaxoSmithKline, is a bivalent vaccine. It is composed of VLPs made with proteins from HPV types 16 and 18. In addition, there is some initial evidence that cervarix provides partial protection against a few additional HPV types that can cause cancer. However, more studies will be needed to understand the magnitude and impact of this effect.

Gardasil is approved for use in females to prevent cervical cancer and some vulvar and vaginal cancers caused by HPV types 16 and 18, and for use in males and females to prevent anal cancer and precancerous anal lesions caused by these HPV types. Gardasil is also approved for use in males and females to prevent genital warts caused by HPV types 6 and 11. The vaccine is approved for these uses in females and males ages 9 to 26. Cervarix is approved for use in females ages 10 to 25 to prevent cervical cancer caused by HPV types 16 and 18.

The FDA has also approved a cancer preventive vaccine that protects against HBV infection. The original

Associated Cancers	Infectious Agents
Hepatocellular carcinoma	Hepatitis B virus (HBV)
Hepatocellular carcinoma	Hepatitis C virus (HCV)
Cervical cancer; vaginal cancer; vulvar cancer; oropharyngeal cancer; anal cancer; penile cancer; squamous cell carcinoma of the skin	Human papillomavirus (HPV) types 16 and 18, as well as other HPV types
Burkitt lymphoma; non-Hodgkin lymphoma; Hodgkin lymphoma; nasopharyngeal carcinoma	Epstein-Barr virus
Kaposi sarcoma	Kaposi sarcoma-associated herpesvirus (KSHV), also known as human herpesvirus 8 (HHV8)
Adult T-cell leukemia/lymphoma	Human T-cell lymphotropic virus type 1 (HTLV1)
Stomach cancer; mucosa-associated lymphoid tissue (MALT) lymphoma	Helicobacter pylori
Bladder cancer	Schistosomes (Schistosoma haematobium)
Liver flukes (Opisthorchis viverrini)	Cholangiocarcinoma (a type of liver cancer)

HBV vaccine was approved in 1981, making it the first cancer preventive vaccine to be successfully developed and marketed. Today, vaccination against Hepatitis B is included in the national immunization schedule.

HAVE OTHER MICROBES BEEN ASSOCIATED WITH CANCER?

The International Agency for Research on Cancer (IARC) has classified several microbes as carcinogenic. Vaccinations against these microbes, if developed, may be preventive for the carcinomas they predispose to.

HOW ARE CANCER TREATMENT VACCINES DESIGNED TO WORK?

Cancer treatment vaccines are designed to treat cancers that have already developed. They are intended to delay or stop cancer cell growth; to cause tumor shrinkage; to prevent cancer from coming back; or to eliminate cancer cells that have not been killed by other forms of treatment.

TUMOR CELL VACCINES

Tumor cell vaccines are made from actual cancer cells that have been removed during surgery, irradiated in the lab, chemicals or new genes may be added, so that they are recognized as foreign. The cells are then injected into the patient. The immune system recognizes antigens on these cells, then seeks out and attacks any other cells with these antigens that are still in the body.

The two basic kinds of tumor cell vaccines are autologous and allogeneic.

Autologous tumor cell vaccines: Tumor cells are taken from the same person in whom they will later be used. Their potential drawbacks are that they are expensive, malignant cells tend to mutate over time, so the vaccine might become less effective later, also if the tumor size is less usable cells in the removed tumor to make a vaccine may not be enough.

Allogeneic tumor cell vaccines: These vaccines use cells of a particular cancer type that originally came from someone other than the patient being treated.

Antigen Vaccines

Antigen vaccines boost the immune system by using only one antigen (or a few), rather than whole tumor cells that contain many thousands of antigens. Antigen vaccines may be specific for a certain type of cancer, but they are not made for a unique patient like autologous cell vaccines are.

Dendritic Cell Vaccines

Dendritic cell vaccines are autologous vaccines. Dendritic cells are the most effective antigen-presenting cells (APCs) known. Dendritic cells are separated from the blood and multiplied in vitro. They are then exposed to cancer antigens and then injected back into the patient.

Anti-idiotype Vaccines

Every B cell or plasma cell makes only one kind of antibody. The unique part of each type of antibody is called an idiotype. Antibodies and antigens fit together like a lock and key. So an antibody to a particular idiotype of another antibody (an anti-idiotype) will usually look like the antigen that triggered cells to make the antibody in the first place. Because the anti-idiotype antibodies look like the antigen and appear foreign, injecting them into the body causes the immune system to attack the anti-idiotypes, along with the antigens themselves.

Lymphomas are the most promising targets for anti-idiotype vaccines, because all lymphoma cells have unique antigen receptors not present on normal lymphocytes or other normal cells of the body.

DNA Vaccines

When tumor cells or antigens are injected into the body as a vaccine, they may cause the desired immune response at first, but soon the immune system recognizes them as foreign and quickly destroys them. Cells can be injected with bits of DNA that code for protein antigens. This DNA might be taken up by cells and instruct them to keep making more antigens. These types of therapies are called DNA vaccines.

Vector-based Vaccines

They aren't really a separate category of vaccine; for example, there are vector-based antigen vaccines and vector-based DNA vaccines. Vectors may be viruses, bacteria or yeast cells.

HAS THE FDA APPROVED ANY CANCER TREATMENT VACCINES?

At this time, only one true cancer vaccine has been approved by the FDA. Sipuleucel-T is used to treat advanced prostate cancer. It is a type of dendritic cell vaccine.

WHAT TYPES OF VACCINES ARE BEING STUDIED IN CLINICAL TRIALS?

Clinical trials of cancer treatment vaccines are focussing mainly on Hodgkin and non-Hodgkin lymphoma, leukemia, bladder cancer, brain tumor, breast cancer, cervical cancer, kidney cancer, lung cancer, melanoma, multiple myeloma and solid tumor.

Clinical trials of cancer preventive vaccines focus on cervical cancer and solid tumor.

WHAT ARE THE REASONS FOR THE HIGH FAILURE RATES OF THERAPEUTIC CANCER VACCINES?

Although general immune activation directed against the target antigens contained within the cancer vaccine has been documented in most cases, reduction in tumor load has not been frequently observed, and tumor progression and metastasis usually ensue, possibly following a slightly extended period of remission. The failure of cancer vaccines to fulfill their promise is due to the very relationship between host and tumor: Through a natural selection process the host leads to the selective enrichment of clones of highly aggressive neoplastically transformed cells, which apparently are so dedifferentiated that they no longer express cancer cell specific molecules. Specific activation of the immune system in such cases only leads to lysis of the remaining cells expressing the particular TAAs in the context of the particular human leukocyte antigen (HLA) subclass and the necessary costimulatory molecules. The most dangerous clones of tumor cells however, lack these features and thus the cancer vaccine is of little use. The use of cancer vaccines seems, at present, destined to remain limited to their

employment as adjuvants to both traditional therapies and in the management of minimal residual disease following surgical resection of the primary cancer mass.

WHAT ARE THE SIDE EFFECTS OF CANCER VACCINES?

The most commonly reported side effect of cancer vaccines is inflammation at the site of injection, including redness, pain, swelling, warming of the skin, itchiness and occasionally a rash. Flu-like symptoms, hypotension, asthma, appendicitis, pelvic inflammatory disease and certain autoimmune diseases, including arthritis and systemic lupus erythematosus may occur. Severe hypersensitivity (allergic) reactions are rare.

CAN CANCER TREATMENT VACCINES BE COMBINED WITH OTHER TYPES OF CANCER THERAPY?

Cancer treatment vaccines may be most effective when given in combination with other forms of cancer therapy. In addition, in some clinical trials, cancer treatment vaccines have appeared to increase the effectiveness of other cancer therapies. Clinical trials are also being designed to test whether a specific cancer treatment vaccine works best when it is administered before, after, or at the same time as chemotherapy.

VACCINE FOR CERVICAL CARCINOMA

Cervical cancer is the third most common cancer of the women. Invasive cervical cancer is a preventable disease, because it has a very long preinvasive stage which could be detected by screening tests, particularly PAP smear. It has been found that infection with Human Pappilloma Virus (HPV) is found to be the causal agent for development of cervical cancer. In nearly 99% of cases of cancer cervix HPV infection is found. Type 16 and 18 HPV are the most notorious in this regard. Prevention of sexually transmitted disease particularly HPV infection appears to be the most effective prevention against cervical cancer. A vaccine against HPV has been developed which becomes a very effective primary prevention for cancer of the cervix.

Two vaccines are namely, cervarix (GlaxoSmithKline) and gardasil (Merck). One of the HPV vaccines, gardasil, also prevents genital warts as well as anal, vulvar and vaginal cancers. Both vaccines are given in 3 injections over 6 months.

WHICH GIRLS/WOMEN SHOULD RECEIVE HPV VACCINATION?

HPV vaccination is recommended with either vaccine for 11 and 12 year-old girls. It is also recommended for girls and women age 13 through 26 years of age who have not yet been vaccinated. HPV vaccine can also be given to girls beginning at age 9 years.

WILL SEXUALLY ACTIVE FEMALES BENEFIT FROM THE VACCINE?

Ideally females should get the vaccine before they become sexually active and exposed to HPV. Females who are sexually active may also benefit from the vaccine, but they may get less benefit from it. This is because they may have already gotten one or more of HPV types targeted by the vaccines. However, few sexually active young women are infected with all HPV types prevented by the vaccines, so most young women could still get protection by getting vaccinated.

SHOULD GIRLS AND WOMEN BE SCREENED FOR CERVICAL CANCER BEFORE GETTING VACCINATED?

Girls and women do not need to get an HPV test or Pap test to find out if they should get the vaccine. However, it is important that women continue to be screened for cervical cancer, even after getting HPV vaccine.

EFFECTIVENESS OF THE HPV VACCINES

The vaccines target the HPV types that most commonly cause cervical cancer. One of the vaccines also protects against the HPV types that cause most genital warts. Both vaccines are highly effective in preventing specific HPV types and the most common health problems from HPV.

HOW LONG DOES VACCINE PROTECTION LAST?

Research suggests that vaccine protection is long-lasting. Current studies (with up to about six years of follow-up data) indicate that the vaccines are effective, with no evidence of decreasing immunity.

WHAT DOES THE VACCINE NOT PROTECT AGAINST?

The vaccines do not protect against all HPV types—so they will not prevent all cases of cervical cancer. About 30% of cervical cancers will not be prevented by the vaccines, so it will be important for women to continue getting screened for cervical cancer (regular Pap tests).

SAFETY OF THE HPV VACCINE

Both vaccines have been licensed by the Food and Drug Administration (FDA) for females aged 9 through 26 years and approved by CDC as safe and effective.

WILL GIRLS/WOMEN WHO HAVE BEEN VACCINATED STILL NEED CERVICAL CANCER SCREENING?

Yes, vaccinated women will still need regular cervical cancer screening (Pap tests) because the vaccines protect against most but not all HPV types that cause cervical cancer. Also, women who got the vaccine after becoming sexually active may not get the full benefit of the vaccine if they had already acquired HPV.

ARE THERE OTHER WAYS TO PREVENT HPV?

For those who are sexually active, condoms may lower the chances of getting HPV, if used with every sex act, condoms may also lower the risk of developing HPV-related diseases (genital warts and cervical cancer).

CANCER VACCINES IN PEDIATRICS

It is said that for any diseases, compared to cure, prevention is better, cheaper and hence preferred. In the modern era of vaccination against so many vaccine preventable infections, growing question is apt to root in the mind of common people, whether there is a vaccine against cancer. Since, cancer itself is not an infectious disease, a vaccine against cancer is a difficult consideration. In the earlier chapters of this textbook, it has been elaborated that cancer roots its origin to diverse etiologies and infection is only one of them. Among so many oncogenic infections, vaccines are available against only two. They are: (1) Human Papilloma Virus causing cervical cancer and cancer of the anogenital area and (2) Hepatitis B virus, causing hepatocellular carcinoma. Besides, vaccines against a few others are under research.

HUMAN PAPILLOMA VIRUS

Human Papilloma Virus (HPV) is primarily a sexually transmitted infection, and most sexually active men and women acquire this infection at some time of their lives. However, of nearly 100 serotypes of HPV discovered so far, only 15–20 are oncogenic and infection caused by the rest is self-limiting and benign. Among the oncogenic serotypes, type 16 is the most prevalent type among the women suffering from carcinoma cervix and pre-cancerous lesions, followed by type 18. Among the non-oncogenic serotypes, type 6 and 11 are responsible for anogenital warts and recurrent respiratory papillomatosis in the vast majority of cases.

Researches for more than a decade have been successful in inventing two vaccines against HPV; one is a quadrivalent vaccine giving protection against HPV serotypes 16, 18, 6 and 11; and the other a bivalent vaccine which confers protection against HPV serotypes 6 and 11. From what have been discussed earlier, it's obvious that the quadrivalent vaccine, in addition to protection against cervical cancer, confers additional protection against anogenital warts as well. Both the vaccines are manufactured by recombinant DNA technology, producing non-infectious virus like particles containing HPV L1 protein with aluminium containing adjuvant. The vaccine confers protection probably by both cell-mediated and IgG antibody-mediated immune response. Since, the lag period between infection with oncogenic strains of HPV and development of cervical cancer is quite long (15–20 years), clinical trials till now with both types of vaccines used efficacy against cervical intraepithelial neoplasia grade 2 and 3 and adenocarcinoma in situ, and the regulatory authorities have also accepted that.

Natural infection caused by various serotypes of HPV does not induce a vigorous immune response. Detectable antibodies, although appear in nearly half of the women acquiring natural infection, that is not necessarily protective against future re-infection even with the same serotypes. Therefore, vaccination should be offered to every woman and before the onset of sexual activity; which is the basis of the recommendation of the age of vaccination between 10–12 years. In this connection it should be noted that vaccination does not give 100% protection against cervical cancer; since the vaccine confers protection from only two most common oncogenic serotypes of HPV, besides the fact that there some other hitherto unknown risk factors for development of cervical cancer as well.

The vaccine is to be preserved between 2-8°C in a refrigerator, and should never be frozen. The dose is 0.5 mL, to be given intramuscularly in the deltoid. The primary series of vaccination is a three-dose schedule; for the tetravalent vaccine the schedule is 0, 2 and 6 months and that for the bivalent vaccine 0, 1 and 6 months. The recommended age of vaccination is 10–12 years, i.e. before the onset of sexual activity. Till date, there is no data regarding the need for booster doses.

HEPATITIS B VACCINE

Hepatitis B virus is a hepatotropic DNA virus, transmitted from man to man through blood and blood products, sexual transmission and by vertical transmission. Infection acquired in adulthood usually results in symptomatic viral hepatitis manifested by jaundice, anorexia, nausea, vomiting, low-grade fever and sometimes skin rash and joint pain; whereas infection during infancy causes the individual to remain clinically silent and harbor the infection (chronicity) which in the long run can cause cirrhosis and hepatocellular carcinoma. Studies have documented that hepatocellular carcinoma, although multifactorial, is caused mainly by hepatitis B virus, and hepatitis B virus infection is the most common cause of hepatocellular carcinoma. Therefore, prevention of transmission of hepatitis B virus infection is expected to prevent incidence of hepatocellular carcinoma to a considerable extent. Besides universal precautions and screening of blood and blood products, vaccination is an important and effective step for prevention of transmission of hepatitis B infection, and thus for prevention of hepatocellular carcinoma.

The vaccine against hepatitis B infection uses the HBsAg, which is again derived by two means. First is from the plasma of chronic carriers of hepatitis B, and the other from recombinant DNA technology. The HBsAg thus obtained is bound to alum adjuvant and appropriate preservative is added. These two types of vaccines are somewhat similar in respect of efficacy and safety, and both these types can be used interchangeably as well. However, most of the hepatitis B vaccines available in the market now are of the latter type.

Since transmission of hepatitis B infection in our community is quite rampant, vaccination should be given at the earliest, i.e. at the time of birth; which obviously contributes to prevent perinatal transmission as well. Babies born to hepatitis B positive mothers at that time, in addition, should be given a dose of hepatitis B immunoglobulin 100–200 IU intramuscularly at different site, away from the site of vaccination. Moreover, studies have found that seroconversion following hepatitis B vaccination is somewhat unpredictable in preterm and low birth weight babies weighing less than 2 kg. Therefore, for babies weighing less than 2 kg at the time of birth, the vaccination may either be started at the age of 6 weeks along with all other vaccines in the immunization schedule, or three more doses of vaccine in addition to the dose given at birth can be given to complete the hepatitis B vaccination schedule.

Dosage schedule: Hepatitis B vaccine is given in a three dose schedule; 0, 1 and 6 months. However, for the sake of administrative convenience, in an attempt to incorporate the vaccine in the routine immunization schedule, the three doses are scheduled at 0, 6 and 14 weeks starting from the time of birth, and results are acceptable. However, if someone misses the first dose at the time of birth, the three doses can be given at 6, 10 and 14 weeks of age, along with other vaccines scheduled in the immunization schedule.

The vaccine is given in a dose of 0.5 mL intramuscularly, which corresponds to 10 μg of the antigenic component. The adult dose is twice the pediatric dose. The dose may be increased further for immunizing immunosuppressed individuals. The injection is to be given in the deltoid, or in neonates and young infants in the anterolateral aspect of thigh. The vaccine should not be injected in the gluteus, since, there it is deposited in the adipose tissue and renders systemic absorption, and hence, seroconversion unpredictable. Following injection, little pain at the injection site, and infrequently, low rise of temperature is noted. Severe anaphylactic reactions are exceptional.

Duration of protection: The recommended schedule of three doses of the vaccine confers lifelong immunity in an immunocompetent individual. Earlier, it was believed that immunity wanes off after 5–7 years of immunization, since the geometric mean titre of antibody falls below the cut off level of 10 mIU/ml. However, it is now known that despite that fall of GMT of antibody, the immunological memory persists, which can result in sudden exodus of enormous amount of protective antibody on subsequent exposure to antigen.

Now since quite a good number of vaccines are scheduled at a time in the different immunization schedules, hepatitis B vaccine has been incorporated in different combination vaccines, viz. combined with DTP, hemophilus influenza B and hepatitis A vaccines in different combinations. The combination vaccines are equally safe and efficacious.

The vaccine is to be stored in a refrigerator between 2–8°C temperature and should never be frozen. Freezing the vaccine decreases its efficacy considerably.

A recent concept regarding hepatitis B infection is development of a mutant strain of hepatitis B virus. The danger related to this strain is that it can lead to chronicity even without exhibiting HBsAg positivity, and hence, infection caused by this mutant strain may not be prevented by the currently available vaccine. Emergence of this mutant strain of hepatitis B virus threatens the world to be resistant to the currently available hepatitis B vaccine around the end of this decade. However, researches are going on to circumvent this emerging problem.

SUGGESTED READING

1. Hong CW, Zenq Q. Awaiting a new era of cancer immunotherapy. Cancer Res. 2012;72:3715-9.
2. IAP guide book on Immunization. Yearle Y, Chondhury P, Thecker N (Eds). IAP committee on immunization, 2009-2011.
3. Lal S, Kriplani A, Bhatla N, Agarwal N. Invasive carcinoma of cervix during pregnancy – a care report and review of literature. JIMA 2011;109:751-3.

43 Biomedical Statistics: A Snapshot

Avijit Hazra

Although application of statistical methods to biomedical research began in earnest only some 150 years ago, statistics is now an integral part of medical research. Knowledge of statistics is becoming mandatory to understand most biomedical literature, including those dealing with cancer epidemiology, treatment and prevention. Biostatistics may be viewed simply as the science of data analysis applied to biomedical research questions and health-related issues. This entails summarizing data and describing patterns in data sets (descriptive statistics) and then comparing datasets to draw conclusions valid in general (inferential statistics). In some cases, one may proceed beyond these routine applications to more advanced relationship analysis situations whereby statistical models are built up that can have predictive value.

DATA TYPES

Data (values of a variable) constitutes the raw material for statistical work. It is important to understand the different types of data and their mutual interconversion. At the most basic level, there are two types of data or variables. The first type includes those, which are defined by some characteristic, or quality and is referred to as qualitative variable. Because qualitative data are best summarized by grouping the observations into categories and counting the numbers in each, they are often referred to as categorical variables. The second type includes those that are measured on a numerical scale and is called quantitative variable. Since quantitative variables always have values expressed as numbers and the differences between values have numerical meaning, they are also referred to as numerical variables.

A qualitative variable can be a nominal variable or an ordinal variable. A nominal variable covers categories that cannot be ranked; and no category is more valuable than another. The data is generated simply by naming the appropriate category to which the observation belongs. An ordinal variable has categories that follow a logical hierarchy and hence can be ranked. We can assign numbers (scores) to nominal and ordinal categories; although the differences among those numbers do not have numerical meaning. However, category counts do have numerical significance. A quantitative variable can be continuous or discrete. A continuous variable can, in theory at least, take on any value within a given range, including fractional values. A discrete variable can take on only certain discrete values within a given range, often these values are integers. Often certain variables, like age or blood pressure, are treated as discrete variables although strictly speaking they are continuous. A special case may exist for both categorical or numerical variables, when the variable in question can take on only one of two numerical values or belong to only one of two categories; these are known as binary or dichotomous data.

To illustrate the above data types, let us consider the human hair as an example. Hair color would be a categorical variable, but hair length would be a numerical one. Since there is no natural hierarchy of hair color, nor is any ranking possible, hair color would be a nominal variable. However, hair loss may be an ordinal variable if it is expressed as none, partial and total, for example.

Hair length would be a continuous variable, but we can treat is as discrete if we are recording it only to the nearest millimeter. It is possible to convert numerical data to categorical. Thus, after recording hair length we may classify the subject into long, medium or short hair category. If we are interested in only two categories of hair length, say long or short, then this becomes a binary variable.

DESCRIPTIVE STATISTICS

Descriptive statistics summarizes data from a sample or population. Categorical data are described in terms of percentages or proportions. With numerical data, individual observations within a sample or population tend to cluster about a central location, with more extreme observations being less frequent. The extent of this clustering is summarized by measures of central tendency such as the mean, median or mode, while the spread is described by measures of dispersion such as range, variance, standard deviation or coefficient of variation.

The confidence interval is an increasingly important measure of precision. When we observe samples, there is no way of assessing true population parameters. We can, however, obtain a standard error from the sample and use it to define a range in which the true population value is likely to lie with a certain acceptable level of uncertainty. This is the confidence interval. Conventionally, the 95% confidence interval is used.

Patterns in data sets, called data distributions, are important component of descriptive statistics. The most common distribution is the normal distribution which is depicted as the well-known symmetrical bell-shaped Gaussian curve. Familiarity with other distributions, such as the binomial distribution and the Poisson distribution, would be also helpful.

Various graphs and plots have been devised to summarize data and trends visually. Pie chart, line diagram, bar chart and the histogram are universally used. Some plots, such as the box-and-whiskers plot (Figure 43.1) and the stem-and-leaf plot, are used less often but provide useful summaries in selected situations. Error bars should be used to depict the variation or the precision of the measurements, wherever applicable.

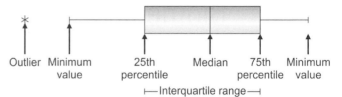

Fig. 43.1: A horizontal box plot depicting the five number summary of numerical data. Note that this particular dataset is not symmetrical but is skewed to the left

MEASURING DISEASE FREQUENCY

Incidence and prevalence are the two basic measures of disease frequency but they are often wrongly used and interpreted. The key to understanding measures of disease frequency is the three elements of N-E-T—number of persons who are observed for occurrence of the event (i.e. the population), the event (i.e. the disease, condition or outcome of interest) and the time period during which such events are observed. Incidence is the number of new cases occurring in a particular time period. In other words, it measures the rate at which people without a disease develop the same over a specified period of time. Average annual incidence, incidence density, cumulative incidence, attack rate and attributable risk are extensions of this concept. Prevalence is the count of existing disease at a single point in time or over a defined period of time. If over a period of time, it will count both new and existing cases. Prevalence may be expressed as point prevalence, period prevalence or cumulative (e.g. lifetime) prevalence.

Mortality, incidence and prevalence may be stated as crude or specific rates. The crude rate refers to the number of occurrences for a whole population and is often expressed as rate per 1000, 10,000 or 100,000 members of the population. It may be more meaningful to state specific rates for factors like age, sex, ethnicity and others.

Standardized rates adjust for differences in structures between populations. Although age is normally used in this process, other factors (e.g. ethnicity) can also be employed. A single statistic is produced, allowing ready comparisons between populations. Standardization can be done by direct or indirect methods. Both compare a specific study population with a 'standard population' (often national population or the standard world population modeled by the World Health Organization). This may be carried out for both sexes individually. Indirect standardization is used more commonly and yields more stable results, than direct standardization, for small populations or small numbers of events. A standardized mortality ratio (SMR) is generated by this method.

DETERMINING SAMPLE SIZE

An adequate sample ensures that a study yields reliable information, regardless of whether it ultimately suggests a clinically important association between the interventions or exposures and the outcomes being studied. The probability of Type I and Type II errors, the expected variance in the sample and the effect size are the essential determinants of sample size for interventional studies.

Any method for deriving a conclusion from experimental data carries with it some risk of drawing a false conclusion. Two types of false conclusion may occur, called type I and type II errors, whose probabilities are denoted by the symbols α and β. A type I error occurs when one concludes that a difference exists between the groups or data sets being compared when, in reality, it does not. This is akin to a false positive result. A type II error occurs when one concludes that a difference does not exist when, in reality, it does, and the difference is equal to or larger than the effect size defined by the alternative to the null hypothesis. This is a false negative result. When considering the risk of type II error, it is more intuitive to think in terms of power of the study or $(1 - \beta)$. Power denotes the probability of detecting a difference when it does exist. When calculating sample size, conventional acceptable values for α and power are maximum 5% and minimum 80%, respectively. Smaller α or larger power will increase sample size. Increasing variance in the sample tends to increase the sample size required to achieve a given power level. The effect size is the smallest clinically important difference that is sought to be detected and, rather than statistical convention, is a matter of past experience and clinical judgment. Larger samples are required, if smaller differences are to be detected.

In the past, sample size determination was difficult due to the need to learn relatively complex mathematics and numerous formulae. However, the task has become much easier of late, owing to improving availability, capability and user-friendliness of power and sample size determination software. Many can execute routines for a wide variety of research designs and statistical tests. Therefore, researchers must now concentrate on applying the principles appropriately and achieving calculated sample size targets so that study conclusions are truly meaningful.

HYPOTHESIS TESTING

Hypothesis testing (the major part of inferential statistics) is one of the major applications of biostatistics. Most studies have a research question that can be framed as a hypothesis. Inferential statistics begins with the null hypothesis that reflects the conservative position of no change or no difference in comparison to baseline or between groups. Usually the researcher has reason to believe that there is some effect or some difference, that is believed in an alternative hypothesis. The researcher therefore proceeds to study samples and measure outcomes in the hope of generating evidence strong enough for the statistician to be able to reject the null hypothesis.

The p value concept is almost universally used in hypothesis testing. It denotes the probability of obtaining by chance a result at least as extreme as that observed, even when the null hypothesis is true and no real difference exists. Usually, if p is < 0.05 the null hypothesis is rejected and sample results are deemed statistically significant. The two-tailed p value is used more commonly, implying that the results would be accepted irrespective of whether they are favoring the test or the control intervention, as against a one-tailed p value that is used when change, if any, would be one direction only for certain.

With the universal availability of computers and increasing access to specialized statistical software, the drudgery involved in inferential statistics calculations is now gone. The researcher is free to devote time to optimally designing the study, carefully selecting the hypothesis tests to be applied and taking care in conducting the study well. Thinking of the research hypothesis in terms of generic research questions helps in selection of the right hypothesis test. In addition, it is important to be clear about the nature of the variables (e.g. numerical vs. categorical; parametric vs. non-parametric) and the number of groups or data sets being compared (e.g. two or more than two) at a time.

Finally, it is becoming the norm that an estimate of the size of any effect, expressed with its 95% confidence interval, is required for meaningful interpretation of results. A large study is likely to have a small (and therefore statistically significant) p value, but a 'real' estimate of the effect would be provided by the 95% confidence interval. If the intervals overlap between two interventions, then the difference between them is not so clear-cut even if $p < 0.05$.

COMPARING GROUPS: NUMERICAL VARIABLES

Numerical data that are normally distributed can be analyzed with parametric tests, that is tests based on the parameters that define a normal distribution curve. If the distribution is uncertain, the data can be plotted as a normal probability plot and visually inspected, or tested for normality using one of a number of goodness of fit tests, such as the Kolmogorov-Smirnov test or the Shapiro-Wilk test.

The widely used Student's t test has three variants. The one-sample t test is used to assess if a sample mean (as an estimate of the population mean) differs significantly from a given population mean. The means of two independent samples may be compared for a statistically significant difference by the unpaired or independent samples t test. If the data sets are related in some way, their means may be compared by the paired or dependent samples t test.

The t test should not be used to compare the means of more than two groups. Applying the t test to compare groups in pairs in such a situation will increase the probability of type I error. The one-way analysis of variance (ANOVA) is employed to compare the means of three or more independent data sets that are normally distributed. However, multiple measurements from the same set of subjects cannot be treated as separate unrelated data sets. Comparison of means in this scenario requires repeated measures ANOVA. It is to be noted that while a multiple group comparison test such as ANOVA can point to a significant difference, it does not identify exactly between which two groups the difference lie. To do this, an appropriate post hoc test is necessary. Examples are the Tukey's test, Student-Newman-Keuls test or Dunnett's test following ANOVA.

If the assumptions for parametric tests are not met, there are non-parametric alternatives for comparing data sets. These include Mann-Whitney U test instead of unpaired Student's t test, Wilcoxon's matched pairs signed ranks test in lieu of paired Student's t test, Kruskal-Wallis test as the non-parametric counterpart of ANOVA and the Friedman's test instead of repeated measures ANOVA. The Dunn's test is used as a post hoc test following Kruskal-Wallis or Friedman's ANOVA.

COMPARING GROUPS: CATEGORICAL VARIABLES

Categorical variables are commonly represented as counts or frequencies. For analysis, such data are conveniently arranged in contingency tables (tables in which counts in individual cells are independent of one another and their sum denotes the total sample). Conventionally, such tables are designated as r × c tables, with r denoting number of rows and c denoting number of columns.

The Chi-squared probability distribution is particularly useful in analyzing categorical variables. A number of tests yield test statistics that fit, at least approximately, a Chi-squared distribution and hence are referred to as Chi-squared tests. Examples include Pearson's Chi-squared test (or simply the Chi-squared test), McNemar's Chi-squared test, Mantel-Haenszel Chi-squared test and others. The Pearson's Chi-squared test is the most commonly used test for assessing difference in distribution of a categorical variable between two or more independent groups. If the groups are ordered in some manner, the Chi-squared test for trend should be used. The Fisher's exact probability test is a test of the independence between two dichotomous categorical variables. It provides a better alternative to the Chi-squared statistic to assess the difference between two independent proportions when numbers are small, but cannot be applied to a contingency table larger than 2 × 2. The McNemar's Chi-squared test assesses the difference between paired proportions. It is used when the frequencies in a 2 × 2 table represent paired (dependent) samples. The Cochran's Q test is a generalization of the McNemar's test that compares more than two related proportions.

The p value from the Chi-squared test or its counterparts does not indicate the strength of the difference or association between the categorical variables involved. This information can be obtained from the relative risk or the odds ratio statistics. Both are measures of dichotomous association obtained from 2 × 2 tables.

ASSOCIATION BETWEEN VARIABLES

Correlation and linear regression are commonly used techniques for quantifying the association between two numeric variables. Correlation quantifies the strength of the linear relationship between a pair of variables, expressing this as a correlation coefficient. If both variables x and y are normally distributed, we calculate Pearson's correlation coefficient (r). The value r^2 denotes the proportion of the variability of y that can be attributed to its linear relation with x, and is called the coefficient of determination. If normality assumption is not met for one or both variables in a correlation analysis, a rank correlation coefficient, such as Spearman's rho (ρ) or Kendall's tau (τ), may be calculated. A hypothesis test of correlation tests whether the linear relationship between the two variables holds in the underlying population, in which case it returns $p < 0.05$. A 95% confidence interval for the population correlation coefficient can also be calculated.

Linear regression is a technique that attempts to link two numerical variables x and y in the form of a mathematical equation (y = a + bx), such that given the value of one variable the other may be predicted. It is a simple modeling technique. Generally, the method of least squares is applied to obtain the equation of the regression line.

Correlation and linear regression analyses are based on certain assumptions and misleading conclusions may be drawn if these are not met. The first assumption is that of linear relationship between the two variables. A scatter plot is essential before embarking on any correlation-regression analysis to show that this is indeed the case. Outliers or clustering (subgroups) within data sets can distort the correlation coefficient value. Finally, it is vital to remember that though strong correlation can be a pointer towards causation, the two are not synonymous.

Association between categorical variables can be depicted by constructing a 2 × 2 contingency table and then calculate the Odds ratio or Relative risk as stated later. This is usually done in epidemiology (analytical observational studies) and sometimes in interventional studies. Chi-square for trend analysis may be applied to contingency tables with more than two rows.

Multiple linear regression models a situation where a single numerical dependent variable is to be predicted from multiple independent numerical variables. It is thus an extension of simple linear regression to more than two numerical variables. Logistic regression is an analogous technique that is used when the outcome variable is dichotomous in nature. In this, the natural logarithm of odds ratios is modeled as a linear function of the explanatory variables. Logistic regression is a versatile technique in the sense that it can accommodate various types of predictors—both numerical and categorical—without any distributional assumptions. The risk attributable to individual predictors can be expressed as adjusted odds ratios with 95% confidence intervals. The log-linear technique models count type of data and can be used to analyze cross-tabulations where more than two variables are included. It can look at three or more variables at the same time to determine associations between them and also show just where these associations lie.

STATISTICS OF DIAGNOSTIC TESTS

Crucial therapeutic decisions are based on diagnostic tests. Therefore, it is important to evaluate such tests before adopting them for routine use. Tests on blood or other biological fluids, radiological imaging and microbial cultures are obvious diagnostic tests. However, even things like specific clinical examination procedures, scoring systems based on physiological or psychological evaluation, ratings based on questionnaires are also diagnostic tests and therefore merit similar evaluation.

In the simplest scenario, a diagnostic test will give either a positive (disease likely) or negative (disease unlikely) result. Ideally, all those with the disease should be classified by a test as positive and all those without the disease as negative. Unfortunately, in practice, no test gives 100% accurate results. Therefore, leaving cost aside, the performance of diagnostic tests is evaluated on the basis of at least four statistical parameters—sensitivity, specificity, positive predictive value and negative predictive value. Likelihood ratios combine information on specificity and sensitivity to express the likelihood that a given test result would occur in a subject with a disorder compared to the probability that the same result would occur in a subject without the disorder.

Not all tests can be categorized simply as 'positive' or 'negative'. Test results may come on a numerical scale and in such cases judgment is required in choosing a cut-off point to distinguish normal from abnormal. Naturally a cut-off value should provide the greatest predictive accuracy but there is a trade-off between sensitivity and specificity here – if the cut-off is too low, it will identify most patients who have the disease (high sensitivity) but will also incorrectly identify many who do not (low specificity). A receiver operator characteristic (ROC) curve plots pairs of sensitivity versus (1 – specificity) values, and helps in selecting an optimum cut-off – the one lying on the 'elbow' of the curve.

The Bland-Altman plot is a graphical method of assessing agreement between two diagnostic tests that measure on a numerical scale. It plots the difference between pairs of observations against their arithmetic mean.

Cohen's kappa statistic is a measure of inter-rater agreement for categorical variables. It is also used to assess how far two tests agree with respect to diagnostic categorization. It is generally thought to be a more robust measure than simple percent agreement calculation since κ takes into account the agreement occurring by chance.

ASSESSING RISK

A basic measurement of risk is the probability of an individual developing an outcome when exposed to a risk factor. This can be simply expressed as proportion (percentage) of those exposed to the risk factor who develop the outcome, along with its 95% confidence interval. However, to assess the importance of an individual risk factor, it is necessary to compare the risk of the outcome in the exposed group with that in the non-exposed group. A comparison between risks in different groups can be made by examining either their ratio or the difference between them. The 2 × 2 contingency table comes in handy in the calculation of ratios.

Odds is the ratio of the probability of occurrence of an event to the probability of non-occurrence of the same event. Odds ratio (OR) or cross-product ratio is the ratio of the odds of an event in the exposed group, to the odds of the same event in the non-exposed group. It can range from zero to infinity. OR > 1, indicates exposure increases risk while OR < 1 indicates that exposure is protecting against risk. The OR should be presented with its 95% CI to enable more meaningful interpretation – if this interval includes 1, then even a relatively large OR will not carry much weight. The relative risk (RR) or risk ratio denotes ratio of probability of event in exposed group to probability of same event in the non-exposed group. Its interpretation is similar (but not identical) to the OR. If the event in question is relatively uncommon, values of OR and RR tend to be similar. However, for common events the value of RR is constrained while the OR may become very large.

Absolute risk reduction (ARR) is a measure of the effectiveness of an intervention with respect to a dichotomous event. It is calculated as proportion experiencing the event in control group minus the proportion experiencing the event in treated group. It is often used to denote the benefit to the individual. The reciprocal of ARR is the number needed to treat (NNT) and this denotes the number of subjects who would need to be treated in order to obtain one more success than that obtained with a control treatment. Alternatively (e.g. in vaccine trials), this could also denote the number that would need treatment in order to prevent one additional adverse outcome as compared to control treatment. Extended to toxicity, the NNT becomes a measure of harm and is then called number needed to harm (NNH). NNT and NNH are important concepts from the policy maker's perspective.

SURVIVAL ANALYSIS

Survival analysis is concerned with 'time to event' data. Traditionally it dealt with cancer death as the event in question, but it can handle any event occurring over a time frame such as complication, recovery, failure, success, etc.

When the outcome of a study is the time to an event, a likely problem is that it is often not possible to wait until events have happened in all the subjects (e.g. till all are dead). Additionally, many subjects may leave the study prematurely or simply be lost to follow-up. Such situations lead to what is called censoring as complete information is not available for some subjects. The data set is thus a mixture of times to the event in question and times after which no more information on the individual is available. Survival analysis methods make no assumption regarding normal distribution of time data and are the only techniques capable of handling censored observations without treating them as missing data.

Descriptive methods for estimating the survival times from a sample include calculation of mean survival or median survival. However, calculation of these measures would mean that the investigators wait till all or half the subjects have died, which may be too long a period to wait. Time-specific mortality rates (e.g. 5-year survival, 10-year survival) are also familiar ways to summarize survival data. Calculating these from a group of subjects is not possible till the specified length of time has passed for all the subjects. Alternatively this calculation can be done ignoring those subjects for whom the observation period has not yet extended to the specified time interval, but this would mean ignoring the survival experience of these subjects.

To circumvent the problems posed by a limited observation period (during which all subjects will not attain the outcome in question) and unequal lengths of observation, methods have evolved to handle these data sets comprising censored observations and unequal lengths of observation. These include the actuarial or life table method and the more recent Kaplan-Meier product limit method. The availability of increasingly user-friendly computer software has made the later method more popular. It is exemplified by the Kaplan-Meier survival plot (Fig. 43.2), which plots the cumulative probability of survival against time. Several techniques are available for comparing survival experience in two or more groups—the log-rank test is popularly used. An advantage of the log rank test is that it can also be used to produce an estimate of risk of the event—this is called a hazard ratio.

The hazard ratio is interpreted in a manner similar to conventional odds ratio. Thus a hazard ratio of 2.0 implies that the odds of the event in one group is twice

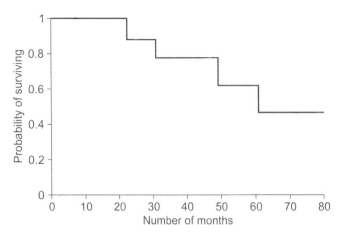

Fig. 43.2: A basic Kaplan-Meier survival plot. Note the staircase pattern. Note also that this is a 'crazy' staircase since neither the height nor the width of the 'stairs' fixed.

that in the reference group at any time. The ratio has to be expressed with its 95% confidence interval to interpret it more convincingly. One caveat in using the hazard ratio is the assumption that the hazard, that is the risk of the event, remains constant throughout the duration of the study. If this is not likely to be true in practice, the Mantel-Haenszel Chi-square statistic or the Gehan's (or generalized Wilcoxon) test may be used to compare two survival distributions.

Finally, survival analysis encompasses different regression models for estimating the relationship of multiple predictor variables to survival. Cox proportional hazards model or Cox regression is a popular regression method that allows the hazard function to be modeled on a set of explanatory variables without making restrictive assumptions concerning the nature or shape of the underlying survival distributions. It can accommodate any number of covariates, whether they are categorical or continuous.

The mathematics of the Cox regression model involves a complicated exponential equation which establishes that the predictors have a multiplicative or proportional effect on the probability of dying—hence the name 'proportional hazards'. Like the adjusted odds ratios in logistic regression, this multivariate technique produces hazard ratios for individual factors that may modify survival, adjusted for the effects of other variables in the equation. The model is being extended to situations when the time-dependent outcome in question is not a binary event like death but can have multiple categories.

THE GENERAL LINEAR MODEL AND OTHER MULTIVARIATE METHODS

Multivariate analysis refers to statistical techniques that look at a number of variables simultaneously, with a view to clarify the relationships between them. Many of them try to build mathematical models that can be used for prediction. The general linear model is not a discrete statistical technique in itself, but rather a strategy for analysis. Its goal is to determine whether and how one or more independent variables relate to or affect one or more dependent variables, assuming that the relationships between them are linear. It is an umbrella concept, that in addition to simple linear regression and one-way analysis of variance (ANOVA), includes several multivariate techniques.

Multiple linear regression, logistic regression and log-linear analysis have already been mentioned. Factor analysis and principal component analysis are a group of related techniques that seek to reduce a large number of predictor variables to a smaller number of factors or components, that are linearly related to the original variables.

Analysis of covariance (ANCOVA) is an extension of ANOVA, in which an additional independent variable of interest for which data is available, the covariate, is brought into the analysis. It tries to examine whether a difference still persists after 'controlling' for the effect of the covariate that can impact the numerical dependent variable of interest. MANOVA and MANCOVA, are multivariate extensions of ANOVA and ANCOVA respectively, and are used when multiple numerical dependent variables have to be incorporated in the analysis.

Structural equation modeling includes a number of advanced statistical techniques and is referred to by a variety of other names. It is the most flexible approach under the general linear model, and is able to deal with multiple dependent and independent variables, whether numerical or categorical in nature. Two analytic techniques that use structural equation modeling, path analysis and confirmatory factor analysis, are considered distinct techniques in their own right.

Path analysis may be regarded as a multivariate statistical technique that makes use of multiple regression to explore causal relationship among variables and depicts this relationship in graphical form called the path diagram. The path diagram can only be constructed if one has formulated a 'causal hypothesis', that is some hypothesis regarding which variables may be related and in what manner. Path diagram conventions allow relationships to be shown with their directions and strengths.

Classification and regression tree (CART) analysis is an alternative to procedures like multiple regression and logistic regression for investigating the relationship between a response or outcome variable and a set of predictor or explanatory variables. The goal is to determine subsets of explanatory variables most important for prediction of the response variable. Rather than fitting a mathematical model to the sample data, the observations are divided recursively into a number of groups, each division being chosen so as to maximize some measure of the difference in the response variable in the resulting two groups. The resulting CART dendrogram often provides easier interpretation than a regression equation, and those variables most important for prediction can be quickly identified. Binary response variables lead to classification trees, while continuous numerical response variables lead to regression trees.

Factor analysis and principal component analysis are a group of related techniques that seek to reduce a large number of predictor variables to a smaller number of factors or components, that are linearly related to the original variables.

Analysis of covariance (ANCOVA) is an extension of ANOVA, in which an additional independent variable of interest for which data is available, the covariate, is brought into the analysis. It tries to examine whether a difference still persists after 'controlling' for the effect of the covariate that can impact the numerical dependent variable of interest. MANOVA and MANCOVA, are multivariate extensions of ANOVA and ANCOVA respectively, and are used when multiple numerical dependent variables have to be incorporated in the analysis.

Structural equation modeling includes a number of advanced statistical techniques and is referred to by a variety of other names. It is the most flexible approach under the general linear model, and is able to deal with multiple dependent and independent variables, whether numerical or categorical in nature. Two analytic techniques that use structural equation modeling, path analysis and confirmatory factor analysis, are considered distinct techniques in their own right.

Path analysis may be regarded as a multivariate statistical technique that makes use of multiple regression to explore causal relationship among variables and depicts this relationship in graphical form called the path diagram. The path diagram can only be constructed if one has formulated a 'causal hypothesis', that is some hypothesis regarding which variables may be related and in what manner. Path diagram conventions allow relationships to be shown with their directions and strengths.

Classification and regression tree (CART) analysis is an alternative to procedures like multiple regression and logistic regression for investigating the relationship between a response or outcome variable and a set of predictor or explanatory variables. The goal is to determine subsets of explanatory variables most important for prediction of the response variable. Rather than fitting a mathematical model to the sample data, the observations are divided recursively into a number of groups, each division being chosen so as to maximize some measure of the difference in the response variable in the resulting two groups. The resulting CART dendrogram often provides easier interpretation than a regression equation, and those variables most important for prediction can be quickly identified. Binary response variables lead to classification trees, while continuous numerical response variables lead to regression trees.

CONCLUSION

All medical persons must evaluate and utilize new information throughout their professional lives. This entails familiarity with the basic tenets of biomedical statistics. The dedicated researcher will also require a more in-depth understanding of the statistical techniques they intend to utilize. In this chapter we have provided only a 'sampling' of the biomedical statistics universe. The onus is upon the reader now on building up the necessary statistical knowledge and skills. The following bibliography would help in this regard.

SUGGESTED READING

1. Biostatistics. In: Parikh MN, Hazra A, Mukherjee J, Gogtay N. Research methodology simplified: Every clinician a researcher. New Delhi: Jaypee Brothers; 2010;80-175.
2. Cox TF. An introduction to multivariate data analysis. London: Hodder Education; 2005.
3. Dawson B, Trapp RG. Basic & clinical biostatistics. 4th edn. New York: McGraw-Hill; 2004.
4. Everitt BS. Medical statistics from A to Z: A guide for clinicians and medical students. Cambridge: Cambridge University Press; 2006.
5. Petrie A, Sabin C. Medical statistics at a glance. 2nd edn. Oxford: Blackwell Publishing, 2005.

44 Childhood Cancer Survivors

Madhumita Nandi

Probably, medical science has not made such rapid strides in any other field as it has done in the field of Pediatric Oncology. We have traveled a long distance from the time when utterance of the word 'cancer' meant sure-shot death-nail for the child. Nothing could have been more grim than this when a young and productive life ahead had to be nipped in the bud because of cancer. Nowadays, most of these children, if treated appropriately and timely, are not only surviving but also are looking forward to a productive and bright future. Nearly 80% of children with cancer can expect to be cured of the disease, an increase of almost 45% from the early 1960s. This tremendous increase in survival rates have resulted in an ever-increasing population of cancer survivors. Though the exact figures from India are not available, about 1 in 1000 young adults in US has been treated for childhood cancer. In absolute terms, approximately 67,000 are childhood cancer survivors in US and about 25,000 survivors in UK. Figure 44.1 shows the overall increase in percentage of cancer survival rates. Figure 44.2 shows increase in survival rates of individual cancers over the years. But, this cancer free survival is not always exactly 'disease-free'. We have to increasingly deal with cases of 'after-effect' of our so-called 'successful treatment'.

TYPES OF LATE EFFECTS

The types of late effects may be anticipated based on the specific therapy on which the patients were exposed, the doses of the therapy and the age at the time of that exposure. These late effects may be as a result of chemotherapeutic, radiotherapeutic, bone marrow transplant or surgical interventions. Lack of cell nourishment, chronic cell injury, death of healthy cells, and scar tissue formation may all contribute to late effects. These late effects may be broadly of two types—psychosocial and medical. Younger children are at the greatest risk because of the effects on their growth, fertility and neuropsychological functions.

Chemotherapy

Cancer chemotherapeutic agents mostly give rise to dose dependent acute toxicities because of its effect on rapidly dividing cells, such as bone marrow, GI mucosa, and epidermis (Fig. 44.3). Least susceptible are those that either do not replicate or those which do so very slowly, such as neurons, muscle cells and connective tissue. As children tend to tolerate more doses or dose intensities of therapeutic agents, they often receive chemotherapy in higher doses. This higher threshold for acute toxicities in childhood results in higher rate of delayed or chronic toxicities that may become apparent only years after the exposure. So chemotherapy may sometimes have late effects on even the least susceptible tissues, such as vinca alkaloids, methotrexate, cisplatin, ifosfamide and high dose cytosine arabinoside may cause neural damage, adverse effects of methotrexate and corticosteroids on bones, myocardial dysfunction after anthracycline exposure. Injuries to these tissues with low repair potential tend to be long lasting or permanent.

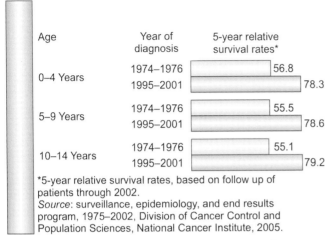

Fig. 44.1: Trends in survival, children 0-14 years, all sites combined 1974–2001

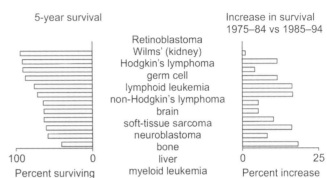

Fig. 44.2: Childhood cancer survival rates (SEER Pediatric Monograph, 1999)

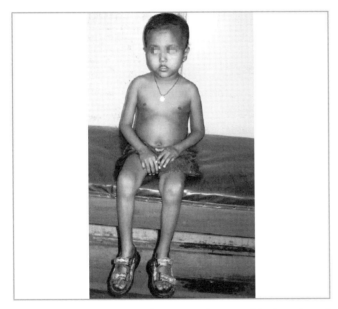

Fig. 44.3: ALL patient on maintenance therapy with alopecia and muscle wasting

Radiation

Radiation therapy involves the use of high-energy rays to kill or shrink cancer cells. The radiation may come from outside of the body (external radiation) or from radioactive materials placed directly in the tumor (internal or implant radiation). Radiation therapy may be used to reduce the size of a cancer before surgery, to destroy any remaining cancer cells after surgery, or, in some cases, as the main treatment. As with chemotherapy, radiation therapy can

affect normal cells as well as cancerous ones. Late effects of irradiation again are site and dose specific. Like cranial irradiation may result in short stature, learning disabilities and second malignancies, head and neck irradiation may give rise to alopecia, cataracts, facial deformities, mediastinal radiation to cardiomyopathy, vaso-occlusive disease, radiation to spine may result in short stature and scoliosis, pelvic and gonadal irradiation may give rise to azoospermia and amenorrhea, and bone irradiation may lead to avascular necrosis, osteoporosis and osteochondromas.

Surgery

Late effects of surgical interventions include long-term consequences of splenectomy, thoracotomy giving rise to scoliosis, coping with amputation, enucleation leading to blindness, malabsorption following bowel surgery and metabolic complications of ureteral diversions.

How Specific Parts of the Body React

Brain: Chemotherapy delivered into the spinal column has been linked to learning disabilities in children. These effects are more common in children who are under age 5 at the time of treatment, and usually show up within 2 to 5 years of treatment. Learning disabilities are most common in children who receive both IT chemotherapy and radiation therapy to the brain.

Cognitive impairments are typically seen as declines of 10 to 20 points in IQ and in academic achievement scores, as well as specific problems in visual motor skills, memory, and attention.

Eyesight and hearing: Vision may be affected in a number of ways resulting from treatment, particularly if the tumor was on or near the eye. Certain medicines can be toxic to the eye and may lead to problems, such as blurred vision, double vision, and glaucoma..

Radiation in the area of the eye can sometimes cause cataracts. Radiation therapy to the bones near the eye may also slow bone growth, possibly leading to facial deformity.

Certain chemotherapy agents like cisplatin and antibiotics may cause high-frequency hearing loss. In addition, radiation therapy given to the brain or ear can lead to hearing loss.

Typically, careful evaluation of hearing and vision during treatment may allow for early changes in therapy should vision or hearing loss occur. After therapy, annual exams will help identify potential problems. Ultimately, treatments such as cataract removal, eyeglasses, or hearing aids may be needed.

Growth and development: Decreased growth during childhood cancer therapy is a common problem. A certain amount of catch-up growth may occur after treatment, but in some instances, short stature is permanent. Chemotherapy may contribute to a slow-down in growth, but when given alone, without radiation, it is usually temporary. Many patients eventually catch up to a normal growth pattern. Certain chemotherapy medications, however, when given in high enough doses, may have more lasting effects. Some of the long-term effects of intensive chemotherapy without radiation are still unclear.

Radiation therapy has a direct effect on the growth of bones that are within the radiation field. Cranial radiation also contributes to slower growth. Exactly how cranial radiation affects growth is not completely understood. Growth hormone deficiency is one of the factors. Early onset of puberty in girls with ALL (acute lymphocytic leukemia) may result in shorter final height. The effects of cranial irradiation appear to be age and dose related. Treatment with growth hormone may reverse some of these damaging effects of radiation therapy.

Thyroid: Thyroid function may be at risk when head and neck radiation is given. With annual check-ups of thyroid function, thyroid hormone replacement can be given if needed. Hyperthyroidism is less likely, but may occur. Yearly thyroid check-ups can help detect these problems. They may be needed for more than 10 years after treatment.

Sexual Development

Males: Radiation therapy and chemotherapy are both capable of reducing sperm production. Low doses of radiation or certain chemotherapy medications may cause temporary reduction in sperm production. Higher radiation doses and many chemotherapy regimens which include high dose alkalyting agents and procarbazine lead to permanent reduction of sperm count.Specific late effects vary depending on the dose of the therapeutic agent. This is an important concern to consider before starting cancer treatment in the older child. Sperm banking may be offered, so that the patient can still father children through alternative means later in life.

While radiation therapy may be necessary, some patients can have the testicles moved out of the radiation field during treatment. For some, the decrease in sperm count is reversible. This reversal can take place as many as 15 years after treatment. The very young male, who is treated prior to puberty, is less of a risk.

Other effects that may occur as a result of radiation damage to the brain include altered testosterone levels, which can lead to failure to complete puberty, accelerated puberty, decreased sexual desire, and impotence. Careful monitoring and handling of these effects, in close collaboration with an endocrinologist, can produce better outcomes.

Females: Ovarian function can be affected by both chemotherapy and radiation to the abdomen. The degree of dysfunction largely depends on the age and stage of puberty at diagnosis. Girls who have not yet been through puberty are less affected. Protecting the ovaries is a major concern when abdominal radiation is necessary. Some chemotherapy drugs may allow for puberty to progress normally after treatment, but girls who receive these are still at risk for delayed menses, premature menopause, and reduced fertility.

Radiation treatment to the head can interfere with the hormones needed for ovarian function. Such alterations can lead to irregular menstrual bleeding, changes in the release of eggs, and early puberty.

Reproduction: Many survivors of childhood cancer have concerns related to their ability to parent a child, support a pregnancy, and produce healthy offspring. Most survivors of childhood cancer can go on to produce healthy children, though risks do exist. Decreased fertility issues, early menopause, and other treatment-related problems could affect pregnancy outcome. Some women are encouraged to try and get pregnant during the early childbearing years to improve the chances of a successful conception. Individual circumstances vary. Genetic counseling may be helpful.

Radiation therapy to the abdomen or testicles can reduce or eliminate sperm production in males. Abdominal radiation in females interferes with the quality of eggs and may reduce the ability of the uterus to carry a fetus to term.

Studies continue to monitor the risk of congenital anomalies in the offspring of cancer survivors. While recent studies have shown no significant link, treatment protocols may involve different medicines or doses not yet proven safe to future offspring.

Cardiovascular system: Anthracyclines, have been linked with decreased heart function in childhood cancer survivors. Other medications have also been linked, though not as strongly, with the risk of heart problems. Radiation to the chest area is also considered a risk to the heart. Total dose delivered, type of delivery, and age of the patient at the time of treatment all contribute to this risk. Late cardiotoxic effects in long-term survivors include pericarditis, myocarditis, left ventricular failure, arrhythmias, coronary artery disease, myocardial infarction, heart failure and even death. Careful monitoring is especially important in these patients because often there are no symptoms. Echocardiography can identify hidden problems. With routine physical examinations and testing, such complications may be found early and treated, if necessary. Echocardiography every 2 years is indicated for patients treated with a cumulative dose of 300 mg/m^2 or more of anthracyclines or lower doses with mediastinal irradiation. Percutaneous endomyocardial biopsy is also undertaken in some centers as the most direct evidence of anthracycline cardiotoxicity.

Studies are now underway to determine if medications proven to protect the heart in adults, such as ICRF-187 during similar chemotherapy may also help children.

Respiratory: Respiratory problems, such as decreased lung volume and lung fibrosis, are most common in children who have received radiation therapy to the chest. Such therapy is used for patients with Hodgkin disease or cancers that have spread to the lung from other primary sites. Other lung problems may include pneumonitis and reduced lung compliance.

Certain chemotherapy drugs, such as bleomycin, may also lead to these problems. The problems may be worse if both radiation and certain chemotherapy drugs are given. These changes can occur even years after treatment, but for many, problems are first seen within 1 to 2 years.

Treatments are available to help reduce the symptoms of fibrosis and pneumonitis. Careful clinical follow-up and investigations, such as chest radiography and pulmonary function tests will help to identify those at risk. Lung biopsy may also be indicated if chest radiograph suggests fibrosis.

Muscle and bone: Radiation therapy can have serious effects on the proper growth of bone and muscle in young people. Very young children have much growth ahead of them, and radiation therapy can slow the growth of any given area. Bones, soft tissue, muscle, and blood vessels are very sensitive to radiation during times of rapid growth. Therefore, children under the age of 6 or children undergoing a growth spurt at puberty are at risk, and there may be unequal growth of body parts. In addition to stunted bone growth, osteoporosis and joint problems can occur.

Teeth: Radiation therapy given to an area that involves the teeth may cause a reduced salivation, leading to dry mouth and/or cavities. When given to the very young child, tooth development may be delayed. Routine dental exams are important to identify problems early.

Second cancers: Childhood cancer survivors have a small but increased risk of developing a second cancer during their lifetime. This risk is 10–20% times than the general population. This risk is not the same for all survivors. Many factors affect risk, such as the type of the first cancer, type of treatments received, and genetics. Those survivors who received radiation therapy tend to show a higher risk of second cancers in the areas that were irradiated. As childhood cancer survivor lives longer into adulthood, they are at higher risk of developing cancers usually seen in adults. One such example is increased incidence of breast cancer in women who have received radiation to the chest due to malignancy in childhood like Hodgkin's Disease. Radiotherapy also increases the chances of thyroid cancer, skin cancer, brain tumors and bone and soft tissue sarcomas. Chemotherapeutic agents like alkalyting agents and topoisomerase II inhibitors increase the chances of secondary leukemia.

As these children grow up and age, lifestyle influences, environmental exposures, and personal choices all play a part in their cancer risk. It is important to remember and keep permanent, detailed records of the cancer treatments that were received during childhood. Sharing this information with their doctors will help those who had cancer as children to make better screening choices throughout their lives.

Psychosocial consequences: The anxiety felt during the therapy is often replaced by concerns about disease recurrence, future well-being, physical disabilities and psychosocial adjustments. They are more likely to show agitation, restlessness and hyperactivity. Specific educational and occupational achievements may be affected by intellectual deficits and learning problems. The learning problems along with school disruptions may have a bearing on the child's academic performance.

In adulthood, they may also face workplace discrimination, ineligibility for health and life insurance and adverse employers' attitude.

Recommendations for intervention include baseline assessment and periodic neuropsychological monitoring. A multidisciplinary approach to the psychosocial care of these children and their families is of utmost importance for optimum outcome.

Care of Cancer Survivors

Survivors of childhood cancers should undergo follow-up throughout the rest of their lives. Carers should strike a balance between reassurance to the patient and his family and watchful vigilance for occurrence of serious side-effects like second malignancies or relapse. Ideally, every pediatric oncology unit must have a protocol for follow-up programs to fulfill medical and social obligations towards children cured of cancer. As these children graduate to the care of non-pediatric medical specialists, the late-effects clinic should include appropriate transitional programs involving medical oncologist, family practitioner, psychologist and obstetrician-gynecologist. Table 44.1 gives the salient information to be obtained during follow-up visits.

- History of any intercurrent illness
- Educational and academic performance
- Employment status
- Marital, menses and sexual activity
- Pregnancy outcome.

In addition to the continued vigilance for late-effects of cancer treatment, the preventive health considerations directed to the population, in general, are also warranted in case of these special children. These include avoidance of smoking, excessive alcohol consumption, and routine cancer related screening tests like breast self-examination, etc.

The population of childhood cancer survivors presents researchers with both an opportunity and an obligation:

- The *opportunity* to gain new knowledge about the long-term effects of cancer and therapy, knowledge that can be used to help design treatment protocols and intervention strategies that will increase survival and minimize harmful health effects.

Table 44.1: The patient evaluation should include the following during each visit

- Growth monitoring
- Assessment of pubertal development and fertility counseling
- Neuropsychological and social status assessment. IQ examination
- Measurement of blood pressure
- Cardiac evaluation
- Complete blood count and urine analysis.
- Thyroid and other endocrine evaluation as indicated
- Monitoring for relapse and second malignancies
- Postsplenectomy precautions
- Genetic counseling when indicated such as in survivors of retinoblastoma.

- The *obligation* to educate survivors about the potential impacts of cancer diagnosis and treatment on their health, and to provide follow-up care, for example, by creating and implementing programs for the prevention and early detection of late effects.

The Childhood Cancer Survivor Study (CCSS) in USA was created to take advantage of this opportunity and obligation. The CCSS is a component of the long-term follow-up study, which is a collaborative, multi-institutional study funded by the National Cancer Institute,USA. The CCSS is composed of individuals who survived five or more years after treatment for cancer, leukemia, tumor, or similar illness diagnosed during childhood or adolescence between 1970 and 1986. It is coordinated through St. Jude Children's Research Hospital in Memphis, Tennessee.

In UK, the Childhood Cancer Study Group (UKCCSG) is collaborating with British Children Cancer Survival Study (BCCSS), which is examining the health of about 16,000 survivors diagnosed with cancer during their childhood between 1947 and 1991. These patients were identified through the records of the National Registry of Childhood Tumors housed at Children Cancer Reasearch Group (CCRG) in Oxford.

Childhood cancer follow-up programs are yet to gain momentum in a systematic way in India. Tata Memorial Hospital was the first to initiate a childhood cancer survival clinic in the year 1991. It was named after completion of therapy (ACT) clinic. It aims to monitor growth, development, sexual maturation, the late effects of therapy and proper rehabilitative measures to help these children have a productive adulthood. Table 44.2 shows the follow-up statistics of 370 surviving children with childhood cancers from the ACT clinic.

For all survivors, while late effects may offer significant problems, they are the result of lifesaving treatment. Researchers will continue to search for ways to reduce long-term effects. Meanwhile, the gift of life may involve coping with the late effects of treatment as the quest for 'disease free' survival continues (Figs 44.4 to 44.6).

Additional Resources

Candlelighters Childhood Cancer Foundation Internet Address: http://www.cancer.org/docroot/ipg.asp?sitename=Candlelighters+Childhood+Cancer+Foundation&url=http://www.candlelighters.org

National Cancer Institute Internet Address: http://www.cancer.org/docroot/ipg.asp?sitename=National+Cancer+Institute&url=http://www.cancer.gov (search for "late effects of childhood cancer")

CureSearch, a combined effort of National Childhood Cancer Foundation and Children's Oncology Group http://www.cancer.org/docroot/ipg.asp?sitename=CureSearch&url=http://www.curesearch.org (look for "after treatment" section)

National Dissemination Center for Children with Disabilities (NICHCY) http://www.cancer.org/docroot/

Table 44.2: Statistics of 370 surviving children with childhood cancers from the ACT clinic

Condition of survivors	No.	%
Completely normal	162	44%
Asymptomatic laboratory changes detected by study protocol	89	24%
Moderate symptomatic changes corrected by interventions	30	8%
Severe impairments (impaired reproduction learning disabilities, etc.	74	20%
Life threatening problems like recurrence and second malignancy	15	4%
Total	370	100%

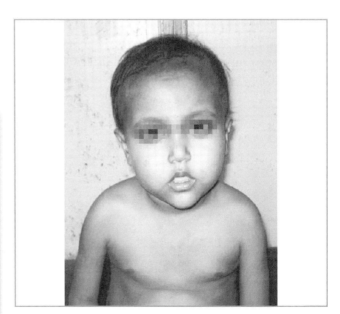

Fig. 44.4: ALL survivor

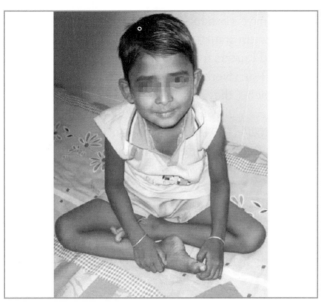

Fig. 44.5: ALL survivor maintaining remission in continuation phase

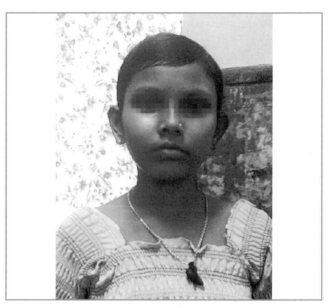

Fig. 44.6: ALL survivor in remission following completion of maintenance therapy

ipg.asp?sitename=National+Dissemination+Center +for+ Children+with+Disabilities&url=http://http:// www.nichcy.org

SUGGESTED READING

1. Dreyer ZE, Blatt J, Bleyer A. Late effects of childhood cancer and its treatment. In: Principles and Practice of Pediatric Oncology. (Editors-Pizzi PA, Poplack DG). Fourth Edition. Lippincott, Williams and Wilkins Philadelphia. 2002;1431-61.

2. Hobbie W, Ruccione K, Harvey J, Moore IM. Care of survivors. In: Baggott CR, Kelly KP, Fochtman D, Foley GV (Eds). Nursing Care of Children and Adolescents with Cancer. WB Saunders; Philadelphia: 2002;426-65.

3. Kurkure P, Achrekar S, Dalvi N, Goswami S. Childhood Cancer survivors-Living beyond cure. Indian J Pediatr. 2003;70:825-8.

4. Kurkure PA. Childhood cancer survivors. In: Practical Pediatric Oncology. Agarwar BR (Ed);PHO:2:154-7.

5. Marina N. Long-term survivors of childhood cancer: The medical consequences of cure. P Clin N Am. 1997;44:1021-42.

6. Robison, Green, Hudson, et al. Long-term outcomes of adult survivors of childhood cancer. In: Cancer-Survivorship: Resilience Across the Lifespan. Supplement to Cancer. American Cancer Society. 2005;2557-664.

45 Evidence-based Pediatric Oncology Practice

Madhumita Nandi

In this era of rapidly expanding medical information, it is really difficult to keep oneself up-to-date with all the latest developments. It has been calculated that a clinician would have to read at least 19 articles a day, 365 days a year just to keep himself abreast with the latest developments. For a pediatrician, this figure is 1694 articles a year or at least 5 articles a day. So to make this task somewhat easier, a system is gradually evolving since the past few decades which can give scientifically validated medical information in a short time and which is also easily retrievable and reproducible. This system is called Evidence-based Medicine (EBM). In the system of EBM, a busy clinician has to devote minimum reading time to access maximum possible, selective and patient-driven medical information.

Evidence-based Medicine (EBM) is integrating individual clinical expertise with the best available external evidence from systematic research. It has made rapid strides in the last ten years. Many EBM centers, books and agencies are coming up. Some of the important ones relevant to child health are the Evidence-based Pediatrics (book with updates), ACP Journal Club/Evidence-based Medicine Online (Best Evidence and Ovid EBM reviews), Bandolier, Clinical Evidence, Evidence-based On-Call, Cochrane Database of Systematic Reviews, Cochrane Controlled Clinical Trials Register, Archives of Disease of Childhood—Archimedes section, Archives of Pediatric and Adolescent Medicine—evidence-based journal club, Journal of Pediatrics—Abstracts from the Literature, etc. Most of these are based in the western world. Our side of

the world is yet to catch up with it, though a sincere effort is being made by a few Indian centers. A new section has been started in Indian Pediatrics called EURECA (Evidence that is Understandable, Relevant, Extendible, Current and Appraised), which carries evidence based discussions on issues relevant to child health. But, for EBM to be truly relevant in the Indian settings, the systematic reviews should be carried out on studies conducted only in our settings because the results of western studies cannot always be extrapolated to our settings. But, still IAP has made a commendable beginning.

The supporters of EBM claim that it is the best and most objective system of medicine. Its opponents criticize it for many reasons like it is a 'cook-book' medicine, it is the fad of epidemiologists, etc. So, rather than allowing EBM to rule over us, we can make it our friend keeping all its caveats in mind. We should have a balance between clinical experience and acumen and knowledge gained from EBM. As Sackett, the pioneer of EBM, has himself said, "We should build upon rather than disparage or neglect the knowledge gained from good clinical skills and sound clinical experience. Rather, it needs a high level of clinical acumen to arrive at a sound evidence based therapeutic decision."

Keeping all these in mind, following is a discussion on evidence-based practice on different issues related to pediatric oncology. As the Cochrane studies are considered the 'Gold-Standard" of evidence-based medicine, most of the following evidences have been taken from the Cochrane Libraries.

EFFECTS OF RADIATION ON TESTICULAR FUNCTION IN LONG-TERM SURVIVORS OF ALL

In a Cochrane contolled clinical trial, the author studied the long-term effects of radiation on the testicular function in 60 survivors of acute lymphoblastic leukemia. All the patients were treated on two consecutive Children Cancer Study Group protocols and received identical chemotherapy and either 18 or 24 Gy radiation therapy (RT) to one of the following fields: craniospinal plus 12 Gy abdominal RT including the gonads (group 1); craniospinal (group 2); or cranial (group 3). The median age at the time of their last evaluation was 14.5 years (range, 10.5 to 25.7), which took place a median of 5.0 years (range, 1 to 10.3) after discontinuing therapy. The incidence of primary germ cell dysfunction as judged by raised levels of follicle-stimulating hormone (FSH) and/ or reduced testicular volume was significantly associated with field of RT; 55% of group 1, 17% of group 2, and 0% of group 3 were abnormal (P = .002). Leydig cell function, as assessed by plasma concentrations of luteinizing hormone (LH) and testosterone, and pubertal development, was unaffected in the majority of subjects regardless of RT field. These data indicate that in boys undergoing therapy for ALL, germ cell dysfunction is common following testicular irradiation and can occur following exposure to scattered irradiation from craniospinal RT. In contrast, Leydig cell function appears resistant to direct irradiation with doses as high as 12 Gy.

Sklar CA, Robison LL, Nesbit ME, Sather HN, Meadows AT, Ortega JA, Kim TH, Hammond GD. Effects of radiation on testicular function in long-term survivors of childhood acute lymphoblastic leukemia: a report from the Children Cancer Study Group. The Cochrane Central Register of Controlled Trials (CENTRAL), 2008, Issue 2.

EFFECTS OF RADIATION ON OVARIAN FUNCTION IN LONG-TERM SURVIVORS OF CHILDHOOD ACUTE LYMPHOBLASTIC LEUKEMIA

In a Cochrane controlled clinical trial, the author assessed serum follicle-stimulating hormone (FSH), luteinizing hormone (LH), and pubertal development in 97 long-term female survivors of childhood acute lymphoblastic leukemia (ALL). All patients received identical induction and maintenance therapy with either 18 or 24 Gy of radiation therapy (RT) to one of the following fields: cranial, craniospinal, or craniospinal plus 12 Gy abdominal RT including the ovaries. Thirty-six percent (35 patients) were found to have above normal levels of FSH and/or LH. The percentages of elevated values for RT fields were 93% for craniospinal plus abdominal RT, 49% for craniospinal RT, and 9% for cranial RT (P less than .001). A dose-response relationship was observed between 18 Gy and 24 Gy in females receiving only craniospinal RT (P = .01). Craniospinal plus abdominal RT and abnormal FSH/LH levels were significantly associated with lack of pubertal development and delayed onset of menses. Duration of maintenance chemotherapy was not associated with abnormal gonadotropin levels or the development of secondary sexual characteristics.

Hamre MR, Robison LL, Nesbit ME, Sather HN, Meadows AT, Ortega JA, D'Angio GJ, Hammond GD. Effects of radiation on ovarian function in long-term survivors of childhood acute lymphoblastic leukemia: a report from the Childrens Cancer Study Group. The Cochrane Central Register of Controlled Trials (CENTRAL), 2008, Issue 2.

LONG-TERM NEUROPSYCHOLOGIC SEQUELAE OF CHILDHOOD LEUKEMIA: COMPARISON

In a Cochrane controlled clinical trial, the author, compared the late neuropsychologic toxicities of CNS prophylaxis in childhood acute lymphoblastic leukemia (ALL), a transversal assessment was performed in two groups of ALL patients and two control groups. The ALL patients had received one of the following CNS prophylaxes: cranial irradiation, 24 Gy and i.t. MTX 10 mg/m^2, 6 doses (RT group, n = 25) or i.t. Ara-C 30 mg/m^2 and i.t. MTX 10 mg/m^2, 10 doses (ChT group, n = 29). The two control groups were: Siblings (Sb, n = 24) and solid tumors (ST, n = 22). Intelligence quotient (IQ), memory, learning, attention and frontal tasks were studied. Comparative analyses between ChT and RT showed no differences in any of the tests. When RT was compared with ST or Sb, RT showed a 10-point lower mean IQ (p greater than 0.05). The results of ChT versus ST or versus Sb were worse in the ChT group. In many tests, the differences were statistically significant. Analyses of the 54 ALL patients compared with the 46 controls showed significant differences in all tests except verbal memory and verbal learning. The author concluded that prophylactic CNS therapy definitely cause cognitive dysfunctions.

Giralt J, Ortega JJ, Olive T, Verges R, Forio I, Salvador L. Long-term neuropsychologic sequelae of childhood leukemia: comparison of two CNS prophylactic regimens. The Cochrane Central Register of Controlled Trials (CENTRAL), 2008, Issue 2.

LONG-TERM EFFECTS OF CRANIAL RADIATION THERAPY ON ATTENTION FUNCTIONING IN SURVIVORS OF CHILDHOOD LEUKEMIA

The author retrospectively examined the long-term effects of cranial radiation therapy (CRT) on attention functioning. Fifty-six survivors of childhood leukemia who had been randomly assigned to a treatment regimen of chemotherapy with or without 1,800 cGy CRT were administered a neuropsychological test battery. Significant differences were found between the irradiated and nonirradiated groups on three of four attentional components. An interaction between treatment type and age at diagnosis was significant on one attentional component. Further, the mean scores of participants irradiated in early childhood were significantly low relative to published norms for age-standard scores on the majority of task variables, while the other groups showed rare deviations from average scores. Findings from this study indicate that irradiation in early childhood is associated with significant impairment in attentional filtering, focusing, and automatic shifting

Lockwood KA, Bell TS, Colegrove RW Jr. Long-term effects of cranial radiation therapy on attention functioning in survivors of childhood leukemia. The Cochrane Central Register of Controlled Trials (CENTRAL), 2008, Issue 2.

PROPHYLACTIC CRANIAL IRRADIATION DOSE EFFECTS ON LATE COGNITIVE FUNCTION IN CHILDREN TREATED FOR ACUTE LYMPHOBLASTIC LEUKEMIA

Long-term neuropsychological sequelae are documented in children who received 2400 cGy prophylactic cranial irradiation. The dose was reduced to 1800 cGy. This study assesses radiation dose effects on cognitive function in children with leukemia who received central nervous system prophylaxis with 2400 cGy versus 1800 cGy whole brain radiotherapy. All leukemic children also received intrathecal methotrexate. A control group of children (treated for Wilms' tumor) received no central nervous system therapy. Nineteen children were treated with 2400 cGy, 16 children with 1800 cGy. The 12 control children received no irradiation. All patients were off therapy for at least 70 months. The 1800 cGy and 2400 cGy patient groups were off therapy for equivalent periods of time (range 70-123 mo) at follow-up testing standardized psychological tests were administered. Full-scale, verbal, and performance IQ were measured with the Wechsler intelligence scale for children-revised. Wide Range Achievement Testing evaluated reading, spelling, and arithmetic abilities. Children treated with 1800 cGy performed significantly better than those who received 2400 cGy, and at the same level as controls. There were statistically significant differences between the 1800 cGy and 2400 cGy subjects in all measures. 2400 cGy patients had deficiencies in IQ and academic performance. 1800 cGy patients scored approximately 12 points higher than 2400 cGy children. Eleven children, two in the control group, two in the 1800 cGy, and seven in the 2400 cGy group had IQ scores of less than 90. Eight of the nine irradiated children with deficits had radiotherapy before age 5. These results indicate a mild, but diffuse information processing deficit in children who received 2400 cGy, but not in children who received 1800 cGy. These findings with a minimum of 6 years of follow-up provide new information on late effects of CNS prophylaxis in ALL. Reducing the cranial RT dose from 2400 cGy to 1800 cGy reduced neurotoxicity to acceptable levels.

Halberg FE, Kramer JH, Moore IM, Wara WM, Matthay KK, Ablin AR. Prophylactic cranial irradiation dose effects on late cognitive function in children treated for acute lymphoblastic leukemia. The Cochrane Central Register of Controlled Trials (CENTRAL), 2008, Issue 2.

INTERMEDIATE-DOSE METHOTREXATE VERSUS CRANIAL IRRADIATION IN CHILDHOOD ACUTE LYMPHOBLASTIC LEUKEMIA

With the improving cure rate, the quality of life and avoidance of second cancers have become important concerns in the management of ALL. 596 children and adolescents with ALL were randomized between 1976 and 1979 to receive intermediate-dose methotrexate (IDM) plus intrathecal methotrexate (IT MTX) or cranial radiation (CRT) plus IT MTX. After 10 additional years of follow-up, the pattern and significance of the results reported in 1983 are confirmed. IDM offered better hematologic protection (P < 0.0006), better testicular protection (P = 0.002), but CRT offered better central nervous system (CNS) protection (P < 0.0001). There was no evidence of an excessive number of second primaries over the general population of children. It was concluded that CRT offered better CNS protection, but IDM offered better systemic and testicular protection. A small risk of second cancers or cardiac dysfunction may be acceptable with therapies, which produce long-term documented survival benefits.

Freeman AI, Boyett JM, Glicksman AS, Brecher ML, Leventhal BG, Sinks LF, Holland JF. Intermediate-dose methotrexate versus cranial irradiation in childhood acute lymphoblastic leukemia: a ten-year follow-up. The Cochrane Central Register of Controlled Trials (CENTRAL), 2008, Issue 2.

EFFICACY OF POST–INDUCTION INTENSIFICATION CHEMOTHERAPY REGIMENS IN PREVENTING RELAPSE IN ALL

Four hundred thirty patients with high-risk acute lymphoid leukemia were entered on the acute leukemia in childhood protocol (AlinC 12) of the Pediatric Division of the Pediatric Oncology Group. This study was a prospective randomized comparison of two regimens that had as their primary differences: (1) an intensification period with Cytoxan (cyclophosphamide) and asparaginase after induction; (2) a period of intravenous methotrexate before initiating maintenance; and (3) in the regimen that had those two additions, triple-drug chemoprophylaxis of the central nervous system (CNS) using methotrexate, hydrocortisone, and cytosine arabinoside as compared to cranial irradiation and intrathecal methotrexate. All patients received vincristine and prednisone induction, 6-mercaptopurine and methotrexate maintenance, and vincristine and prednisone pulse intensification. There was no significant difference in the rate of bone marrow relapse. However, overall disease-free survival favored the arm with intensification and chemoprophylaxis because of a lesser incidence of extramedullary relapse. Thus, for treatment 1 versus treatment 3, the two-sided P values were for overall disease-free survival 0.16; bone marrow relapses 0.13; all CNS relapses 0.04; and all extramedullary disease relapses 0.013. It is concluded that post-induction intensification protects against testicular relapse and that chemoprophylaxis is adequate prophylaxis against isolated CNS relapse.

Van Eys J, Berry D, Crist W, Doering E, Fernbach D, Pullen J, Shuster J, Wharam M. A comparison of two regimens for high-risk acute lymphocytic leukemia in childhood. A Pediatric Oncology Study Group. The Cochrane Central Register of Controlled Trials (CENTRAL), 2008, Issue 2.

COLONY STIMULATING FACTORS FOR CHEMOTHERAPY INDUCED FEBRILE NEUTROPENIA

Febrile neutropenia is a frequent event for cancer patients undergoing chemotherapy and it is potentially a life-threatening situation. The current treatment is supportive care plus antibiotics. Colony stimulating factors (CSF) are cytokines that stimulate and accelerate the production of one or more cellular lines in bone marrow. Some clinical trials addressed the question of whether the addition of CSF to antibiotics (ATB) could improve the outcomes of patients with febrile neutropenia. A Cochrane metanalysis included all RCTs that compared CSF plus antibiotics versus antibiotics alone for the treatment of established febrile neutropenia in adults and children. The author concluded that the use of CSF in patients with febrile neutropenia due to cancer chemotherapy does not affect overall mortality, but reduces the amount of time spent in hospital and the neutrophil recovery period. It was not clear whether CSF has an effect on infection-related mortality.

Clark OAC, Lyman G, Castro AA, Clark LGO, Djulbegovic B. Colony stimulating factors for chemotherapy induced febrile neutropenia. Cochrane Database of Systematic Reviews 2000, Issue 4. Art. No. CD003039. DOI: 10.1002/14651858.CD003039.

COLONY STIMULATING FACTORS FOR PREVENTION OF MYELOSUPPRESSIVE THERAPY INDUCED FEBRILE NEUTROPENIA IN CHILDREN WITH ACUTE LYMPHOBLASTIC LEUKEMIA

Febrile neutropenia is a potentially life-threatening side effect of treatment of acute leukemia of childhood. Current treatment consists of supportive care plus antibiotics. Clinical trials have attempted to evaluate the use of colony-stimulating factors (CSF) as additional therapy to prevent febrile neutropenia in children with ALL. The individual trials do not show whether there is significant benefit or not. Systematic review provides the most reliable assessment and the best recommendations for practice. The author tried to evaluate the safety and effectiveness of the addition of G-CSF or GM-CSF to myelosuppressive chemotherapy in children with ALL, in an effort to prevent the development of febrile neutropenia. Evaluation of number of febrile neutropenia episodes, length to neutrophil count recovery, incidence and length of hospitalization, number of infectious disease episodes, incidence and length of treatment delays, side effects (flu-like syndrome, bone pain and allergic reaction), relapse and overall mortality (death) were undertaken.

Six studies were included with a total of 332 participants in the analysis. There were insufficient data to assess the effect on survival. The use of CSF significantly reduced the number of episodes of febrile neutropenia episodes (Rate ratio = 0.63; 95% confidence interval (CI) 0.46 to 0.85; p = 0.003, with substantial heterogeneity), the length of hospitalization (weighted mean difference (WMD) = – 1.58; 95% CI – 3.00 to – 0.15; p = 0.03), and number of infectious diseases episodes (Rate ratio = 0.44; 95% CI 0.24 to 0.80; p = 0.002). In spite of these results, CSF did not influence the length of episodes of neutropenia (WMD = – 1.11; 95% CI – 3.55 to 1.32; p = 0.4) or delays in chemotherapy courses (Rate ratio = 0.77; 95% CI 0.49 to 1, 23; p = 0.28). The author concluded that children with ALL treated with CSF benefit from shorter hospitalization and fewer infections. However, there was no evidence for a shortened duration of neutropenia nor fewer treatment delays, and no useful information about survival.

Sasse EC, Sasse AD, Brandalise SR, Clark OAC, Richards S. Colony stimulating factors for prevention of myelosuppressive therapy induced febrile neutropenia in children with acute lymphoblastic leukemia. Cochrane Database of Systematic Reviews 2008 DOI: 10.1002/14651858.CD004139.pub2

THE EFFECT OF CYTOKINES G-CSF AND GM-CSF IN THERAPY OF CHILDHOOD MALIGNANCIES

The increase in the intensity of oncologic treatment leads to the improvement of therapeutic results and increased number of permanent complete remissions in children with malignant tumors and lymphoproliferative diseases. The negative side of intensive chemotherapy and radiotherapy is the high-risk of serious side effects the most frequent of which is complication of a drug dependent bone marrow suppression observed in more than 70% patients. The author assessed the influence of G-CSF and GM-CSF on the duration of neutropenia and the number of infectious complications in oncologic patients. The group of 43 children with malignant solid tumors and lymphoproliferative diseases were included in the study and 10 patients selected at random who received no cytokines formed the control group. The clinical indication to cytokines administration was the decrease in neutrophils number below 500/mm^3 and leukocytes number below 1000/mm^3. The increase of leukocytosis above 1000/mm^3 was described as a positive therapeutic effect and only in 5 of 116 therapeutic cycles a positive effect was not achieved. The beneficial effect of cytokines was a 4 days reduction in the duration of neutropenic period in comparison with the control group. None of the patients died from infections during the cytokines administration. Both cytokines were all tolerated and the only side effects were observed: parainfluenzal symptoms, local inflammatory infiltration in the site of the drug administration and generalized allergic skin. These symptoms appeared occasionally and were completely reversible.

Balcerska A, Ploszynska A, Polczynska K, Maciejka-Kapuscinska L, Wlazlowski M, Drozynska E, Stefanowicz J, Szalewska M, Klejnotowska J. The effect of cytokines G-CSF and GM-CSF in therapy of childhood malignancies. The Cochrane Central Register of Controlled Trials (CENTRAL) 2008, Issue 2.

IMPROVEMENT IN TREATMENT OF CHILDHOOD ACUTE LYMPHOBLASTIC LEUKEMIA: A 10-YEAR STUDY BY THE CHILDREN'S CANCER AND LEUKEMIA STUDY GROUP

The Children's Cancer and Leukemia Study Group (CCLSG) has conducted, since 1981, a series of protocols for treatment of acute lymphoblastic leukemia (ALL) in childhood. In a randomized control study of the 811 protocol (1981-1983) for standard-risk ALL, an intermittent cyclic regimen of an intermediate-dose of methotrexate (MTX) plus 6-mercaptopurine (6 MP) showed significant superiority for maintenance chemotherapy as compared with conventional continuous administration of a low dose of the two drugs. The event-free survival (EFS) rate at 10 years was 65.4% for the intermittent cyclic regimen, while the EFS rate of continuous regimen was 36.1% (P < 0.01). The intermittent cyclic regimen may

also be effective in preventing extramedullary relapses. In the 841 protocol (1984-1987), the three-drug induction therapy consisting of vincristine (VCR), prednisone (PDN) and L-asparaginase (L-ASP) improved the EFS rate (94.1% at 8 years) as compared with the two-drug therapy consisting of VCR and PDN (64.1%, P < 0.05). In the 874 protocol (1987-1990), two regimens with or without cranial irradiation for standard-risk patients were compared with respect to their ability to prevent central nervous system (CNS) leukemia and to improve overall outcome of ALL. The regimen with cranial irradiation showed a 79.9% EFS rate at 5 years, whereas the regimen without cranial irradiation demonstrated a 69.1% EFS rate (not significantly). Life-table analysis of serial CCLSG protocols for ALL in which the cyclic administration of intermediate-dose MTX plus 6 MP has been standardized as maintenance therapy revealed that the outcome of all over ALL has gradually improved with increase of the EFS rate; 41.4% for the 811 protocol, 51.4% for the 841 protocol to 54.4% for the more recent 874 protocol.

Koizumi S, Fujimoto T. Improvement in treatment of childhood acute lymphoblastic leukemia: a 10-year study by the Children's Cancer and Leukemia Study Group. The Cochrane Central Register of Controlled Trials (CENTRAL) 2008, Issue 2.

TREATMENT STRATEGY AND RESULTS IN CHILDREN TREATED ON THREE DUTCH CHILDHOOD ONCOLOGY GROUP ACUTE MYELOID LEUKEMIA TRIALS

This report describes the long-term follow-up data of three consecutive Dutch Childhood Oncology Group acute myeloid leukemia (AML) protocols. A total of 303 children were diagnosed with AML, of whom 209 were eligible for this report. The first study was the AML-82 protocol. Results were inferior (5-year probability of overall survival (pOS) 31%) to other available regimes. Study AML-87 was based on the BFM-87 protocol, with prophylactic cranial irradiation in high-risk patients only, and without maintenance therapy. This led to a higher cumulative incidence of relapse than that reported by the Berlin-Frankfurt-Münster (BFM), but survival was similar (5-year pOS 47%), suggesting successful retrieval at relapse. The subsequent study AML-92/94 consisted of a modified BFM-93 protocol, that is, without maintenance therapy and prophylactic cranial irradiation. However, all patients were to be transplanted (auto- or allogeneic), although compliance was poor. Antileukemic efficacy was offset by an increase in the cumulative incidence of nonrelapse mortality, especially in remission patients, and survival did not improve (5-year pOS 44%). The results demonstrated that outcome in childhood AML is still unsatisfactory, and that further intensification of therapy carries the risk of enhanced toxicity.

Kardos G, Zwaan CM, Kaspers GJ, de-Graaf SS, de Bont ES, Postma A, Bökkerink JP, Weening RS, van der Does-van den Berg A, van Wering ER, Korbijn C, Hählen K-Treatment strategy and results in children treated on three Dutch Childhood Oncology Group acute myeloid leukemia trials. The Cochrane Central Register of Controlled Trials (CENTRAL) 2008, Issue 2.

DIFFERENT ANTHRACYCLINE DERIVATIVES FOR REDUCING CARDIOTOXICITY IN CANCER PATIENTS

The use of anthracycline chemotherapy is limited by the occurrence of cardiotoxicity. The primary objective of this Cochrane database of systematic reviews study was to determine the occurrence of cardiotoxicity with the use of different anthracycline derivatives (doxorubicin, daunorubicin, epirubicin) in cancer patients. The authors found that for the use of many different combinations of anthracycline derivates there was no high quality evidence available and it was impossible to draw conclusions.

For the use of epirubicin versus doxorubicin, there was some suggestion of a lower rate of clinical heart failure in patients treated with epirubicin. There is no evidence, which suggests a difference in anti-tumor response rate and survival between epirubicin and doxorubicin. No conclusions can be made regarding adverse effects. There are no data for children and patients with leukemia. Further research is needed. For the use of doxorubicin versus liposomal-encapsulated doxorubicin, the author found a significantly lower

rate of both clinical heart failure and subclinical heart failure (i.e various cardiac abnormalities, diagnosed with different diagnostic methods like echocardiography in asymptomatic patients) in patients treated with liposomal-encapsulated doxorubicin. There is no evidence which suggests a difference in anti-tumor response rate and survival between doxorubicin and liposomal-encapsulated doxorubicin. A lower rate of adverse effects was identified in patients treated with liposomal-encapsulated doxorubicin. There are no data for children and patients with leukemia. Further research is needed.

Van Dalen EC, Michiels EMC, Caron HN, Kremer LCM. Different anthracycline derivates for reducing cardiotoxicity in cancer patients. Cochrane Database of Systematic Reviews 2006, Issue 4. Art. No. CD005006. DOI: 10.1002/14651858.CD005006.pub2.

DIFFERENT DOSAGE SCHEDULES FOR REDUCING CARDIOTOXICITY IN CANCER PATIENTS RECEIVING ANTHRACYCLINE CHEMOTHERAPY

In yet another Cochrane database of systematic reviews, different anthracycline dosage schedules (i.e. peak doses and infusion durations) have been studied, to compare their efficacy, response rates, survival rates and cardiotoxicity. Six RCTs involving 625 patients (both children and adults) were included in the meta-analysis. The author found that an anthracycline infusion duration of six hours or longer reduced the risk of clinical heart failure, and it seemed to reduce the risk of subclinical cardiac damage. There is no evidence, which suggests a difference in response rate and survival between both treatment groups. Since there is only a small amount of data for children and also because data obtained in adults cannot be extrapolated to children, different anthracycline infusion durations should be evaluated further in children. For different anthracycline peak doses no high quality evidence was available and therefore, no definitive conclusions can be made about the occurrence of cardiotoxicity in patients treated with different anthracycline peak doses.

Van Dalen EC, Van der Pal HJH, Caron HN, Kremer LCM. Different dosage schedules for reducing cardiotoxicity in cancer patients receiving anthracycline chemotherapy. Cochrane Database of Systematic Reviews 2006, Issue 4. Art. No. CD005008. DOI: 10.1002/14651858.CD005008.pub2.

INTERVENTIONS FOR EARLY STAGE HODGKIN'S DISEASE IN CHILDREN

Hodgkin's disease is one of the most curable cancers in children, particularly at the early stages. However it is not clear which combinations of treatment strategies are most effective at maintaining high cure rates and minimizing long-term harmful effects or sequelae of treatment. A Cochrane meta-analysis tried to assess the effects of radiotherapy, chemotherapy or combined radiotherapy and chemotherapy on relapse free survival and overall survival rates in children with early (stage I to IIA) Hodgkin's disease. Four randomized controlled trials of involved field radiotherapy, extended field radiotherapy, anthracycline based chemotherapy regimens, or alkylating chemotherapy agents in children to 19 years of age with Hodgkin's disease involving 334 children were included. The trials were of variable quality.

One trial comparing radiotherapy alone showed no discernible difference in relapse free survival (relative risk 0.73, 95% confidence interval 0.49 to 1.09) or overall survival (relative risk 0.92, 95% confidence interval 0.79 to 1.07) between involved field and extended field radiotherapy. No discernible difference was found between involved field radiotherapy plus chemotherapy and extended field radiotherapy and chemotherapy (based on one small trial). In another trial, involved field radiotherapy plus chemotherapy appeared to increase relapse free survival compared to either involved field or extended field radiotherapy alone, although a discernible difference was found for overall survival. Extended field radiotherapy alone appeared to increase relapse free survival compared to extended radiotherapy plus chemotherapy (relative risk 0.34, 95% confidence interval 0.14 to 0.83) but no discernible difference was apparent for overall survival (based on one trial).

The review found there was not enough evidence from trials to show which treatments are best for children with Hodgkin's disease. Involved field radiotherapy, though, may be better than extended field radiotherapy.

Louw G, Pinkerton CR. Interventions for early stage Hodgkin's disease in children. Cochrane Database of Systematic Reviews 2002, Issue 2. Art. No. CD002035. DOI: 10.1002/14651858.

CHEMOTHERAPY, RADIOTHERAPY AND COMBINED MODALITY FOR HODGKIN'S DISEASE, WITH EMPHASIS ON SECOND CANCER RISK

Second malignancies (SM) are a major late effect of treatment for Hodgkin's disease (HD). Reliable comparisons of SM risk between alternative treatment strategies are lacking. Radiotherapy (RT), chemotherapy (CT) and combined chemo-radiotherapy (CRT) for newly-diagnosed Hodgkin's disease were compared with respect to SM risk, overall (OS) and progression-free (PFS) survival. Further, involved-field (IF-)RT is compared to extended-field (EF-)RT. 37 trials (9312 patients) were analysed: 15 (3343) for RT vs CRT, 16 (2861) for CT vs CRT, 3 (415) for RT vs CT and 10 (3221) for IF-R ' vs EF-RT. CRT was superior to RT in terms of OS (OR = 0.76, CI = 0.66 to 0.89, p = 0.0004), PFS (OR = 0.49, CI = 0.43 to 0.56, p < 0.0001) and SM (OR = 0.78, CI = 0.62 to 0.98, p = 0.03). The superiority of CRT also applied to early and advanced stages (mainly IIIA) separately. Excess SM with RT is due mainly to ST and is apparently caused by greater need for salvage therapy after RT. CRT was superior to CT in terms of PFS (OR = 77, CI 0.68 to 0.77, p < 0.0001). OS was better with CRT for early stages only (OR = 0.62, CI 0.44 to 0.88, p = 0.006). SM risk was higher with CRT (OR = 1.38, CI 1.00 to 1.89, p = 0.05), although not significant for early stages alone. This effect, also seen in AL and ST separately, was due directly to first-line treatment. Data were insufficient to compare RT to CT. EF-RT was superior to IF-RT (each additional to CT in most trials) in terms of PFS (OR = 81, CI 0.68 to 0.95, p = 0.009) but not OS. No significant difference in SM was observed. The author concluded that CRT seems to be optimal for most early stage (I-II) HD patients. For advanced stages (III-IV), CRT better prevents progression/relapse but CT alone seems to cause less SM. RT alone gives a higher overall SM risk than CRT due to increased need for salvage therapy. Reduced SM risk after

IF-RT instead of EF-RT could not be demonstrated. Due to the large number of studies excluded because no IPD were received, to the inclusion of many outdated treatments and to the limited amount of long-term data, one must be cautious in applying these results to current therapies.

Franklin JG, Paus MD, Pluetschow A, Specht L. Chemotherapy, radiotherapy and combined modality for Hodgkin's disease, with emphasis on second cancer risk. Cochrane Database of Systematic Reviews 2005, Issue 4. Art. No. CD003187. DOI: 10.1002/14651858.CD003187.pub2.

THERAPEUTIC INTERVENTIONS FOR BURKITT'S LYMPHOMA IN CHILDREN

Burkitt's lymphoma (BL) is a small non-cleaved cell lymphoma, which commonly presents as jaw swellings. Uncertainty remains as to the most effective form of management. Different regimens have been used to treat this condition with varied success rates. Randomized controlled trials (RCTs) of any duration were included to assess the evidence of any therapeutic strategy in the treatment of BL in this Cochrane analysis. Data could only be reviewed for ten studies but results were difficult to collate due to study and reporting quality, with differing outcome measures, small trial sizes, and each addressing a different question. There is need for further research on treatment options.

Okebe JU, Lasserson TJ, Meremikwu MM, Richards S. Therapeutic interventions for Burkitt's lymphoma in children. Cochrane Database of Systematic Reviews 2006, Issue 4. Art. No. CD005198. DOI: 10.1002/14651858. CD005198.pub2.

PROSPECTIVE STUDY OF 90 CHILDREN REQUIRING TREATMENT FOR JUVENILE MYELOMONOCYTIC LEUKEMIA OR MYELODYSPLASTIC SYNDROME: A REPORT FROM THE CHILDREN'S CANCER GROUP

The findings of first large prospective study of children with myelodysplastic syndrome (MDS) and juvenile myelomonocytic leukemia (JMML) treated in a uniform fashion on Children's Cancer Group protocol 2891 are reported in this Cochrane Central study. Ninety children with JMML, various forms of MDS, or acute myeloid leukemia (AML) with antecedent MDS were treated with a five-drug induction regimen (standard or intensive timing). Patients achieving remission were allocated to allogeneic bone marrow transplantation (BMT) if a matched family donor was available. All other patients were randomized between autologous BMT and aggressive nonmyeloablative chemotherapy. Results were compared with patients with de Novo AML. Patients with JMML and refractory anemia (RA) or RA-excess blasts (RAEB) exhibited high induction failure rates and overall remission of 58% and 48%, respectively. Remission rates for patients with RAEB in transformation (RAEB-T) (69%) or antecedent MDS (81%) were similar to de Novo AML (77%). Actuarial survival rates at 6 years were as follows: JMML, 31% +/− 26%; RA and RAEB, 29% +/− 16%; RAEB-T, 30% +/− 18%; antecedent MDS, 50% +/− 25%; and de Novo AML, 45% +/− 3%. For patients achieving remission, long-term survivors were found in those receiving either allogeneic BMT or chemotherapy. The presence of monosomy 7 had no additional adverse effect on MDS and JMML. The study concluded that childhood subtypes of MDS and JMML represent distinct entities with distinct clinical outcomes. Children with a history of MDS who present with AML do well with AML-type therapy. Patients with RA or RAEB respond poorly to AML induction therapy. The optimum treatment for JMML remains unknown.

Woods WG, Barnard DR, Alonzo TA, Buckley JD, Kobrinsky N, Arthur DC, Sanders J, Neudorf S, Gold S, Lange BJ. Prospective study of 90 children requiring treatment for juvenile myelomonocytic leukemia or myelodysplastic syndrome: a report from the Children's Cancer Group. The Cochrane Central Register of Controlled Trials (CENTRAL) 2008, Issue 2.

IMMEDIATE NEPHRECTOMY VERSUS PREOPERATIVE CHEMOTHERAPY IN THE MANAGEMENT OF NON-METASTATIC WILMS' TUMOR

The purpose of this study was to determine if patients receiving preoperative chemotherapy with vincristine and actinomycin D for non-metastatic Wilms' tumor have a more advantageous stage distribution and so need less treatment compared to patients who have immediate nephrectomy, without adversely affecting outcome. One hundred and eighty six patients were randomly assigned either to immediate surgery or to 6 weeks preoperative chemotherapy and then delayed surgery. Both groups of children received postoperative chemotherapy according to tumor stage and histology determined at the time of nephrectomy. The study found that six weeks of preoperative chemotherapy with vincristine and actinomycin D results in a significant shift towards a more advantageous stage distribution and hence reduction in therapy, while maintaining excellent event free and overall survival in children with non-metastatic Wilms' tumor. Around 20% of survivors were, therefore, spared the late-effects of doxorubicin or radiotherapy.

Mitchell C, Pritchard-Jones K, Shannon R, Hutton C, Stevens S, Machin D, Imeson J, Kelsey A, Vujanic GM, Gornall P, Walker J, Taylor R, Sartori P, Hale J, Levitt G, Messahel B, Middleton H, Grundy R, Pritchard J. Immediate nephrectomy versus preoperative chemotherapy in the management of non-metastatic Wilms' tumor. The Cochrane Central Register of Controlled Trials (CENTRAL) 2008, Issue 2.

INFLUENCE OF SURGERY AND RADIO-THERAPY ON GROWTH AND PUBERTAL DEVELOPMENT IN CHILDREN TREATED FOR BRAIN TUMOR

The increasing number of childhood cancer survivors has resulted in a growing interest in the late effects, which depend on type of treatment. Frequently, a brain tumor and its therapy in children are endocrinologically devastating. The aim of study was to compare growth and pubertal development in children after brain tumor therapy treated or not treated with recombinant growth hormone (rGH). Eighteen children were included in this study. Group I—(12/18) not treated with rGH, after total resection of brain tumor: craniopharyngeoma (8/12), astrocytoma (2/12) ependymoma (1/12), germinoma (1/12). Mean time of remission was 5.0 yrs (+/– 0.9). Group II—(6/12) treated with rGH, after subtotal resection of craniopharyngeoma (4/6), ependymoma (1/6), medulloblastoma (1/6) and cranial irradiation with mean total doses 46.5 Gy (+/– 5.65). Children were qualified for rGH replacement according to deceleration of growth and lower growth hormone secretion (< 10 ng/ml) in stimulating tests. Mean time of remission was 6, 5 years (+/– 2.41). Growth, height in centimeters converted to standard deviation score--SDS, body mass index (BMI), pubertal status and hormonal tests, were also evaluated. All patients were treated with surgery with no cranial irradiation in prepubertal age. 100% children of group I needed substitution because of secondary hypothyroidism, 83% due to secondary adrenal insufficiency and 53% of diabetes insipidus. Mean height after brain tumor surgical treatment in group I was – 1.24 SDS (+/– 0.85) and did not significantly change in the time of observation. Two girls needed hormonal substitution for hypogonadotropic hypogonadism. Mean BMI after total resection of brain tumor was 18.09 (+/– 4.20) and significantly increased to 23.73 (+/– 2.82). In group II—all children presented multihormonal pituitary insufficiency. Mean deviation score of height before rGH treatment was – 3.84 SDS (+/– 2.87) and after mean time of rGH therapy of 1.5 years (+/– 1.2) decreased to 2.6 (+/– 1,06). Mean BMI before treatment with rGH 18, 06 (+/– 4.4) increased to 22.41 (+ 0.74) in the time of observation and decreased to 18.5 (+/– 2.87) after 1, 5 years (+/– 1) of rGH treatment. The authors concluded that children treated with surgery for brain tumor need substitution for secondary hypothyroidism, part of them need treatment for secondary adrenal and gonadal insufficiency and diabetes insipidus. Children who were treated with surgery and/or cranial irradiation developed multihormonal pituitary insufficiency, growth failure and replacement rGh therapy was needed. Total resection of brain tumor without chemo- and radiotherapy did not impair growth in first year after surgery.

Birkholz D, Korpal-Szczyrska M, Kamińska H, Bień E, Połczyńska K, Stachowicz-Stencel T, Szołkiewicz A. Influence of surgery and radiotherapy on growth and pubertal development in children treated for brain tumor. The Cochrane Central Register of Controlled Trials (CENTRAL) 2008, Issue 2.

INTERVENTIONS FOR IMPROVING COMMUNICATION WITH CHILDREN AND ADOLESCENTS ABOUT THEIR CANCER

Communication with children and adolescents with cancer about their disease and treatment and the implications of these is an important aspect of good quality care. It is often poorly performed in practice. Various interventions have been developed that aim to enhance communication involving children or adolescents with cancer. In this Cochrane systematic review, the author tried to examine the effects of interventions to enhance communication with children and/or adolescents about their cancer, its treatment and their implications. Nine studies which met the criteria for inclusion were reviewed. They were diverse in terms of the interventions evaluated, study designs used, types of people who participated and the outcomes measured. One study of a computer-assisted education program reported improvements in knowledge and understanding about blood counts and cancer symptoms. One study of a CD-ROM about leukemia reported an improvement in children's feelings of control over their health. One study of art therapy as support for children during painful procedures reported an increase in positive, collaborative behavior. Two out of two studies of school reintegration programs reported improvements in some aspects of psychosocial well-being (one in anxiety and one in depression), social well-being (two in social competence and one in social support) and behavioral problems; and one reported improvements in physical competence. The author concluded that interventions to enhance communication involving children and adolescents with cancer have not been widely or rigorously assessed. The weak evidence that exists suggests that some children and adolescents with cancer may derive some benefit from specific information-giving programs and from interventions that aim to facilitate their reintegration into school and social activities. More research is needed to investigate the effects of these and other related interventions.

Scott JT, Harmsen M, Prictor MJ, Sowden AJ, Watt I. Interventions for improving communication with children and adolescents about their cancer. Cochrane Database of Systematic Reviews 2003, Issue 3. Art. No. CD002969. DOI: 10.1002/14651858.CD002969.

SURVIVING CANCER COMPETENTLY INTERVENTION PROGRAM (SCCIP): A COGNITIVE-BEHAVIORAL AND FAMILY THERAPY INTERVENTION FOR ADOLESCENT SURVIVORS OF CHILDHOOD CANCER AND THEIR FAMILIES

Psychological reactions to having had childhood cancer often continue after treatment ends, for survivors and their parents. The author developed an intervention program for adolescent survivors of childhood cancer, their parents, and siblings. Surviving Cancer Competently: An Intervention Program--SCCIP--is a one-day family group intervention that combines cognitive-behavioral and family therapy approaches. The goals of SCCIP are to reduce symptoms of distress and to improve family functioning and development. Program evaluation data indicated that all family members found SCCIP helpful. Standardized measures administered before the intervention and again at 6 months after SCCIP showed that symptoms of post-traumatic stress and anxiety decreased. Changes in family functioning were more difficult to discern. Overall, the results were promising with regard to the feasibility of the program and its potential for reducing symptoms of distress for all family members

Kazak AE, Simms S, Barakat L, Hobbie W, Foley B, Golomb V, Best M. Surviving cancer competently intervention program (SCCIP): a cognitive-behavioral and family therapy intervention for adolescent survivors of childhood cancer and their families. The Cochrane Central Register of Controlled Trials (CENTRAL) 2008, Issue 2.

SUGGESTED READING

1. Feldman W. Evidence-based pediatrics; BC Decker Inc. 2000.
2. Hadi I. Evidence-based medicine why and how? KMJ. 2006;38:1-2.

3. http://hiru.mcmaster.ca/cochrane/centers/Canadian.

4. http://www.ahrq.gov/clinic/.

5. http://www.cochrane.uottawa.ca/.

6. http://www.ebmny.org/ebmbib.html.

7. http://www.library.utoronto.ca/medicine/ebm.

8. Jadad AR, Moher M, Browman G, et al. Systematic reviews and meta-analyses on treatment of asthma: critical evaluation. BMJ. 2000;320:537-40.

9. Jaeschke R, Guyatt GH. What is evidence-based medicine? Sem Med Practice. 1999; 2:3-7.

10. John W. Evidence-based medicine in Japan. Lancet. 2005;336:112.

11. Sackett D: Evidence-based medicine: In its place. Lancet. 1995;346:785.

12. Sackett DL, RosenbergWMC, GrayL et al. Evidence-based medicine: What is and what it is not. BMJ. 1996;312:71-2.

13. Sackett DL, Straus SE, Richardson WS, Rosenberg W, Haynes RB. Evidence-based medicine: how to practice and teach EBM. Edinburgh, UK: Churchill Livingstone, 2000.

14. Smyth RL. Evidence-based Childhealth. In: Forfar and Arneil's Textbook of Pediatrics-6th Edition. McIntosh N, Helms P, Smyth RL (Eds). Churchill Livingstone. 2003:3-10.

Rakesh Mondal, Biman Roy

Q. Mom, the doctor said that I have cancer. But what is cancer?

Ans. Cancer is not one but a general name for a group of diseases. Just as apples, oranges, strawberries are each different but are given a general name "fruits" so also, a group of individual diseases is called cancer. There are more than 100 types of cancer.

Q. What causes cancer?

Ans. Our body is made up of hundred trillion cells just as a building is made up of millions of bricks. But our body grows (as distinct from a building!) by replacing old cells with new ones. The new cells must be in the right number, in the right place and of the right type.

This process of growth has to be carefully controlled (it wouldn't be nice if our two hands were of different sizes and shapes, or if we continued to gain height throughout our lives!) Interestingly, usually the process is well-controlled.

However all goes awry if accidentally an abnormal cell is produced which goes on producing similar abnormal cells whose growth is both disorganized and uncontrolled.

In response to cancer producing signals, cells start dividing unchecked due to absence of control by 'stop' signals. These cells serve no purpose to the host but live like a parasite draining the host. They not only grow relentlessly but spread to different organs and even travel by blood to reach distant organs and grow there. The site where the cancer originated is called 'primary' and the site of disease away from the primary is the 'metastasis'. Metastasis may occur in one organ or many organs. Bones, liver, lungs and brain are the most common sites of metastasis.

Q. What causes 'Tumor'?

Ans. If the abnormal cells form a lump, it is called a 'tumor' (tumor means a 'lump'); if they are abnormal brain cells it is a brain tumor, if they are abnormal bone cells it is a bone tumor. If the abnormal cells are white blood cells they may occur in lumps called a lymphoma, if they are found in blood and bone marrow it is a leukemia. Tumors which do not spread are called 'benign tumors' ('benign' means 'friendly'); but benign tumors in the wrong place can cause problems e.g. benign brain tumors. Tumors which are able to spread or 'metastasize' are called 'malignant tumors' or 'cancers'.

These days, cancer detected in early stages show good survival rates.

Q. How is cancer treated?

Ans. Cancer may be treated by:
1. Surgery
2. Radiotherapy
3. Chemotherapy.

The treatment that you had or going to have is decided by the doctors according to the disease that you have. It can be either of the three or a combination of these.

Surgery means having an operation. The bad cells are got rid of by cutting them out.

Ionizing radiation is a form of energy, obtained from disintegrating radioactive isotopes or from high energy X-ray machines. The radiation is a form of energy like light but cannot be seen. The radiation on being shined on cancer cells kills them off without causing much damage to the surrounding normal cells. According to the site where the disease is, it may be given to head, legs or tummy. Chemotherapy means treatment with medicines. These are very powerful drugs targeted at the bad cells. These drugs destroy or control the cancer cells. More than 100 chemotherapy drugs are in use either singly or in combination according to the disease.

Q. Are children's cancers same as adults'?

Ans. The most common cancers in adults are cancers of the lining parts of the body like lungs, breast, bowel and prostate cancers and are caused in part by environmental/lifestyle factors. These cancers are almost never seen in children. Many of childhood cancers come from cells which are left over when the baby was still developing in the mother's womb. These are again rarely seen in adults.

Certain tumors like leukemias, lymphomas and brain tumors do occur in both adults and children. However, the disease might behave differently in different age groups. Children often respond better to treatment.

However, there is precious little you could have done to prevent getting the disease. It didn't occur because of your naughtiness or playing pranks with your peers nor because of any faulty upbringing by your parents.

Older kids sometimes develop some nasty habits like smoking, which is the single most important thing linked with cancer. In certain situations like with a group of friends or maybe in a party there is pressure to have a puff. But, this occasional smoking can develop into a habit and makes people more likely to get cancer. This is more true to kids who have had cancer. Smoking clogs up one's lungs and makes the heart work harder, which is more harmful for those whose heart and lungs are weaker as a result of having cancer.

Q. My uncle also had cancer. Does it run in our family?

Ans. Sadly, cancer is a very common disease specially among elders. Hence, it is not uncommon to find an elder member of the family of a child who has cancer to be having cancer also, though at a different site. But often this occurs per chance. Cancer does originate in the genes, in that, cancer is caused by changes in the genes that cause cells to divide abnormally. However, these gene changes will probably have occurred only in that individual.

Very occasionally, childhood cancers do run in families like an eye tumor called retinoblastoma. In that case, other family members need to be checked to be sure that they do not have the condition.

Q. Why should I have to come regularly to the clinic?

Ans. Firstly, to check that there are no side-effects from radiotherapy and chemotherapy. To kill off the bad cells, the chemotherapy drugs have to be really strong. It might per chance kill off some healthy cells too. Radiotherapy can also hurt some healthy ones.

Normally, if only a few healthy cells are hurt they grow back quickly; but in some parts of the body they do not grow back quickly enough and the child may have problems in growth or of the heart, lungs or kidneys. Though this does not occur frequently, still it is a good idea to have it checked by a doctor.

Secondly, since you had cancer once, there is always a possibility of it coming back again. Though you are fit and healthy now, it is always good to have it checked.

Thirdly, by watching you how you are getting better doctors can learn a lot. They then use what they learn from your improvement to treat other children who have cancer.

Fourthly, you may have some questions to ask- like when you can start your normal outdoor activities, when you can attend school or of any other problems that you are having while receiving the drugs. You might feel shy and nervous at first but once you ask it will be easier for you to ask the next time and the doctor will only be happy to explain it to you. You can also ask about the tests that are being done-as to why they are necessary! You need not feel ashamed even if others feel that such questions are silly! The doctor uncle would definitely not feel so and would only be happy to answer your queries.

Fifthly, when you come to the clinic they weigh and measure you to know to be sure that you are growing properly. As a result of treatment sometimes the hormones that make children grow are upset. Though this occurs rarely, if it is detected, corrective steps may be taken by the doctor.

Q. Can cancer ever really be cured?

Ans. Yes, now nearly three quarters of childhood cancers are cured. Till 1960's, it was very unusual for cancer to be treated successfully, unless it was completely removed by the surgeon. Not so nowadays, though many of your elders will find it hard to believe. Today, most children are not only cured of the disease, but go on to live full and active lives.

Still there are certain cancers in children which cannot be cured. For them, treatment can often keep the cancer under control for sometime. For still few, it may be possible to control only the symptoms. Always remember that every cancer patient and each type of cancer is different from others and it carries little meaning as to how another child who had cancer has responded to treatment. Again, continuous progress is being made in developing better treatment.

Q. What are the difficulties that I may face following radiation?

Ans. Most of the time the side-effects of radiation are less than what is anticipated. However,

a. Fever and infection by organisms are to be watched for.

b. Skin irritation in the area of the body being treated can occur. It may be very mild redness to severe peeling of the skin in rare cases.

c. Hair loss may occur at the site where radiation is given. Scalp hair is lost only if there is radiation to the head. In most cases, hair grows back following radiation.

d. A feeling of weariness, weakness or exhaustion or loss of energy may occur while undergoing radiation therapy.

Q. What problems are likely during or after chemotherapy?

Ans. Though the severity of side-effects varies from one child to another, be sure to talk to your doctor when you meet him in the clinic. He may give you some medicines that will help you. You may have—

a. Nausea and vomiting. There also may be loss of appetite and weight loss. Diarrhea and constipation may also occur in some children.

b. Gum or throat problems and increased chance of bruising and bleeding are there.

c. You can also have fatigue, hair loss, anemia and infection.

d. Some have dry skin, nerve and muscle problem and some have irritation of urinary bladder.

However, most side-effects gradually disappear at the end of treatment because the healthy cells recover quickly. The recovery time varies from one child to another and also depends on your overall health and the drugs that you are getting.

Q. What happens at the end of treatment?

Ans. At the end of treatment, the doctor uncle would like to meet you about every 4–6 weeks during the 1st year. At the very beginning he would meet you every 1–2 weeks. With time, the frequency diminishes—about every three months in the 2nd year and may be yearly at about 5 years on completion of treatment.

So many things happen at the end of treatment-you no more feel sick, you don't have to gulp those tablets that you had been taking all through the treatment, you get rid of the line through which drugs were given. You also grow hairs, do not have to spend boring times at the hospital. You may be allowed to go out with your friends more frequently, go back to school, play with your friends and look normal.

You may also plan something special to celebrate the end of the difficult period that you have been through successfully—

a. Have a special meal with your family.

b. Plan a party or celebration evening with your mates.

c. Plan a holiday.

d. Do something which you couldn't do these days like go swimming.

Q. When should my parents contact my cancer doctor apart from my routine visits to the clinic?

Ans. For the first few weeks after treatment stops, you will be neutropenic or still have a central line and will need to come to hospital if there is sign of infection. Once you have a normal blood count, a local practitioner can first evaluate and then decide when to go to hospital.

However, the following things require urgent attention—

a. Many bruises at the same time that is unlikely to have been caused by normal activity.

b. Repeated headache or vomiting that are worse in the morning.

c. Lumps when you are, otherwise, well and is not suffering from viral illness.

Q. What are the restrictions that I would have to abide by?

Ans. When you finish treatment you may feel tired often as you are not as strong as before, have lost weight and are not used to joining in all the usual activities. You should take a good balanced diet and take part in your activities gradually—as you continue to build your stamina. Likely, soon you will be able to attend school full-time and join in sports both in and out of school.

If you are having any difficulty or disability possibly your school will help you in adjusting to it.

Please remember—

- Most cancers in children and young people don't come back ever!
- The chances of the cancer coming back get smaller and smaller the longer you have been out of treatment.
- For some cancers, there is still a chance of cure even if they do come back.

Though, you have suffered from a serious illness which many of your peers have not suffered, you have borne it through. You are braver to have faced such a challenge with a smile and hence are one up than most of the others of your age.

Hence, good luck and keep smiling.

SUGGESTED READING

1. Candlelighters Childhood Cancer Foundation Internet Address: http://www.cancer.org/docroot/ipg.asp?sitename=Candlelighters+Childhood+Cancer+Foundation&url=http://www.candlelighters.org.

2. CureSearch, a combined effort of National Childhood Cancer Foundation and Children's Oncology Group http://www.cancer.org/docroot/ipg.asp?sitename=CureSearch&url=http://www.curesearch.org.

3. Marina N. Long-term survivors of childhood cancer: The medical consequences of cure. Ped Clin North Am. 1997;44:1021-42.

47 Modern Technology and Childhood Cancers—The Interface

Indira Banerjee, Ajay Ghosh, Rakesh Mondal

"Cancer appears to be a modern disease created by modern life."

Professor Rosalie David,
a biomedical Egyptologist at the
University of Manchester

INTRODUCTION

Researchers looking at almost a thousand mummies from ancient Egypt found only a handful suffered from cancer when now it accounts for nearly one in three deaths. The findings suggest that it is modern lifestyles and pollution levels caused by industry are probably the main cause of the disease and that it is not a naturally occurring condition. They showed the disease rate has raised dramatically since the industrial revolution, in particular childhood cancer which proves that the rise is not simply due to people living for long time.

Over the years modern technologies evolved in time making the lifestyle easy. Nobel Prize winner Max Planck had said, "A new scientific truth does not triumph by convincing its opponents and making them see the light, but rather its opponents eventually die and a new generation grows up that is familiar with it." As newer technological gadgets continue to be a part of our everyday lives, it is often overlooked that they carry risk of health hazards.

The list of such gadgets is endless. They have different ways of functioning, but the present concern is mostly confined to a common technology: The use of electromagnetic radiation (EMR). The spectrum of electromagnetic radiation ranges in accordance to its frequency or corresponding wavelength. Quanta are the particles forming electromagnetic waves, and those of higher frequency carry a large amount of energy capable of disrupting chemical bonds and considered as ionizing radiation. It has been quite some time that health professionals have underscored the harmful effects of this ionizing radiation, whose man-made sources include X-rays among many others, and implicated its exposure in the molecular and genetic basis of cancers. Man-made sources of electromagnetic fields that form a major part of industrialized life—electricity (extremely low frequency energy waves or ELF waves), microwaves and radiofrequency fields—are found at the relatively long wavelength and low frequency end of the electromagnetic spectrum and their quanta are unable to break chemical bonds. They affect the human body in various ways. The main biological effect is heating which produces heat stress at the cellular level causing alteration in their normal functioning. Theories suggest that they induce cell stress and damage at the non-thermal level of EMR as well, through molecular vibration, free radical formation and altered protein synthesis. They also alter blood brain permeability affecting the functioning of the pineal gland and melatonin metabolism that has a considerable role in maintaining physiologicai homeostasis in humans. The epigenetic influence of EMR though has not been conclusively established, the health concerns have been addressed by various health activists, as well as the World Health Organization.

TELECOMMUNICATION DEVICES (PROTOTYPE: PHONE)

The most common exposures to radiofrequency energy are from telecommunications devices, etc. In the United States, cell phones currently operate in a frequency range of about 1,800 to 2,200 megahertz (MHz). The electromagnetic radiation produced by them is in the form of non-ionizing radiofrequency energy. Cordless phones often operate at radiofrequencies similar to those of cell phones but, since cordless phones have a limited range and require a nearby base, their signals are generally much less powerful than those of cell phones. Among other radiofrequency energy sources are AM/FM radios and televisions operate at lower radiofrequencies than cell phones, whereas sources such as radar, satellite stations, operate at somewhat higher radiofrequencies. Mobile technology is developed enormously from the 1970's analogue systems through to present day family of digital mobile technologies. Mobile phones continue to develop with more user-friendly features being implemented as new technology is released. The boundaries will blur between internet, broadcast and mobile telecommunications in future. Significantly more radio base stations will be needed as communications technology advances. Though the studies do not find any correlation between radiofrequency exposure and carcinogenesis conclusively, but recent data are alarming. Base stations use radio signal to mobile devices to the network, enabling to send and receive calls. They act as 'transceivers'. Base stations are deployed for two reasons either coverage or capacity. The second factor affecting site numbers is data rate. For a given radio path, a fixed amount of energy is required to deliver each data bit, so the power required is directly proportional to the data rate. The last factor affecting the number of base stations is the transmit power allowed at base station and terminal. Higher power would provide greater coverage, but the design of terminals to have long battery life.

International guidelines recommend limits to the human exposure to radiofrequency fields based on large body of biological science and are designed to avoid health hazards for all people. For the frequencies used in public telecommunications, these guidelines define the maximum Specific Absorption Rate (SAR), the measure of radiation absorbed by the human body when the handset is being used at maximum power and the unit is Watts per kilogram. Different models of cellular phones have different SAR specifications. Since SAR is not directly measurable, the guidelines also include limits in the form of other different field parameters that if met, assure the compliance with the SAR limits. The most internationally applied guidance is provided by the International Commission for Non-Ionizing Radiation Protection (ICNIRP). Another set of guidelines is provided by the Institute of Electric and Electronics Engineer (IEEE) and these are used in the USA and in some other countries. While there are a number of national guidelines, they are often based on ICNIRP which is considered for simplicity. ICNIRP recommends that the general public exposure should be limited to 2 W/kg in any 10g for the head and body, 4 W/kg in any 10g for limbs and in addition 0.08 W/kg for the whole body and all of these subject to an averaging period of 6 minutes.

Radiation from cell phones can possibly cause cancer, according to the World Health Organization. Cell phones emit radiofrequency energy, a form of non-ionizing electromagnetic radiation, which can be absorbed by tissues closest to where the phone is held. The amount of radiofrequency energy a cell phone user is exposed to depend on the technology of the phone, which influences the SAR measure, the distance between the phone's antenna and the user, the extent and type of use, and the user's distance from cell phone towers, etc. The agency now lists mobile phone use in the same "carcinogenic hazard" category as lead, engine exhaust and chloroform. A team of 31 scientists from 14 countries, including the US, made the decision after reviewing peer-reviewed studies on cell phone safety. The team found enough evidence to categorize personal exposure as "possibly carcinogenic to humans." They found possible evidence of increase in glioma and acoustic neuroma brain cancer for mobile phone users, but have not been able to draw conclusions for other types of cancers.

The FDA and FCC have suggested some steps that concerned cell phone users can take to reduce their exposure to radiofrequency energy (a) Reserve the use of cell phones for shorter conversations or for times (b) Use a hands-free device, which places more distance between the phone and the head of the user. Volkow et al shows, in healthy participants and compared with no exposure, 50-minute cell phone exposure was associated with increased brain glucose metabolism in the region closest to the antenna, i.e. orbitofrontal cortex and temporal pole. Zook et al studied detrimental effects of pulsed 860 MHz radiofrequency radiation on the promotion of neurogenic tumors in rats.

The different statement of international agency regarding safety profile of radiofrequency devices are listed below:

a. The International Agency for Research on Cancer (IARC), a component of the World Health Organization, has classified radiofrequency fields as "possibly carcinogenic to humans," based on limited evidence from human studies, limited evidence from studies of radiofrequency energy and cancer in rodents, and evidence from studies of genotoxicity, effects on immune system function, gene and protein expression, cell signalling, oxidative stress, and apoptosis, along with studies of the possible effects of radiofrequency energy on the blood-brain barrier.

b. The American Cancer Society (ACS) states that the IARC classification means that there could be some risk associated with cancer, but the evidence is not strong enough to be considered causal and needs to be investigated further. Individuals who are concerned about radiofrequency exposure can limit their exposure, including using an ear piece and limiting cell phone use, particularly among children.

c. The National Institute of Environmental Health Sciences (NIEHS) states that the weight of the current scientific evidence has not conclusively linked cell phone use with any adverse health problems whereas more research is needed.

d. The US Food and Drug Administration (FDA), which is responsible for regulating the safety of machines and devices that emit radiation, e.g. cell phones, notes that studies reporting biological changes associated with radiofrequency energy have failed to be replicated and that the majority of human epidemiologic studies have failed to show a relationship between exposure to radiofrequency energy from cell phones and health problems.

e. The US Centers for Disease Control and Prevention (CDC) states that, although some studies have raised concerns about the possible risks of cell phone use, scientific research as a whole does not support a statistically significant association between cell phone use and health effects.

f. The Federal Communications Commission (FCC) concludes that there is no scientific evidence that wireless phone use can lead to cancer or to other health problems, including headaches, dizziness, or memory loss.

A large prospective cohort study of cell phone use and its possible long-term health effects was launched in Europe in March 2010. This study, known as COSMOS, will enrol approximately 250,000 cell phone users ages 18 or older and will follow them for 20 to 30 years. Participants in COSMOS will complete a questionnaire about their health, lifestyle, and current and past cell phone use. This information will be supplemented with information from health records and cell phone records. Children have the potential to be at greater risk than adults for developing brain cancer from cell phones. Their nervous systems are still developing and therefore more vulnerable to factors that may cause cancer. Their heads are smaller than those of adults and therefore have a greater proportional exposure to the field of radiofrequency radiation that is emitted by cell phones. And children have the potential of accumulating more years of cell phone exposure than adults do. The first published analysis came from a large case-control study called CEFALO, which was conducted in Denmark, Sweden, Norway, and Switzerland. The study included children who were diagnosed with brain tumors between 2004 and 2008, when their ages ranged from 7 to 19. Researchers did not find an association between cell phone use and brain tumor risk in this group of children. However, they noted that their results did not rule out the possibility of a slight increase in brain cancer risk among children who use cell phones, and that data gathered through prospective studies and objective measurements, rather than participant surveys and recollections, will be key in clarifying whether there is an increased risk. Researchers from the Centre for Research in Environmental Epidemiology in Spain are conducting another international study Mobikids to evaluate the risk associated with new communications technologies including cell phones and other environmental factors in young people ages 10 to 24. Despite all doubts standards have been developed for terminals used. For evaluating exposure against the body, the IEC is developing a standard. In the European Union, work is well advanced in defining base station standards and IEC/ITU is developing global base station standards. Before being put on the market, a new terminal design is tested to confirm that when used according to the manufacturer's operating instructions. The user should not be exposed to radiofrequency fields above the relevant guidelines for the country of sale. Each base station is evaluated and measures defined so as to ensure that people cannot be overexposed. Transmitter power control, capacity dimensioning, discontinuous transmission and use of half-rate all mean that GSM base stations transmit well under their maximum power capability even for the part of the day when usage is highest. At a given time, the transmit power from a base station largely depends on the traffic it is carrying. New technologies use spectrum more efficiently but are getting closer to the physically achievable limits.

WASTE MANAGEMENT

Studies of cancer incidence and mortality in populations around landfill sites or incinerators have been equivocal, with varying results for different cancer sites. Two reports of cancer incidence among persons living near the Miron Quarry site, the third largest in North America found increased incidence of cancers of the liver, kidney, pancreas and non-Hodgkin's lymphomas. Studies focusing on a single waste incinerator suggested some relationship between distance from the site and mortality or incidence from some cancers, for example, laryngeal and lung cancers, childhood cancers and leukemias and soft-tissue sarcoma and non-Hodgkin's lymphoma. A series of studies in the UK of multiple sites compared observed cancer incidence rates in bands of increasing distance from each incinerator with rates based on national data.

FULL BODY SCANNER USED FOR AIR PASSENGERS

Millimeter wave machines represent one of two primary technologies currently being used for the "digital strip searches" being conducted at airports around the world.

"The Transportation Security Administration utilizes two technologies to capture naked images of air travelers – backscatter X-ray technology and millimeter wave technology. In order to generate the nude image of the human body, these machines emit in the tetrahertz range high-frequency energy "particles" that can pass through clothing and body tissue. Alamos National Laboratory in New Mexico showed that these terahertz waves could unzip double-stranded DNA, creating bubbles in the double strand that could significantly interfere with processes such as gene expression and DNA replication. It can damage DNA and can cause cancer.

NUCLEAR POWER PLANT

A government-sponsored study of childhood cancer in the proximity of German nuclear power plants found that children < 5 years living < 5 km from plant exhaust stacks had twice the risk for contracting leukemia as those residing > 5 km. The researchers concluded that since "this result was not to be expected under current radiation-epidemiological knowledge" and confounders could not be identified, the observed association of leukemia incidence with residential proximity to nuclear plants "remains unexplained."

DIAGNOSTIC RADIOLOGY

A study presented at the annual meeting of the Radiological Society of North America (RSNA) last winter conclusively showed that low-dose radiation from annual mammography screening significantly increases breast cancer risk in women with a genetic or familial predisposition to the disease. Comparison of mammography with Breast-Specific Gamma Imaging (BSGI) or Positron Emission Mammography (PEM) examinations shows one single BSGI or PEM carries a lifetime risk of inducing fatal cancer that is far greater than the cancer risk associated with having annual screening mammograms starting at age forty.

MICRO-OVEN

In Comparative Study of Food Prepared Conventionally and in the Microwave Oven, published by Raum & Zelt in 1992, showed Microwaved food contains both molecules and energies not present in food cooked in the way humans have been cooking food since the discovery of fire. Artificially produced microwaves, including those in ovens, are produced from alternating current and force a billion or more polarity reversals per second in every food molecule they hit. Production of unnatural molecules is inevitable. Naturally occurring amino acids have been observed to undergo isomeric changes as well as transformation into toxic forms, under the impact of microwaves produced in ovens. One short-term study found significant and disturbing changes in the blood of individuals consuming microwaved milk and vegetables. Eight volunteers ate various combinations of the same foods cooked different ways. All foods that were processed through the microwave ovens caused changes in the blood of the volunteers. Hemoglobin and lymphocyte levels decreased and overall white cell levels and cholesterol levels increased. Luminescent (light-emitting) bacteria were employed to detect energetic changes in the blood. Significant increases were found in the luminescence of these bacteria when exposed to blood serum obtained after the consumption of microwaved food. An article stated that the consumption of food cooked in microwave ovens had cancerous effects on the blood.

As a device for domestic use microwave ovens operates at very high power levels. Effective 'shielding' is necessary to reduce leakage outside the ovens. Furthermore microwave leakage falls very rapidly with increasing distance from the oven. There are manufacturing standards to specify maximum leakage. Adherence to the guidelines is necessary, as well as estimation of effect of long-term use or accidental improper handling on this 'shielding' are required to minimize harmful exposure.

CONCLUSION

The effect of regular handling of such gadgets of daily necessity causes exposure to radiation that is invisible, imperceptible and inappreciable to the individual. The challenge of establishing irrefutable scientific proof of harm is tedious as primarily, the precise mechanism of injury cannot be highlighted. The conclusionily primary depends on epidemiological studies as RCTs are often deemed unethical for this purpose. In a cause-effect statistical analysis, establishing causality requires the

investigator to consider factors like consistency and strong association between exposure and effect, a clear dose-response relationship, a credible biological explanation, support provided by relevant animal studies, and above all, consistency between studies. Studies involving electromagnetic fields and cancer have not been able to outline these factors conclusively. Scientists thus have refrained from quoting that these technological devices which have now become a part and parcel of modern life and their associated weak electromagnetic radiation have an effect on human body, harmful or not. However, there is a possibility that the adverse effects of EMR might be misdiagnosed and ineffectively managed. Hence it is important to have a clear understanding of the existence of such a scenario while in health practice.

SUGGESTED READING

1. Aydin D, Feychting M, Schüz J, et al. Mobile phone use and brain tumors in children and adolescents: a multicenter case-control study. Journal of the National Cancer Institute. 2011;103:1-13.

2. Electromagnetic fields (EMF): World Health Organization; Available from: http://www.who.int/peh-emf/en/ Accessed on 15th June 2015.

3. Elliott P, Eaton N, Shaddick G, Carter R. Cancer incidence near municipal solid waste incinerators in Great Britain. Part 2: Histopathological and case-note review of primary liver cancer cases. Br J Cancer. 2000; 82:1103-6.

4. Elliott P, Hills M, Beresford J, Kleinschmidt I, Jolley D, Pattenden S, et al. Incidence of cancers of the larynx and lung near incinerators of waste solvents and oils in Great Britain. Lancet. 1992;339:854-8.

5. Elliott P, Shaddick G, Kleinschmidt I, Jolley D, Walls P, Beresford J, et al. Cancer incidence near municipal solid waste incinerators in Great Britain. Br J Cancer. 1996;73: 702-10.

6. EN 50361:2001. Basic standard for the measurement of specific absorption rate related to human exposure to electromagnetic fields from mobile phones (300 MHz - 3 GHz) 2001.

7. EN 50383:2002, Basic standard for the calculation and measurement of electromagnetic field strength and SAR related to human exposure from radio base stations and

fixed terminal stations for wireless telecommunications system (110 MHz - 40 GHz), 2002.

8. Full-body scanners used on air passengers may damage human DNA Adams M available at file:///F:/technology/Fullbody%20scanners%20used%20on%20air%20passengers%20may%20damage%20human%20DNA.htm accessed, 2012.

9. Goldberg MS, Al-Homsi N, Goulet L, Riberdy H. Incidence of cancer among persons living near a municipal solid waste landfill site in Montreal, Quebec. Arch Environ Health. 1995;50:416-24.

10. Goldberg MS, DeWar R, Desy M, Riberdy H. Risk of developing cancer relative to living near a municipal solid waste landfill site in Montreal, Quebec, Canada. Arch Environ Health. 1999;54:291-6.

11. Hirose H, Suhara T, Kaji N, et al. Mobile phone base station radiation does not affect neoplastic transformation in BALB/3T3 cells. Bioelectromagnetics. 2008;29:55-64.

12. http://www.who.int/docstore/peh-emf/EMFStandards/who-0102/Worldmap5.htm accessed Sept 2005.

13. IEEE 1528, IEEE Recommended Practice for Determining the Peak Spatial-Average Specific Absorption Rate (SAR) in the Human Head from Wireless Communications Devices: Measurement Techniques, 2003.

14. IEEE Std C95.1, Standard for Safety Levels with Respect to Human Exposure to Radiofrequency Electromagnetic Fields, 3 kHz to 300 GHz, 1999.

15. International Commission on Non-Ionizing radiation Protection (ICNIRP), Guideline for limiting exposure to time-varying electric, magnetic, and electromagnetic fields. Health Physics. 1998;74:494-522.

16. Microwave oven Wayne A, Newell L available at file:///F:/technology/Microwave%20oven%20health%20risk%20-%20cancer%20risk.htm accessed, 2012.

17. New nuclear imaging technology causes breast cancer available at http://www.naturalnews.com/027641_mammograms_brst_cancer.html accessed, 2012.

18. Nussbaum R. Childhood Leukemia and Cancers Near German Nuclear Reactors: Significance, Context, and Ramifications of Recent Studies INT J Occup Environ Health. 2009;15:318-23.

19. US Federal Communications Commission. Wireless. Washington DC. Retrieved, 2011.

20. Volkow ND, Tomasi D, Wang GJ, et al. Effects of cell phone radiofrequency signal exposure on brain glucose metabolism. JAMA. 2011;305:808-13.

21. WCDMA for UMTS – Radio Access For Third Generation Mobile Communication Editor: Halma, H. and Toskala A. John Wiley & Sons LTD, ISBN 0 471 72051 8, 2000.

22. Zook BC, Simmens SJ. The effects of pulsed 860 MHz radiofrequency radiation on the promotion of neurogenic tumors in rats. Radiation Research. 2006; 165:608-15.

Annexures

HODGKIN'S DISEASE

Protocol: ABVD

Doxorubicin	25 mg/m^2 IV bolus	Days 1 & 15
Bleomycin	10,000 IU/m^2 200 ml N. saline/30 mins	Days 1 & 15
Vinblastine	6 mg/m^2 IV bolus	Days 1 & 15
Dacarbazine	375 mg/m^2 250 ml N. saline/1 hour	Days 1 & 15

Cycle frequency: Every four weeks, Total number of cycles: 6-8

Protocol: ChlVPP

Chlorambucil	6 mg/m^2 od oral	Days 1-14
Vinblastine	6 mg/m^2 (max 10 mg) IV	Days 1 & 8
Procarbazine	100 mg/m^2 od oral	Days 1-14
Prednisolone	40 mg od oral	Days 1-14

Cycle frequency: Every four weeks, Total number of cycles: 6-8

NON-HODGKIN'S LYMPHOMA

Protocol: CHOP

Cyclophosphamide	750 mg/m^2 IV	Day 1
Doxorubicin	50 mg/m^2 IV	Day 1
Vincristine	1.4 mg/m^2 (max 2 mg) IV	Day 1
Prednisolone	100 mg oral	Days 2-5

Cycle frequency: Every two to three weeks, Total number of cycles: 6-8

R-CHOP

Rituximab	375 mg/m^2 500 ml N. saline	Day 1
Cyclophosphamide	750 mg/m^2 IV	Day 1
Doxorubicin	50 mg/m^{2}IV	Day 1
Vincristine	1.4 mg/m^2 (max 2 mg) IV	Day 1
Prednisolone	100 mg oral	Days 2-5

Cycle frequency: Every two to three weeks, Total number of cycles: 6-8

LYMPHOMA - RECURRENT

R-ICE (Carboplatin/Ifosfamide/Etoposide)

Rituximab	375 mg/m^2 500 ml N. saline	Day 1
Ifosfamide	5,000 mg/m^2 1L N. saline/24 hours	Day 2
Carboplatin	AUC 5 500 ml 5% dextrose/1 hour	Day 2
Etoposide	100 mg/m^2 500 ml N. saline/2 hours	Days 1-3
Cycle frequency: Every 2 weeks, Total number of cycles: 3		

ESHAP

Cisplatin	25 mg/m^2 IV continuous infusion	Days 1-4
Etoposide	40 mg/m^2 500 ml N. saline/1 hour	Days 1-4
Methylprednisolone	500 mg 100 ml N. saline/30 mins	Days 1-5
Cytarabine	2000 mg/m^2 500 ml N. saline/2 hours	Day 5
Cycle frequency: Every three-four weeks, Total number of cycles: 6		

ACUTE MYELOID LEUKEMIA

Cytarabine and Idarubicin (7 + 3)		
Cytarabine	100 mg/m^2/day IV	Days 1-7
Idarubicin	12 mg/m^2/day IV	Days 1-3
Cycle does not repeat. If the bone marrow does not show complete remission by day 28, reinduction with 5 or 7 days of cytarabine and 2 or 3 days of idarubicin is usually used.		
Cytarabine and Daunorubicin (5 + 2)		
Cytarabine	100 mg/m^2/day IV	Days 1-5
Daunorubicin	45 mg/m^2/day IV	Days 1-2
Cycle does not repeat. If the bone marrow does not show complete remission by day 28, reinduction with other regimes may be tried.		

NEUROBLASTOMA (OPEC)

Vincristine	1.4 mg/m^2 (max 2 mg) IV	Day 1
Cyclophosphamide	600 mg/m^2 IV	Day 1
Cisplatin	100 mg/m^2 IV	Day 2
Etoposide	40 mg/m^2 500 ml N. saline/1 hour	Day 4
Cycle frequency: Every three-four weeks, Total number of cycles: 6-8		

RETINOBLASTOMA (VAC)

Vincristine	1.4 mg/m^2 (max 2 mg) IV	Day 1
Dactinomycin	0.015 mg/kg/day	Day 1-5
Cyclophosphamide	200 mg/m^2 IV	Days 1-5
Cycle frequency: To be adjusted as per staging of the tumor		

RHABDOMYOSARCOMA (VAC MODIFIED)

Induction

Vincristine	1.4 mg/m^2 (max 2 mg) IV	Weekly for 12 weeks
Dactinomycin	0.015 mg/kg/day	Days 1-5 Repeat every 3 wks for 3 cycle
Cyclophosphamide	10 mg/kg/day IV	Days 1-3 Repeat every 3 wks for 5 cycle
Followed by continuation cycle with modification		

ACUTE LYMPHOBLASTIC LEUKEMIA–THE MULTICENTER PROTOCOL (MCP-841)

Induction 1

L1

Prednisolone	40 mg/m^2 PO	Days 1-28
Vincristine	1.4 mg/m^2 (max 2 mg) IV	Days 1, 8, 15, 22
Methotrexate	12 mg /m^{2}IT	Days 1, 8, 15, 22
L-asparaginase	6000 u/m^2 IM on alternate days (10 doses)	Days 2-20
Daunorubicin	30 mg/m^2 IV	Days 8, 15, 29

Induction 2

L2

Mercaptopurine	75 mg/m^2 PO daily	Days 1-7 and Days 15-21
Cyclophosphamide	750 mg/m^2 IV	Days 1, 15
Methotrexate	12 mg/m^2 IT	Days 1, 8, 15, 22
Cranial irradiation	180 cGy daily for 10 days[total 1800cGy]	
Repeat induction	Same as L1	

Consolidation

Cyclophosphamide	750 mg/m^2 IV	Day 1
Vincristine	1.4 mg/m^2 (max 2 mg) IV	Days 1, 15
Mercaptopurine	75 mg/m^2 PO daily	Days 1-7 and 15-21
Cytarabine	100 mg/m^2 SC every 12 hours × 6 doses	Days 1-3 and 15-17
Daunorubicin	30 mg/m^2 IV	Days 15

Maintenance (6 cycles)

Prednisolone	40 mg/m^2 PO	Days 1-7
Vincristine	1.4 mg/m^2 (max 2 mg) IV	Day 1
Daunorubicin	30 mg/m^2 IV	Day 1
L-asparaginase	6000 u/m^{2}IM	Days 1, 3, 5, 7
Methotrexate	15 mg/m^{2}PO once a wk, missing every 4th for a total of 12 wks begin on Day 15	
Mercaptopurine	75 mg/m^2 PO daily, 3 wks out of every 4 for a total of 12 wks begin on Day 15	

Annexure 2: Antiemetic Principles

ANTI-EMETIC PRINCIPLES IN PEDIATRIC ONCOLOGY

Nausea and vomiting are common side effects of anti-neoplastic medication. Nausea occurs at a higher frequency than vomiting and is more difficult to control.

The most common patterns of emesis are:

Acute chemotherapy-induced emesis: Occurs within the initial 24 hours of drug administration with maximum risk is from 1 to 6 hours after chemotherapy.

Delayed emesis: It begins 24 hours or more after chemotherapy and commonly seen with platins, cyclophosphamide, etc. However, this problem may begin somewhat earlier than 24 hours in some patients.

Anticipatory emesis: This is a conditioned vomiting response following inadequate antiemetic protection with prior courses of chemotherapy.

Breakthrough nausea/Vomiting: Vomiting that occurs despite prophylactic treatment, and/or requires rescue with antiemetic agents.

General principles for management:

Prophylaxis is better and must be administered prior to chemotherapy. Titration of the antiemetic dose may be required as the tolerance to drugs differs. In severe cases, combination of antiemetics of different groups may be required.

For most children, receiving any chemotherapy that has emetogenic potential ondansetron or other 5-HT3 receptor antagonist should be of initial choice. If not controlled or breakthrough occurs or for moderately emetogenic regimes, a combination of steroid (dexamethasone) and metoclopramide (dopamine blocker) is effective. For highly emetogenic drugs, ondansetron, steroid combining with antihistamines (prochlorperazin, diphenhydramine) and benzodiazepines (lorazepam) should be tried.

Emesis unrelated to chemotherapy

Patients receiving anticancer drugs may also develop emesis for other reasons or medications like analgesics, anti-infectives, or bronchodilators. Tumor-related complications (such as intestinal obstruction or brain metastases) may also be responsible. In such situations, adjustment of medication or treatment of tumor-related complications are more important than administering an antiemetic agent.

Annexure 3: Safe Handling of Hazardous Drugs

SAFE HANDLING OF HAZARDOUS ANTI-NEOPLASTIC DRUGS

Drugs that meet one or more of the following criteria should be called hazardous:

a. Carcinogenicity

b. Teratogenicity or developmental toxicity

c. Reproductive toxicity

d. Organ toxicity

e. Genotoxicity

The caregivers might be exposed to hazardous drugs by inhalation of aerosolized drug, dermal absorption, ingestion or injections.

Caregiver should take following personal protection during handling of the hazardous drugs:

Disposable gowns –low-permeability to the hazardous drugs

Latex gloves – powder-free, safe for use with chemotherapy drugs

Face and eye protection as splashing of drugs may occur

Management of accidental exposure of the hazardous drugs:

Skin exposure: Remove contaminated clothing and immediately wash affected area thoroughly with soap and water

Eye exposure: Flush eyes with water or isotonic solution for 15 minutes

Exposure by inhalation or ingestion: Acute symptoms may require emergency intervention.

In case of accidental exposure, drug specific instructions are to be consulted. The incidence is to be informed to the employer with a complete report of injury/exposure.

Annexure 4: Management of Drug Extravasations

MANAGEMENT OF DRUG EXTRAVASATIONS

Anti-neoplastic drugs can be categorized as:

Irritant: Agent causing pain, tightness with or without inflammation

Vesicant: Agents causing tissue destruction. Most of the drugs fall into this group but dactinomycin, doxorubicin, daunorubicin, vinblastine and vincristine are notable.

Sclerosant: Agent having sclerosing property

Unintentional leakage of drug out of a blood vessel into the surrounding tissue is called extravasations.

Vesicant extravasations cause pain, necrosis and tissue sloughing. Sometimes it causes local nonpainful, allergic flare.

Management principles:

Prevention-Large veins with good flow should be selected and patency of the IV catheter should always be ensured by flushing with saline beforehand. Central venous line is preferable whenever possible.

When extravasations occur following measures are to be taken:

a. Stop the infusion
b. Do not remove the IV catheter initially.
c. Aspirate the fluid from the extravasated site.
d. Do not flush the line.
e. Remove the IV catheter later once the inflammation subsides

Index

Page numbers followed by *f* refer to figure and *t* refer to table.